Principles of Geriatric Critical Care

Principles of Geriatric Critical Care

Edited by

Shamsuddin Akhtar
Yale University School of Medicine

Stanley Rosenbaum
Yale University School of Medicine

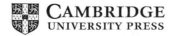

CAMBRIDGE
UNIVERSITY PRESS

University Printing House, Cambridge CB2 8BS, United Kingdom

One Liberty Plaza, 20th Floor, New York, NY 10006, USA

477 Williamstown Road, Port Melbourne, VIC 3207, Australia

314-321, 3rd Floor, Plot 3, Splendor Forum, Jasola District Centre, New Delhi - 110025, India

79 Anson Road, #06-04/06, Singapore 079906

Cambridge University Press is part of the University of Cambridge.

It furthers the University's mission by disseminating knowledge in the pursuit of education, learning and research at the highest international levels of excellence.

www.cambridge.org
Information on this title: www.cambridge.org/9781316613894
DOI: 10.1017/9781316676325

© Cambridge University Press 2018

First published 2018

A catalogue record for this publication is available from the British Library

Library of Congress Cataloging in Publication data
Names: Akhtar, Shamsuddin, editor. | Rosenbaum, Stanley H., editor.
Title: Principles of geriatric critical care / edited by Shamsuddin Akhtar, Stanley Rosenbaum.
Description: Cambridge, United Kingdom ; New York, NY : University Printing House, 2018. | Includes bibliographical references and index.
Identifiers: LCCN 2018018156 | ISBN 9781316613894 (paperback)
Subjects: | MESH: Geriatrics | Critical Care | Critical Illness | Aged
Classification: LCC RC952.5 | NLM WT 100 | DDC 618.97/029–dc23
LC record available at https://lccn.loc.gov/2018018156

ISBN 978-1-316-61389-4 Paperback

....

Contents

Contributors

Steven R. Allen MD, FACS
Penn State Milton S. Hershey Medical
Center, Hershey, PA, USA

Shamsuddin Akhtar MD
Department of Anesthesiology, Yale School
of Medicine, New Haven, CT, USA

Ruben J. Azocar MD, MHCM, FCCM
Department of Anesthesiology and
Perioperative Medicine, Tufts
University School of Medicine, Boston,
MA, USA

Amit Bardia MD
Department of Anesthesiology, Yale School
of Medicine, New Haven, CT, USA

Jeffrey F. Barletta PharmD, FCCM
Department of Pharmacy Practice,
Midwestern University, Glendale, AZ, USA

Nicole Bryan MD, PhD
Department of Medicine, Section of
Infectious Diseases, West
Virginia University, Morgantown,
WV, USA

David S. Geller, MD PhD
Department of Medicine, Yale School of
Medicine, New Haven, CT

Susan T. Crowley MD
Department of Internal Medicine, Yale
School of Medicine, New Haven, CT, USA

Kimberly A. Davis MD, MBA, FACS, FCCM
Department of Surgery, Yale School of
Medicine, New Haven, CT, USA

John W. Devlin PharmD, FCCM, FCCP
School of Pharmacy, Northeastern
University and Division of Pulmonary,

Critical Care and Sleep Medicine, Tufts
Medical Center, Boston , MA, USA

Brenda G. Fahy MD, MCCM
Department of Anesthesiology, University
of Florida College of Medicine, Gainesville,
FL, USA

Sasha Grek MD
Department of Anesthesiology, University
of Florida College of Medicine, Gainesville,
FL, USA

Nazish K. Hashmi MD
Division of Cardiothoracic Anesthesia
and Critical Care, Department of
Anesthesiology, Duke University
School of Medicine, Durham, NC,
USA

Christopher G. Hughes MD
Department of Anesthesiology, Division of
Anesthesiology Critical Care Medicine,
Vanderbilt University Medical Center,
Nashville, TN, USA

Mazyar Javidroozi MD, PhD
Departments of Anesthesiology, Critical
Care Medicine, and Pain Management,
Englewood Hospital and Medical
Center and Team Health Research
Institute, Englewood, NJ, USA

Lewis J. Kaplan MD, FACS, FCCM
Perelman School of Medicine, University of
Pennsylvania, and the Corporal Michael J.
Crescenz VA Medical Center, Philadelphia,
PA, USA

Felix Y. Lui MD, FACS
Section of General Surgery, Trauma and
Surgical Critical Care, Yale School of
Medicine, New Haven, CT, USA

Linda L. Maerz MD, FACS, FCCM
Section of General Surgery, Trauma and
Surgical Critical Care, Department of
Surgery, Yale School of Medicine, New
Haven, CT, USA

Tracy J. McGrane MD
Department of Anesthesiology, Division of
Anesthesiology Critical Care Medicine,
Vanderbilt University Medical Center,
Nashville, TN, USA

Kristin Oliveira MD
Section of General Surgery, Trauma and
Surgical Critical Care, Department of
Surgery, Yale School of Medicine, New
Haven, CT, USA

Pratik P. Pandharipande MD
Department of Anesthesiology, Division of
Anesthesiology Critical Care Medicine,
Vanderbilt University Medical Center,
Nashville, TN, USA

Ronald Pauldine MD
Department of Anesthesiology and Pain
Medicine, University of Washington
School of Medicine, Seattle, WA, USA

Margaret A. Pisani MD
Section of Pulmonary, Critical Care and
Sleep Medicine, Yale School of Medicine,
New Haven, CT, USA

Mihai V. Podgoreanu MD
Division of Cardiothoracic Anesthesiology
and Critical Care Medicine, Duke
Anesthesiology, Duke University
School of Medicine, Durham, NC, USA

Arif R. Sarwari MD, MSc, MBA
Department of Medicine, Section of
Infectious Diseases, West Virginia
University School of Medicine,
Morgantown, WV, USA

Aryeh Shander MD
Departments of Anesthesiology, Critical
Care Medicine and Pain Management,
Englewood Hospital and Medical Center
and Team Health Research Institute,
Morgantown, NJ, USA

Jonathan M. Siner MD
Section of Pulmonary, Critical Care and
Sleep Medicine, Yale School of Medicine,
New Haven, CT, USA

Faraz Syed DO
Departments of Anesthesiology, Critical
Care Medicine and Pain Management,
Englewood Hospital and Medical Center
and Team Health Research Institute,
Englewood, NJ, USA

Arturo G. Torres MD
Department of Anesthesiology, University
of Florida School of Medicine, Gainesville,
FL, USA

Andrea Tsai MD
Department of Anesthesiology and
Perioperative Medicine, Tufts University
School of Medicine, Boston, MA, USA

Gail A. Van Norman MD
Department of Anesthesiology and Pain
Medicine, University of Washington
School of Medicine, Seattle, WA, USA

Preface

The "aging tsunami" is on us. This is no longer a Western or a developed world problem, but a global problem. Elderly patients, especially those who are more than 80 years old, are one of the fastest growing segments of the population. Population demographics are changing, and the proportion of elderly patients who are being treated for critical illness continues to increase rapidly. Increasing numbers of elderly patients are undergoing surgical procedures that decades ago would have been considered prohibitively high risk and would not be offered to elderly patients. Thus many elderly patients require intensive monitoring and postoperative care in critical care units.

Geriatric patients develop significant physiologic changes with aging, including an increased incidence of frailty and diminished physiologic reserve. Complicating the care of geriatric patients are concurrent multiple comorbidities and a high rate of polypharmacy. Elderly patients are more likely to develop chronic critical illness and cognitive dysfunction and to consume significant healthcare resources. Recovery from critical illness not only implies physical recovery and survival but also successful return to baseline function and quality of life. Unfortunately, many elderly patients are unable to achieve these goals after acute illness.

This book addresses special considerations in geriatric patients who require critical care. It addresses topics related to chronic critical illness, pharmacologic considerations, immunologic considerations, cognitive issues, and organizational concepts necessary to an ideal geriatric critical care unit. The editors hope that this book will be a useful resource for practitioners and will foster further investigation and the development of evidence-based guidelines focused on the management of geriatric critically ill patients.

Chapter

1

Epidemiology of Critical Illness in the Elderly

Kristin Oliveira and Linda L. Maerz

Key Points

- Caring for the aging population is one of the most important challenges of the twenty-first century. A key component of medical care delivery in the elderly is the provision of critical care services.
- In addition to chronologic age, disability, comorbidity, and frailty are components of defining the elderly population. Frailty is a clinical syndrome characterized by multiple factors, including weight loss, fatigue, weakness, low activity level, slow motor performance, balance and gait abnormalities, and cognitive decline. A combination of age, function, and social definitions is key to precisely defining the elderly population.
- The demographics of the global and US populations have changed dramatically over the course of the last two centuries as a consequence of demographic transition, which defines a transition in a population from high birth and death rates to low birth and death rates as a result of economic development.
- The world population reached 7.3 billion in 2015 and has aged at unprecedented rates. By 2050, the number of elderly in the world will, for the first time in history, be greater than the number of young individuals.
- The sharp increase in the US birth rate between 1946 and 1964 is termed the *baby boom*. This has resulted in a drastic shift in the age distribution of the population. In 2015, the median age in the United States was 37 years, and it is estimated that this will increase to 42 years by 2050. Conversely, the total fertility rate in the United States has been declining and was 1.89 in 2015. Therefore, the growth rate of the elderly population is far higher than that of the younger population.
- Chronic medical conditions are expensive to treat. Multimorbidity is the presence of two or more chronic diseases and is common in the elderly, with a prevalence of 40 to 80 percent. It has a substantial impact on mental health, quality of life, and overall health outcomes and is associated with a significant increase in mortality. Disability in the elderly may have an even greater impact on mortality than multimorbidity.
- The elderly population comprises an increasing proportion of patients admitted to intensive care units (ICUs), and the mortality rate for these patients is high. Equally important is the significantly decreased physical function and overall health of ICU survivors.

- The United States spent nearly $3 trillion in healthcare expenses in 2014, which is 17.5 percent of the gross domestic product (GDP), a percentage higher than that of any other country. The elderly use a large portion of the total healthcare expenditure in the United States due to the high hospitalization and institutionalization rate. Healthcare spending increases proportionally with age.
- Areas of opportunity for improvement in the allocation of healthcare resources to the elderly include enhanced awareness and education, studies that precisely define and stratify the elderly, and changing focus from survival to mitigation of cognitive impairment, improvement in quality of life, and an increase in functional autonomy. Identification of the best approach to provide multidisciplinary care ranging from surgical and critical care to palliative care in a manner that enhances communication and achieves desired outcomes will improve the quality of care and reduce healthcare expenditures.

Introduction

Caring for the aging population is one of the most important challenges of the twenty-first century. Media outlets, political figures, books, and television programming frequently elaborate on the difficulties the world will face as the age of the population increases [1]. Studies also indicate that not only are people living to an older age, but they may also have an increased number of quality years, as defined by better cognitive function and self-perceived health at the end of life [2]. Therefore, the aging population has become a topic that deserves attention from the medical community.

As the population age increases, so does the body of medical literature examining the best medical practices to care for the elderly. However, to understand the literature, we must first define the elderly population, evaluate the impact this population has on the medical system, and understand its significance in the current medical culture. A key component of medical care delivery in the elderly is the provision of critical care services.

Definition of the Elderly

In order to understand the unique complexities of the elderly patient, we must first define the elderly population. One way to define elderly age is based on lifespan. In nineteenth-century Britain, the Friendly Societies Act defined old age as "any age after 50." At that time, the average life expectancy at birth was only 47.3 years. Therefore, population groups older than 50 years of age represented a minority of the population [3]. Today, most epidemiologists would argue that the definition of the elderly should be fluid and adjusted in accordance with the ever-increasing life expectancy. According to the Centers for Disease Control and Prevention (CDC), the expected lifespan for Americans at birth in 2013 was 78.8 years, which is a two-year increase from the year 2000 [4]. As healthcare continues to change and life expectancy continues to rise, it becomes necessary to use a metric other than chronologic age to define the elderly.

Medicare Definition

President Johnson passed the Medicare law under Title XVIII of the Social Security Act in 1965. Medicare aimed to provide health insurance to the elderly (people 65 years of age and older) regardless of their sociodemographic status [5]. Because of the significant impact this act had on the medical world, and because of the large number of patients covered by Medicare, much of the medical literature defines elderly age using the chronologic age of 65 years or older. Medicare covered nearly 40 million elderly individuals in 2010 and financed an estimated 15.3 million hospital admissions in 2011, which accounted for almost 47 percent of the total inpatient hospital costs in the United States in 2011 [6].

Global Definition

According to the World Health Organization (WHO), 71 years was the average life expectancy of the global population in 2013. However, the average life expectancy in developing countries is as low as 50 years [7]. Most developed countries use the age of 65 years as the cutoff to define an older person, but in developing countries this definition does not necessarily correlate.

Aging is a chronologic biologic certainty, but it is also subject to the social constructs of cultures. In developed countries such as the United States, chronologic age plays a paramount role. However, in developing countries, the change in social roles plays a far more important part in defining the elderly [8]. In most developed countries, 60 or 65 years is the age of retirement and is therefore often the cutoff for the definition of old age. In contrast, in developing countries, where retirement is less common, social roles and loss of social station due to physical decline play a far more important part in dictating the definition of old age. Therefore, in developing countries, old age commences at the stage of life where one is no longer able to contribute to one's assigned role in society [9].

Frailty or Biologic Age

In developed countries such as the United States, there has historically been inconsistent correlation between chronologic and physiologic age. Multiple attempts have been made to categorize patients as elderly based not only on their age but also on their functional status. Fried et al. distinguishes between disability, frailty, and comorbidity by defining frailty as a clinical syndrome characterized by multiple factors, including weight loss, fatigue, weakness, low activity level, slow motor performance, balance and gait abnormalities, and cognitive decline [10]. While many studies have attempted to create an index to predict biologic age based on frailty, comorbidity, and disability, none have completely captured the complexity that defines the elderly patient [11]. A study by Jacobs et al. evaluated a large cohort of elderly patients who had a favorable overall health profile at the age of 70 years but had progressive deterioration at the age of 78 years and older and more profoundly so at the age of 85 years and older [12]. As a consequence of these data, many suggest that a cutoff of 70 years of age may be a better definition of the elderly; however, there is still a need for further research to differentiate between the aging process and disease morbidity [13].

Because of the varying perspectives pertaining to the definition of the elderly, most would agree that a simple characterization such as age or functional status does not answer the complex question of the definition of old age. It may be more appropriate to use a combination of age, function, and social definitions.

Demographics of the Aging World

Demography comes from the two Greek words, *dēmos*, which means "the people," and *graphō*, which means "measurement." Historically, demography has been defined as the study of changes in human populations over time [14]. The global population has changed dramatically over the last two centuries as a consequence of demographic transition. This concept, described by Warren Thompson, defines a transition in a population from high birth and death rates to low birth and death rates as a consequence of economic development [15]. Pre-industrialized societies have high birth rates because children can contribute to individual household economy. In these societies, however, mortality remains relatively high. Accordingly, the population of the pre-industrialized society is predominantly young. Conversely, as countries begin to industrialize, death rates decline due to improved health and augmented resources. As a consequence, the populations of industrialized countries grow exponentially. Birth rates eventually decrease in post-industrialized societies given improved access to contraception, urbanization, and literacy and increased rates of employment in women. Subsequently, the age distribution in post-industrialized societies shifts to a predominantly elderly population [16].

Global Aging

According to the UN *World Population Prospects* in 2015, the world population reached 7.3 billion, an increase of nearly 1 billion over the last 12 years [17]. It is estimated that the world population is growing at an average rate of 1.18 percent per year [18]. Population growth has been particularly high in the least developed countries; continents with high fertility rates, such as Africa, have had the highest rate of population growth in the last decade (2.5 percent annually) [17].

Given the increased number of industrialized countries in the world, the population has aged at unprecedented rates. Predictably, over the last 10 years, life expectancy has increased globally by 3 years (from 67 to 70 years). The greatest increase in life expectancy occurred in Africa. However, this increase is still significantly lower than the North American life expectancy (60 versus 79 years) [17]. As a result of increased life expectancy, the population group older than 60 years of age has had the largest annual growth rate at a global level (3.2 percent per year), nearly three times that of the population as a whole [17]. In 2015, the United Nations reported that globally, there were 901 million people older than 60 years of age, which comprised nearly 12 percent of the world population. The United Nations estimates that by 2050, the number of elderly in the world will, for the first time in history, be greater than the number of young individuals.

National Aging

The United States has seen similar changes in the age structure of its population. After World War II, there was a historic increase in the annual birth rate, with 3.4 million babies born in 1946, 20 percent higher than the year before. The sharp increase in the birth rate was maintained for nearly 18 years, until 1964, at which point there had been 76 million babies born [19]. This sharp rise in the American birth rate has been termed the *baby boom*. As a consequence, the age structure of the population has been continuously and drastically shifting. In 2015, the United Nations reported that the median age in the United States was 37 years, seven years higher than that in 1980. It is estimated that the median age will continue to increase to 42 years in 2050. According to the most recent US Census of 2010, the median age in the United States varies substantially based on both geography and gender. Northeastern states have the highest and western states the lowest median age (39.2 versus 35 years, respectively). Women have the highest median age throughout the country [20]. Accordingly, life expectancy in the United States has increased from 75 years in 1990 to 79 years in 2015.

In contrast, in United States the total fertility rate (average number of children per woman) has been slowly declining. In 2015, the total fertility rate in the United States was 1.9, 8 percent lower than that documented in 2005. It is estimated that the United States has one of the lowest fertility rates in the world [21]. As expected, these data have substantial ramifications for the age distribution. According to the 2010 US Census, the population of Americans under 18 years of age comprised up to 24 percent of the population, with annual growth rates of 2.6 percent per year. In contrast, the 65 years of age and older population comprised only 13 percent of the total population but had a growth rate nearly six times higher than that of the population group younger than 18 years of age [20].

Outcomes and Trends

Many studies have documented the increased prevalence of chronic medical conditions and lower physiologic reserve in the elderly compared with their younger counterparts [22]. The cost of treating chronic conditions is close to five times higher than that of nonchronic illnesses [23]. Kodner et al. suggest that treatment of chronic diseases represents the highest-cost and fastest-growing segment of US healthcare [24]. Multimorbidity, the presence of two or more chronic diseases, is becoming common among the elderly, with a prevalence of 40 to 80 percent, which is eight times higher than the rate seen in the younger than 19 years of age group [25]. Cognitive impairment and cardiovascular disease are the most common disorders among the elderly. In the elderly population, the prevalence of chronic neurologic disorders increases proportionally with age, beyond that seen with cardiovascular disease, with the oldest-old (>85 years of age) having a prevalence of neurologic disorders as high as 36 percent [26]. Many studies have demonstrated that multimorbidity has a substantial impact on mental health, quality of life [27, 28], and overall health outcomes in the elderly population [29]. Multimorbidity in the elderly population has been associated with substantial increases in the risk of mortality, with some studies reporting risks as high as 53 percent [30]. However, more important than comorbidity is the impact of disability on quality of life and mortality among the elderly. According to the most recent CDC estimates, nearly 36 percent of persons older than 65 years of age have evidence of disability [31]. Several studies have demonstrated that disability plays an important role in mortality in the elderly. Landi et al. suggest that the effect of disability on the risk of death was higher than, and independent of, multiple comorbidities. However, the combination of both multiple comorbidities and disability greatly increases the risk of mortality in this population group [32].

Outcomes in Critical Care

The elderly population comprises an increasing proportion of the patients admitted to ICUs. Approximately one-half of all patients admitted to the ICU are over age 65, even though this same age cohort comprises only approximately 12 percent of the population [33]. Despite advances in medical and surgical care, the mortality rate for elderly patients admitted to the ICU is unacceptably high. A study by Tabah et al. demonstrated that the one-year mortality rate was 67 percent in the subgroup of elderly patients being admitted to the ICU for unscheduled surgery [34]. Consistent with these results, de Rooij et al. demonstrated that the one-year mortality rate for both medical and unplanned surgical admissions in the elderly was 89 percent [35].

Equally important is the consideration of how patients who survive their ICU admission will function after discharge. Roch et al. suggest that the two-year mortality rate of patients over 80 years of age who are admitted to the ICU remains unacceptably high compared with the general population. Approximately 50 percent of the elderly discharged from the hospital after their ICU stay were not be alive after two years. Moreover, the physical function and overall health of the survivors were significantly decreased compared with younger populations [36].

Cost of Elderly Healthcare

The ratio of dependent people (children <18 years of age and adults >64 years of age) to 100 working-age people (18 to 64 years of age) is termed the *age-dependency ratio*. This can provide estimates of the economic burden the nonworking population places on the working population. In the United States, the total age-dependency ratio dropped from 2000 to 2010 (61 to 59), signifying that there were 2.7 fewer "dependent-age" people for every 100 working-age people [37]. However, these calculations include both the young and the elderly. The youth age-dependency ratio (<18 years of age) is not expected to increase significantly in the next two decades. However, all the baby boomers will have transitioned to the elderly population over the course of the next two decades. As a consequence, the elderly age-dependency ratio (>64 years of age) is projected to climb rapidly from 22 to 35 in the next two decades [38]. The anticipated increase in the elderly age-dependency ratio is of particular concern in the context of rising healthcare costs in the United States. According to the most recent estimates from the Centers for Medicare and Medicaid Services (CMS), the United States spent nearly $3 trillion in healthcare expenses in 2014, a historical high. This represents approximately 17.5 percent of the US GDP, higher than for any other country in the world [39].

The elderly use a large portion of the total healthcare expenditure in the United States. This is primarily due to the high hospitalization and institutionalization rate among the elderly. Rice et al. suggest that in any given year, 20 percent of the elderly will be hospitalized, and almost a quarter of the elderly will become institutionalized in a nursing home during their lifetimes [40]. According to the CDC, close to 96 percent of the elderly population incurs some healthcare expense every year. CMS estimated that in 2010, the healthcare spending for people older than 64 years of age was $18,424 per person, which is five times higher than the spending per child ($3,628) and three times higher than the spending per working-age person ($6,125) [41].

The increases in healthcare spending increase proportionally with age, nearly doubling between 70 and 90 years of age and peaking at age 96 before tapering off. The mean Medicare spending per person in 2011 was more than double for individuals 96 years of age compared with those 70 years of age ($16,145 versus $7,566, respectively) [42]. Among the elderly, the oldest-old (those ≥80 years of age) comprised 24 percent of the Medicare population and up to a third of total Medicare spending. In contrast, the younger elderly (aged 65 to 69 years) comprised 26 percent of the Medicare population and only 15 percent of Medicare spending [43]. These spending patterns are of particular concern given the disproportionate growth of the oldest-old. It is estimated that from 2010 to 2050, the US population aged 65 and older will nearly double, but the population aged 80 and older will triple [44].

Assuming no drastic changes in the mortality rate of the elderly, it is uniformly accepted that the total cost of healthcare for the elderly will continue to increase. The Agency for Healthcare Research and Quality (AHRQ) estimated that the total healthcare expenses for the elderly in 2011 were $414.3 billion, which was over $100 billion higher than inflation-adjusted expenses for 2001 [45].

The demographic transition that began in both the United States and the world in the nineteenth century continues to have an impact on the age structure of the world. The increasing life expectancy and decreasing fertility rates have drastically modified the age distribution of all countries. The unprecedented reversal in the proportion of young and older population groups will continue to have significant ramifications for healthcare spending and the economies of both developing and developed countries.

Areas of Opportunity for Improvement

Given the staggering statistics regarding the increased numbers of the aging population, it is important for the medical community to focus efforts on improving healthcare for the elderly. Some of the promising areas of opportunity for improvement include awareness and education, studies to define and stratify the elderly more precisely, and a changing focus from survival to mitigation of cognitive impairment, improvement in quality of life, and increases in functional autonomy.

Currently, there is a paucity of data on clinical outcomes in very elderly population (>80 years of age) because many of the previous studies have categorized the elderly as anyone over the age of 65. Many new studies, however, now focus attention on the stratification of age and the difference in needs and outcomes for those individuals who are *extremely elderly*, the *very elderly*, and the *eldest elderly*. The exact ages at which these terms are used varies by study and may apply to individuals older than 70 to 90 years of age [46]. As the population continues to age, it will become increasingly important to define the extreme elderly and to focus research on the specific medical needs and prognoses of this population.

Another area of opportunity for improvement is in the culture of clinical practice, where the focus has traditionally been on improving disease-specific outcomes. Much improvement and data are needed to encourage the shift of focus to overall and long-term goals. As mentioned earlier, mortality for older patients after discharge from the hospital is substantial, and morbidity of the survivors is unacceptably high. Several studies have emphasized the importance of counseling to help prepare patients and families for the difficulties they will face once patients leave the hospital [36]. Equally important is education and preparation for end-of-life discussions in this high-risk group. Literature is emerging to develop guidelines to identify patients who benefit most from palliative care services in the ICU [47]. It will become increasingly important to identify the best approach to provide multidisciplinary care ranging from surgical and critical care to palliative care in a manner that enhances communication and achieves desired outcomes.

Conclusion

The aging of the population in the United States and worldwide will have a substantial impact on healthcare and will create many new challenges and opportunities for medical professionals. The medical community must embrace the changing demographics of our patient populations and focus our efforts not only on improving the life expectancy of our patients but also on improving the quality of life and care, especially for those in the later decades of life. We look forward to the growing body of literature focused on the older population, which will allow us to better understand the very specific needs and concerns of this unique population. It is important to remember that most persons will at some point become elderly, and clinicians should embrace the mentality espoused by Tia Walker in her book about caregivers, "[t]o care for those who once cared for us is one of the highest honors" [48].

References

1. Gusmano MK, Allin S. Framing the issue of ageing and health care spending in Canada, the United Kingdom and the United States. *Health Econ Policy Law* 2014; **9**:313–28.

2. Jagger C, Matthews FE, Wohland P, et al. A comparison of health expectancies over two decades in England: results of the Cognitive Function and Ageing Study I and II. *Lancet* 2015; **387**:779–86.

3. Center for Diseases Control and Prevention. Life expectancy at birth, at age 65, and at age 75, by sex, race, and Hispanic origin: United States, selected years 1900–2010, 2011, available at www.cdc.gov/nchs/data/hus/2011/022.pdf (accessed February 12, 2016).

4. Center for Diseases Control and Prevention. Deaths: final data for 2013, 2016, available at www.cdc.gov/nchs/data/hus/hus14.pdf–016 (accessed February 21, 2016).

5. Oliver TR, Lee PR, Lipton HL. A political history of medicare and prescription drug coverage. *Milbank Q* 2004; **82**:283–54.

6. Torio CM, Andrews RM. National inpatient hospital costs: the most expensive conditions by payer, 2011, 2013, available at www.hcup-us.ahrq.gov/reports/statbriefs/sb160.pdf (accessed February 10, 2016).

7. World Health Organization. Global health observatory data: life expectancy, 2013, available at www.who.int/gho/mortality_burden_disease/life_tables/situation_trends_text/en/ (accessed February 10, 2016).

8. Glascock AP, Feinman S, Holocultural A. Analysis of old age. *Comp Soc Res* 1980; **3**: 311–33.

9. Shah E. The ageing and development report 1999: poverty, independence and the world's older people. *BMJ* 2000; **321**:517.

10. Fried LP, Ferrucci L, Darer J, et al. Untangling the concepts of disability, frailty, and comorbidity: implications for improved targeting and care. *J Gerontol A Biol Sci Med Sci* 2004; **59**:255–63.

11. Rockwood K, Mitnitski A. Frailty defined by deficit accumulation and geriatric medicine defined by frailty. *Clin Geriatr Med* 2011; **27**:17–26.

12. Jacobs JM, Maaravi Y, Cohen A, et al. Changing profile of health and function from age 70 to 85 years. *Gerontology* 2012; **58**:313–21.

13. Newman AB, Ferrucci L. Aging versus disease. *J Gerontol A Biol Sci Med Sci* 2009; **64**:1163–64.

14. Fitzgerald JF. An introduction to the practice of preventive medicine. *Am. J Public Health* 1923; **19**:47–48.

15. Demeny PG, McNicoll G. *Encyclopedia of Population*. New York: Macmillan Reference USA, 2003.

16. Holmes KK. Human ecology and behavior and sexually transmitted bacterial infections. *Proc Natl Acad Sci USA* 1994; **91**:2448–55.

17. United Nations Department of Economic and Social Affairs. World population prospects: the 2015 revision, 2015, available at http://esa.un.org/unpd/wpp/ (accessed February 10, 2016).

18. American Statistical Association. World population likely to surpass 11 billion in 2100: US population projected to grow by 40 percent over next 85 years, 2015, available at www.sciencedaily.com/releases/2015/08/150810110634.htm (accessed February 10, 2015).

19. Tice C, Perkins K. Case management for the baby boom generation: a strengths perspective. *J Case Manag* 1998; **7**:31–36.

20. United States Census Bureau. 2010 Census, 2012, available at www.census.gov/ipc/

www/usinterimproj (accessed January 29, 2016).

21. Jensen MB, Priskorn L, Jensen TK, et al. Temporal trends in fertility rates: a nationwide registry based study from 1901 to 2014. *PLoS One* 2015; **10**:e0143722.

22. Milzman DP, Boulanger BR, Rodriguez A, et al. Pre-existing disease in trauma patients: a predictor of fate independent of age and injury severity score. *J Trauma* 1992; **32**:236–43.

23. Schlesinger M, Mechanic D. Challenges for managed competition from chronic illness. *Health Aff* 1993; **12**:123–37.

24. Kodner DL, Kyriacou CK. Fully integrated care for frail elderly: two American models. *Int J Integr Care* 2000; **1**:e08.

25. Akker MV, Buntinx F, Metsemakers JF, et al. Multimorbidity in general practice: prevalence, incidence, and determinants of co-occurring chronic and recurrent diseases. *J Clin Epidemiol* 1998; **51**:367–75.

26. Marengoni A, Winblad B, Karp A, et al. Prevalence of chronic diseases and multimorbidity among the elderly population in Sweden. *Am J Public Health* 2008; **98**:1198–200.

27. Fortin M, Bravo G, Hudon C, et al. Psychological distress and multimorbidity in primary care. *Ann Fam Med* 2006; **4**: 417–22.

28. Fortin M, Bravo G, Hudon C, et al. Relationship between multimorbidity and health-related quality of life of patients in primary care. *Qual Life Res* 2006; **15**:83–91.

29. St John PD, Tyas SL, Menec V, et al. Multimorbidity, disability, and mortality in community-dwelling older adults. *Can Fam Physician* 2014; **60**:272–80.

30. Lu FP, Chang WC, Wu SC. Geriatric conditions, rather than multimorbidity, as predictors of disability and mortality among octogenarians: a population-based cohort study. *Geriatr Gerontol Int* 2016; **16**: 345–51.

31. Courtney-Long EA, Carroll DD, Zhang QC, et al. Prevalence of disability and disability type among adults. *MMWR Morb Mortal Wkly Rep* 2015; **64**:777–83.

32. Landi F, Liperoti R, Russo A, et al. Disability, more than multimorbidity, was predictive of mortality among older persons aged 80 years and older. *J Clin Epidemiol* 2010; **63**:752–9.

33. Adelman RD, Berger JT, Macina LO. Critical care for the geriatric patient. *Clin Geriatr Med* 1994; **10**:19–30.

34. Tabah A, Philippart F, Timsit JF, et al. Quality of life in patients aged 80 or over after ICU discharge. *Crit Care* 2010; **14**:R2.

35. Rooij SE, Govers AC, Korevaar JC, et al. Cognitive, functional, and quality-of-life outcomes of patients aged 80 and older who survived at least one year after planned or unplanned surgery or medical intensive care treatment. *J Am Geriatr Soc* 2008; **56**: 816–22.

36. Roch A, Wiramus S, Pauly V, et al. Long-term outcome in medical patients aged 80 or over following admission to an intensive care unit. *Crit Care* 2011; **15**:R36.

37. Lindsay JAM, Howden M. Age and sex composition: 2010 US Census briefs, 2010, available at www.census.gov/population/age/data/2010comp.html (accessed January 29, 2016).

38. Grayson K, Velko VA. The next four decades: the older population in the United States: 2010 to 2050. *Curr Pop Reps US Census* 2010; **186**:1–16.

39. Martin AB, Hartman M, Benson J, et al. National health spending in 2014: faster growth driven by coverage expansion and prescription drug spending. *Health Aff* 2016; **35**:150–60.

40. Rice T, Gabel J. Protecting the elderly against high health care costs. *Health Aff* 1986; **5**:5–21.

41. Centers for Medicare and Medicaid Services. Medicare data for the geographic variation: a methodological overview, 2010, available at www.cms.gov/research-statistics-data-and-systems/statistics-trends-and-reports/medicare-geographic-variation/downloads/geo_var_puf_methods_paper.pdf (accessed January 29, 2016).

42. Neuman P, Cubanski J, Damico A. Medicare per capita spending by age and

service: new data highlights oldest beneficiaries. *Health Aff* 2015; **34**:335–39.

43. Anderson GF, Steinberg EP. Hospital readmissions in the Medicare population. *N Engl J Med* 1984; **311**:1349–53.

44. Ortman JM, Velkoff VA, Hogan H. An aging nation: the older population in the United States, 2014, available at www.census.gov/content/dam/Census/library/publications/2014/demo/p25-1140.pdf (accessed January 29, 2016).

45. Lisa KC, Mirel B. Trends in health care expenditures for the elderly, age 65 and over: 2001, 2006, and 2011, 2014, available at www.meps.ahrq.gov/mepsweb/data_

files/publications/st429/stat429.pdf (accessed January 29, 2016).

46. Greenwald PW, Stern ME, Rosen T, et al. Trends in short-stay hospitalizations for older adults from 1990 to 2010: implications for geriatric emergency care. *Am J Emerg Med* 2014; **32**:311–14.

47. Bradley CT, Brasel KJ. Developing guidelines that identify patients who would benefit from palliative care services in the surgical intensive care unit. *Crit Care Med* 2009; **37**:946–50.

48. Speers P, Walker T. *The Inspired Caregiver: Finding Joy While Caring for Those You Love.* Charlston, NC: CreateSpace Independent Publishing Platform, 2015.

Chronic Critical Illness in Geriatric Patients

Amit Bardia and Shamsuddin Akhtar

Key Points

- Chronic critical illness is used to describe patients who survive the initial acute episode of critical illness but persistently remain dependent on intensive care.
- It is typically defined as need for mechanical ventilation for more than 6 hours per day for more than 21 consecutive days with concurrent neurologic changes, endocrine alterations, muscle wasting, predisposition to infection, and changes in body composition, including loss of lean body mass.
- Elderly patients are especially vulnerable to develop chronic critical illness, with its prevalence peaking from 75 to 79 years of age.
- Chronic critical illness involves systemic derangement of immunologic function, persistent inflammation, neurocognitive issues, endocrine imbalance, malnutrition, and muscle wasting.
- Due to elevated levels of catecholamine and glucocorticoids, the metabolism is shifted to the catabolic phase. There is a marked decrease in the pulsatile secretion of anterior pituitary hormones.
- A majority of critically ill patients suffer from neuromuscular weakness, which is broadly classified into critical illness polyneuropathy (CIP), critical illness myopathy (CIM), and combined CIM/CIP.
- Despite the significant burden on the healthcare system afforded by chronic critical illness, there is a lack of guideline-based recommendations regarding management of this patient cohort.

Introduction

Over the last few decades, with significant advances in the field of critical care, the overall mortality of acutely critically ill patients has decreased. These advances include life-sustaining measures that provide artificial support to organs while the patient is recovering from the acute insult [1]. However, a new patient population has emerged that remains dependent on intensive services for their survival for prolonged periods of time. This population is referred to as *chronically critically ill.*

The term *chronically critically ill* was first used by Girard et al. in 1985 to describe patients who survived the initial acute episode of critical illness but persistently remained dependent on intensive care [2,3]. Despite wide recognition of this syndrome, there seems to be a lack of consensus regarding its concrete definition [4]. However, most experts agree that prolonged mechanical ventilation, defined as the need for mechanical ventilation for more than 6 hours per day for more than 21 consecutive days, is a hallmark of this disease [1,5]. Other manifestations of this syndrome include neurologic changes, endocrine alterations, muscle wasting, predisposition to infection, and changes in body composition, including loss of lean body mass.

Epidemiology

With improving survival from acute critical illness, the overall incidence of chronic critical illness (CCI) is on the rise. According to recent estimates, CCI has an overall population-based prevalence of 34.4 per 100,000 [6]. Elderly patients are especially vulnerable to develop CCI, with its prevalence peaking from 75 to 79 years of age. There is a decline of CCI among patients older than 80 years because of a higher early mortality among otherwise eligible patients (Figure 2.1).

Chronic critical illness incurs a tremendous clinical and financial burden, with estimated healthcare cost of $10 billion [7]. Despite meticulous and highly skilled care, CCI is associated with poor long-term survival [8], with 20 percent of surviving patients having residual physical and cognitive impairments and less than 10 percent ever returning home after hospitalization [9]. Moreover, with a rise in the aging population and improvements in management of acute illnesses, the incidence of CCI is expected to increase further [10]. Not surprisingly, CCI has been receiving increasing attention from researchers, healthcare providers, and health policymakers. However, strategies to prevent and improve outcomes in patients with CCI still remain clinically challenging.

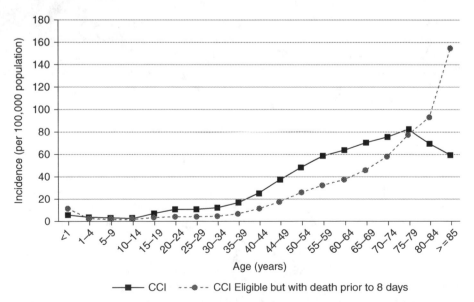

Figure 2.1 Age-specific population-based prevalence of CCI (dark line) and CCI-eligible conditions but with death prior to 8 days (dashed line). Data are for the five-state sample, all years. (*Source:* From Kahn et al. [6].)

Pathophysiology of Chronic Critical Illness

It is estimated that between 5 and 10 percent of patients with acute critical illness who require mechanical ventilation progress to CCI [3,11,12]. The presence of declining baseline organ function and multiple comorbidities predisposes geriatric patients to prolonged mechanical ventilation and CCI. Although various risk factors [11,13–15] and models [12,16,17] for predicting prolonged mechanical ventilation have been described, their applicability in the geriatric population remains to be validated. Additionally, there are no biomarkers to predict CCI. CCI involves systemic derangement of immunologic function, persistent inflammation, neurocognitive issues, endocrine imbalance, malnutrition, and muscle wasting.

Persistent Inflammation, Immunosuppression, and Catabolism

Patients who develop CCI show signs of persistent systemic inflammatory state. They develop a dysregulated response after an acute insult, which leads to the release of pro-inflammatory cytokines such as interleukin-6 and interleukin-8, which continue to be elevated even after resolution of the initial insult [9]. There are persistently increased levels of circulating glucocorticoids, catecholamines, and prostaglandins, leading to further amplification of the inflammatory milieu.

Enhanced levels and prolonged inflammation lead directly to immunosuppression [18]. There is a marked downregulation of antigen receptors at the cell surface and cell signaling pathways, chemotaxis, antigen presentation, and phagocytosis, which hamper the efficacy of the immune response [19–23]. Not surprisingly, CCI patients have been shown to have absolute lymphocyte depletion, decreased antibody per bound cell, and T-cell downregulation, which manifest clinically as an increased incidence of pneumonia and other nosocomial infections [24].

Due to elevated levels of catecholamine and glucocorticoids, the metabolism is shifted to the catabolic phase [25,26]. This leads to a profound change in body composition and a reduction in lean body mass despite adequate nutritional supplementation [27].

This model of maladaptive body response leading to persistent inflammation, immunosuppression, and catabolic syndrome (PICS) was proposed by Gentile et al. [28]. They proposed that a patient meets PICS criterion if residing in the intensive care unit (ICU) for at least 10 days and having persistent inflammation defined by a C-reactive protein concentration of greater than 150 µg/dl and a retinol-binding protein concentration of less than 10 µg/dl, immunosuppression crudely defined by a total lymphocyte count of less than 800/mm^3, and a catabolic state defined by a serum albumin concentration of less than 3.0 g/dl, a creatinine height index of less than 80 percent, and weight loss greater than 10 percent or body mass index (BMI) less than 18, during the current hospitalization.

Geriatric patients are extremely susceptible to developing PICS. They have a abnormal inflammatory state at baseline, often referred to as *inflamm-aging* [29], and are particularly prone to this dysfunctional cytokine response after an acute insult [30]. This is further exacerbated by immunosenescence, which is characterized by multiple immune-related disorders concomitant with aging [31] (see Chapter 10). It includes decreased number of Langerhans cells, impaired neutrophil and macrophage function, decreased T-cell activation, and decreased cytotoxicity by natural killer (NK) cells [32–38]. Finally, underlying nutritional deficiencies in the elderly are further exacerbated by this state of catabolism accelerating sarcopenia and leading to cachexia [27] (Figure 2.2).

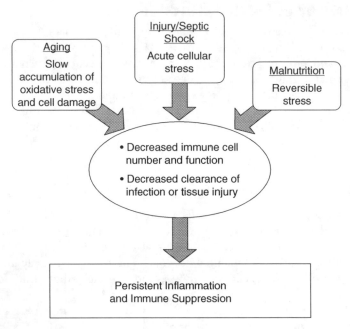

Figure 2.2 Hypothetical representation of the interaction of aging, severe injury, sepsis, and malnutrition and the development of persistent inflammation and immune suppression. (*Source:* From Nomellini et al. [9].)

Clinical Manifestations

In addition to respiratory failure requiring prolonged mechanical ventilation, this syndrome is characterized by a distinct pattern of multiorgan dysfunction. This includes neurologic changes, endocrine alterations, myopathy, loss of lean body mass, and increased susceptibility to infection.

Neurologic Changes

Most patients with CCI suffer from severe neurocognitive dysfunction, with half the survivors being comatose or delirious at hospital discharge [39]. Of these, a majority continue to have neurocognitive deficits at six-months (79 percent) and one-year (71 percent) follow-up [40]. In addition to delirium, neurocognitive issues in patients with CCI include impairments in attention, memory, and executive function [41]. Elderly patients, those with a longer duration of delirium in the acute phase and increased severity of illness, and those affected by multiple complications constitute the patient population at highest risk of developing brain dysfunction [41,42]. Patients with advanced age often have preexisting neurocognitive issues, altered pharmacodynamics, and coexisting diseases, which increase their susceptibility to CCI. The exact mechanism behind the development of these neurocognitive deficits is currently unknown, but it is believed that hypotension, hypoxia, metabolic derangements, and iatrogenic causes such as sedatives may play a role.

In addition, CCI patients incur extreme mental and emotional stress. The presence of tracheostomy (or endotracheal) tubes makes communication difficult. Not surprisingly, more than 40 percent of these patients suffer from anxiety, posttraumatic stress disorder

(PTSD), and depressive disorders [43–47]. The inability to perform activities of daily living (ADLs), difficulty in communication, the need for mechanical ventilation, and poorly treated pain are among the many factors that contribute to psychiatric issues in this patient population.

Endocrine Changes

Patient with CCI experience endocrinopathies that are often a continuation or sequela of the initial acute critical illness. There is a marked decrease in the pulsatile secretion of anterior pituitary hormones [48–50]. This pulsatile loss of growth hormone correlates with decreased anabolism and promotes catabolic metabolism. Similarly, decreased pulsatile thyroid-stimulating hormone (TSH) secretion leads to low plasma T_3 and T_4 levels [1]. The peripheral conversion of T_4 to T_3 is also decreased [51]. Low T_3 plasma levels correlate with muscle weakness and bone loss. Although the adrenocorticotropic hormone (ACTH) levels are low, cortisol levels remain high. High cortisol levels are probably secondary to decreased cortisol clearance in the chronic inflammatory milieu [52]. High cortisol levels contribute to muscle wasting, hyperglycemia with insulin resistance, decreased wound healing, and increased susceptibility to secondary infection. They also contribute to fluid retention and anasarca, which is commonly seen in patients with CCI. Increased peripheral insulin resistance seen in patients with CCI often leads to prolonged hyperglycemia, which has been shown to correlate with mortality [53]. Male CCI patients have been shown to have extremely low levels of testosterone and have high levels of estrogen, indicating increased aromatization of androgens [54,55]. These abnormalities in the gonadal axis may play a role in promoting a catabolic state in CCI patients because testosterone is the most potent endogenous anabolic steroid [56].

Malnutrition

The stress from critical illness, chronic inflammation and the catabolic state increases the nutritional requirements of CCI patients. Unfortunately, these patients often have poor mentation along with swallowing dysfunction. Consequently, they are unable to meet their dietary requirements, which can lead to profound nutritional deficiencies. Geriatric patients with poor preexisting nutritional state, malabsorption, and poor nutritional reserve are prone to malnutrition after critical illness.

Due to the catabolic state, there also is a shift toward proteolysis and gluconeogenesis. The body preferentially uses muscle proteins as an energy substrate, which leads to substantial muscle breakdown. This has profound effects on respiratory muscle strength, ventilatory capacity, and maximal inspiratory effort, which further complicate weaning from the ventilator in patients with CCI [57,58]. In addition, malnutrition has also been shown to blunt the ventilatory drive [59].

Synthetic function of the liver is impaired. as reflected by hypoalbuminemia, leading to low intravascular oncotic pressure and the development of anasarca [60,61]. Patients with CCI often have deficiency in both micro- and macronutrients. Patients often have vitamin D deficiency, leading to bone resorption [62,63]. Similarly, lack of micronutrients such as carnitine has been linked to mitochondrial dysfunction and multiorgan failure during CCI [64]. Elderly patients with CCI often also have electrolyte imbalances, leading to hypernatremia, hypophosphatemia, and hypomagnesemia, which can further impair mentation and respiratory function [65]. Malnutrition also predisposes patients to have abnormal hematopoiesis and immune dysfunction, leading to chronic anemia and increased propensity to have nosocomial infections [66].

Neuromuscular Alterations

A majority of critically ill patients suffer from neuromuscular weakness [67]. Broadly, these disorders are classified into critical illness polyneuropathy (CIP), critical illness myopathy (CIM), combined CIM/CIP, and prolonged neuromuscular blockade. This adversely affects the respiratory muscles, which complicates ventilator weaning, the muscles involved in deglutition, leading to swallowing difficulties and increased risk of aspiration, and the muscles of the extremities, which impairs mobility [68].

Critical illness polyneuropathy is characterized by symmetrical involvement usually of the limbs, especially the lower extremities, weakness of proximal neuromuscular regions (shoulder and hip girdle), and involvement of the respiratory muscles [69]. It usually spares the oculofacial muscles and cranial nerves [70]. Although patients with CIP may exhibit distal sensory loss, it may be difficult to elicit because a significant number of patients with CCI have altered mental status.

Critical illness polyneuropathy is a distal axonal sensorimotor polyneuropathy believed to be secondary to disruption of the blood-brain barrier and neuronal injury by inflammatory mediators [1,71,72]. Electrophysiology studies are generally consistent with a generalized axonal sensorimotor polyneuropathy with low motor and sensory amplitudes [73].

Chronic critical illness patients with CIM have flaccid quadriparesis (proximal greater than distal muscles), difficulty weaning from mechanical ventilation, and often facial muscle weakness [74,75]. Unlike CIP, CIM may be associated with a rise in serum creatine kinase (CK) levels. Muscle histopathologic findings are of myopathy with myosin loss. Electrophysiology studies reveal normal to low motor amplitudes with occasional prolongation of compound muscle action potential [76,77]. Sensory responses are usually preserved.

Critical illness myopathy and CIP can coexist in patients with CCI [78,79]. Patients with CIM have quicker resolution of weakness compared with those with CIP or combined CIM/CIP [80]. Prolonged neuromuscular blockade is a rare form of weakness seen in patients who underwent prolonged neuromuscular junction blockade and had compromised liver or renal function [81]. Train of Four monitoring usually is diagnostic of this form of weakness, although formal testing sometimes may be necessary.

Management of Chronic Critical Illness

Management of CCI patients is an emerging challenge for today's healthcare systems. Despite the significant burden on the healthcare system afforded by CCI, there is a lack of guideline-based recommendations regarding management of this patient cohort.

One of the major challenges remains early identification of patients who meet the definition of CCI. There can also be various venues where these patients receive care, including ICUs, step-down units, weaning units, and floors in acute care hospitals, as well as specialized centers such as long-term acute care hospitals (LTACHs). Variation in care is affected not only by the venue but also by the staffing ratios. The composition of a care team ideally should be multidisciplinary, including physicians, nurses, respiratory therapists, physical therapists, and speech and language specialists, as well as nutritionists who continue to deliver critical care in a manner similar to most ICUs. The goal is to create a comprehensive care plan for the patient with the goal of targeting a return to a functional status, as close to before the illness as possible. In many ways, this might be more of a challenge than in the acute care setting, given not only the resource-intensive patient needs but also a background of multiple chronic illnesses, more limited resources, and continued proclivity for clinical decompensation. In fact, the outcomes for these patients remain grim, with a high 1-year mortality rate of 50 to 77 percent [82,83], significant debilitation at discharge [84], multiple transitions in care following incident hospitalization [8], and increased caregiver fatigue and stress [82].

Tracheostomy and Mechanical Ventilation (MV)

Liberation from mechanical ventilation becomes one of the cornerstones of management. The timing of tracheostomy placement in the acute care setting is becoming shorter, with an average recommendation of about 10 days of mechanical ventilation [85]. Patients with tracheostomies often get admitted to chronic care facilities for weaning from ventilator support. Ventilator dependence is an independent cause of diaphragmatic muscle fiber atrophy [86], and mechanical ventilator for as few as 6 days is shown to cause a 30 percent decline in pressure differentials created by diaphragmatic contraction [87], which predisposes to prolonged mechanical ventilation. As in the acute care setting, adherence to a protocol-driven approach for weaning has been shown to decrease days on mechanical ventilation [88]. Despite the absence of evidence specific to chronic care facilities, formulating a daily multidisciplinary plan of care with adherence to objective data points and constant team and family communication can shorten the duration of mechanical ventilation. In this regard, implementing the ABCDEF bundle (i.e., *Assess*, prevent, and manage pain; *Both* spontaneous awakening trials and spontaneous breathing trials; *Choice* of sedation and analgesia; assess, prevent, and manage *Delirium; Early* mobility and exercise; and *Family* engagement and empowerment [89,90]) is likely to improve time to liberation from mechanical ventilation in this patient cohort. Weaning protocols can be effectively managed by respiratory therapists, and in coordination with bedside nursing, physical therapy, and a speech and language specialist, patients can make a robust clinical improvement. Various methodologies, e.g., use of the Rapid Shallow Breathing Index (RSBI) [91] and use of 50 percent lower ventilator support or T-piece trials for spontaneous breathing trials for as long as tolerated by the patient (often >120 minutes) used in the acute setting are routinely part of the process of weaning patients [5]. Patients who prove to be difficult to wean off ventilator support often require a more thorough assessment of barriers to liberation from the ventilator. Integration of bedside ultrasound in the assessment of diaphragmatic contractility in difficult-to-wean patients can be a useful tool to identify and follow such patients [92]. Once weaned from mechanical ventilation, a standardized approach to tracheostomy decannulation is pursued. In chronic care facilities, management of dysphonia as well as dysphagia after tracheostomy requires engagement of a dedicated speech and language specialist to assist patients in regaining normal function.

Analgesia, Sedation, and Delirium

Assessment of pain in geriatric patients with CCI can be quite challenging. While obvious in patients who have undergone surgical procedures (e.g., trauma, neurologic, or surgical ICU patients), pain is probably significantly underestimated in other patients. Overreliance on clinical markers of pain (hypertension, tachycardia, sweating, frowning), inability of patients to communicate (due to mechanical ventilation, altered consciousness, and pre-existing conditions such as visual and hearing impairment), and lack of validated nonverbal pain assessment tools in patients in the CCI population further complicate management. Routine clinical activities including turns, repositioning, and catheter placement/exchange/removal are all recurrent stimuli of pain. In addition, most patients in the acute care setting likely will be exposed to analgesics (continuous or intermittent infusions during ventilation), and it is important for clinicians to remember to address this in formulating care plans for CCI patients. It is recommended that these patients be treated with a scheduled opiate taper of at least a week's duration if they have been exposed to opiate infusions in their incident hospitalization [90]. While continuous opiate infusions should not be routinely used in most CCI facilities [90], multimodality enteral opiate and nonopiate pain management strategies should be used to manage pain in CCI patients. The goal of analgesia should be such that patients can participate in mobilization and physical therapy while minimizing the side effects of analgesics, including nausea, constipation, sedation, respiratory depression, and the potential for dependence.

Use of sedatives such as propofol, benzodiazepines, and dexmedetomidine is a frequent part of ICU care, especially in mechanically ventilated patients. Despite quality evidence favoring light sedation [93], practice patterns can vary significantly between ICUs. It is therefore not uncommon to see CCI patients who have received high-dose sedatives during their incident hospitalization. Standard recommendations include strict adherence to daily spontaneous awakening trials and use of sedatives only if indicated, starting at half the original dose. Nonbenzodiazepine sedatives are preferred over benzodiazepines [94].

Similar to the acute care setting, delirium in CCI patients has been associated with significantly worse outcomes. It is especially prevalent in geriatric CCI patients given their advanced age, comorbidities, and baseline use of psychotherapeutics. The majority of delirium is hypoactive and goes largely unrecognized, necessitating the use of validated tools such as CAM-ICU [95] in the CCI population. Again, clinicians need to be mindful of the fact that sedatives used in acute care settings, especially benzodiazepines, can increase the risk of delirium significantly. A conservative strategy could include tapering doses of benzodiazepines (if they have been used in acute care setting) in patients with CCI. Significant attention should be paid to delirium prevention, including maintenance of day-night cycle, use of appropriate light cues to promote wakefulness during the day, minimizing noise and clinical interruptions at night to promote sleep, use of restorative visual and hearing aids as soon as the patient is able, and involvement of family visitation and interaction to promote the well-being of patients. Routine use of pharmacologic interventions for the management of delirium is not recommended, and such use should be limited to severe manifestations (e.g., hallucinations, psychosis). Use of daily diaries (written by patients or family members) documenting the patient's stay in a LTACH setting has been shown to help patients with PTSD.

Nutrition

Nutritional assessment and management form the cornerstone for treating geriatric patients with CCI. A specialized approach involving daily assessments by clinicians, nursing staff, and dietitians is of paramount importance in this setting.

Nutritional Assessment. All CCI patients should undergo periodic nutritional assessment, including one at the time of admission to LTACHs. Commonly used nutritional assessment measures involve anthropometric measures (preadmission dry adjusted weight), comprehensive physical examination (temporal wasting, sarcopenia), evaluation of hypoalbuminemic state with fluid status (ascites, pleural effusion, sacral, scrotal, and pedal edema), daily calorie counts, and laboratory indices such as prealbumin, transferrin, and retinol-binding protein levels [96]. In addition, these measures can be used to determine response to nutritional interventions in CCI patients. Although various screening tools such as the Nutritional Risk Index (NRI), subjective global assessment (SGA), and Mini Nutritional Assessment have been described to assess nutritional risk [97–99], currently no clinically validated tool exists for patients with CCI. Determination of nutritional status thus relies on the multidisciplinary team taking care of the CCI patient [61].

Nutritional Goals. The key strategy of nutritional supplementations in patients with CCI is to replenish the nitrogen deficit by ensuring adequate protein intake, preventing underfeeding/overfeeding, and minimizing nutritional interruptions. Both overfeeding and underfeeding are associated with poor outcomes and increased mortality [100–102]. However, determination of adequate energy requirements in geriatric CCI patients is clinically challenging. Given the difficulties associated with indirect calorimetry, the lack of consensus with regard to the use of predictive equations, and the variability of pathophysiologic states in CCI patients, a target of 20 to 25 kcal/kg adjusted dry weight per day is often recommended by experts [61]. It is important to recognize that this "one size fits all" strategy may not hold true for all CCI patients, especially the elderly, and does not replace the requirement of periodic nutritional assessment in these patients. Similarly, a daily protein intake of 1.5 g/kg is recommended [103]. Patients with impaired wound healing, decubitus ulcers, high ostomy outputs, and undergoing renal replacement therapy usually have higher protein requirements. Overfeeding protein can result in hyperammonemia and azotemia, leading to encephalopathy, hypertonic dehydration, and hypernatremia [96]. Periodic measurement of serum blood urea nitrogen (BUN) and sodium thus is recommended to avoid such "protein overfeeding" scenarios.

Chronic critical illness patients often develop *refeeding syndrome* after reintroduction of carbohydrate-based diets. The key features of this syndrome include acute hypophosphatemia, reduction of thiamine and electrolytes such as magnesium and potassium, acute volume expansion, impaired oxygen delivery, and myocardial injury [51,104]. Hypophosphatemia may affect diaphragmatic muscle function and further impair attempts at weaning from mechanical ventilation. Interruptions in diet thus should be minimized, and a high clinical suspicion of refeeding syndrome should be maintained on resumption of feeding. If patients do develop symptoms indicative of refeeding syndrome, feeds should be restricted to about 1,000 kcal/day with slow increments over time and close electrolyte monitoring.

Chronically ventilated patients often require supplemental feeding because tracheotomy affects the muscles of deglutition. Enteral feeding is often preferred over parenteral feeding due to its lower costs and lower invasiveness [105–108]. Enteral feeding has the advantages of preserving gastrointestinal integrity, reducing bacterial translocation, and modulating immunologic and catabolic responses [61,109,110]. However, enteral feeding is commonly associated with interruptions in feeding, especially for procedures, leading to underfeeding. Semi-elemental feeds are preferred over whole-protein formulations. Choice of appropriate enteral formulations should be based on the patient's underlying pathophysiology, sodium status, renal status, and tolerance to a particular formulation [61]. Routine use of "pulmonary formulations" may lead to delayed gastric emptying [111].

Parenteral nutrition is often reserved for patients who are unable to meet their caloric requirements with enteral nutrition alone. Parenteral nutrition is associated with a higher risk of infectious complications than enteral nutrition [108]. Special care should be undertaken to ensure sterility of the central line site, and electrolytes should be monitored closely for patients undergoing parenteral nutrition.

In addition to macronutrients, judicious replenishment of micronutrients is of paramount importance, especially in the geriatric CCI patient population. Vitamin D and pamidronate help with decreasing bone resorption, calcitriol promotes calcium uptake by gastrointestinal tract, vitamin C and zinc sulfate promote wound healing, and carnitine helps in fatty acid oxidation. In addition, pharmacologic supplementation with megesterol, methylphenidate, or mirtazapine may help in stimulating appetite in CCI patients. Thyroid supplementation is often required in these patients based on thyroid function tests. Judicious glycemic control with insulin supplementation forms an integral part of patient management. In addition to intensive insulin management, serial blood sugar checks should be performed to avoid hypoglycemia.

Additional Management Strategies

Early mobilization along with muscle training has been shown to be beneficial in intubated patients [112]. Early physical therapy and mobilization help in decreasing the incidence of pressure ulcers, limb contractures, and deep venous thrombosis in CCI patients. Similarly, whole-body rehabilitation including limb strengthening exercises, trunk control, body posture maintaining exercises, and subsequently ambulation with a wheeled walking aid has been shown to be effective in successful ventilator weaning in patients receiving prolonged mechanical ventilation [113–115]. In addition, such measures enable CCI patients to recover from critical illness myopathies and regain muscle strength and enable them to perform the activities of daily living (ADLs) in the long run. This is especially important for geriatric patients in whom the performance of ADLs is an important milestone toward independent function. Thus early involvement of physical and occupational therapy forms an integral part of CCI management.

Pressure ulcer prevention and aggressive treatment are pivotal in the management of CCI patients because pressure ulcers may progress to osteomyelitis and further complicate the clinical course if left untreated. Pressure ulcer prevention requires daily assessment by the clinical team, timely postural changes, special pressure-reducing mattresses, and barrier ointment application [116,117].

Patients with CCI often have indwelling catheters and intravenous lines. Similar to acute critical care management, daily assessments of the position, functioning, and utility of these lines should be made. Every attempt at early removal of these catheters should be made to prevent further line-related complications.

Communication with Patient and Family Members

Because patients are often unable to participate in decision making regarding continuity of care, families frequently get involved as surrogate decision makers. This can be an emotionally difficult time for most. Depending on the age, quality of life prior to critical illness, and burden of chronic health conditions, the decision to continue intensive care or focus on comfort, often comes to the forefront. In the case where a patients' wishes are clearly known, the burden of this decision is somewhat eased for surrogates. However, there is still a significant proportion of the elderly, that might not have communicated their wishes to their family. The nature of modern day nuclear families can further increase the stress of providing care to a chronic critical ill patient, not just from an emotional, but also a financial and caregiver stress perspective. The transformation of a patient from an independent functional status to being ventilator dependent often with concomitant weakness, delirium and skin breakdown can be a traumatic experience for patients and family alike. Not surprisingly, posttraumatic stress disorder is also common amongst caregivers of patients with CCI [118]. In addition, the experiences of individual patients and families are colored by their cultural and religious backgrounds, belief systems, and health literacy. An inclusive and respectful approach is therefore needed to address the needs of this population.

Communication with CCI patients (when cognizant) and their families is of utmost importance in ongoing care. This can occur in varied settings between patient surrogates and the healthcare team, e.g., daily communication at the bedside or a more formalized conference approach. In many cases, clinicians often find themselves in a unique role of providing information, predicting the course of a patient's clinical trajectory, providing emotional support to the family, and eliciting the goals of care from the surrogate decision makers for a patient. This often requires a multidisciplinary approach from the clinical team (including ICU physicians, palliative care physicians, nursing staff, chaplaincy, social work, etc.) and can be even more challenging when dealing with end-of-life decision making in CCI patients [119]. It is also important to anticipate conflicts in decision making and have a consistent approach to deal with such situations as and when they arise. Palliative care should be an integral part of the care plan for CCI patients [3]. An integrated approach by ICU and palliative care teams with repeated contacts to guide patients and families through simple as well as more complex decisions is likely to have better outcomes than a "same size fits all" structured approach [120].

References

1. Marchioni A, Fantini R, Antenora F, Clini E, Fabbri L. Chronic critical illness: the price of survival. *Eur J Clin Invest* 2015; **45**:1341–49.

2. Girard K, Raffin TA. The chronically critically ill: to save or let die? *Respir Care* 1985; **30**:339–47.

3. Nelson JE, Cox CE, Hope AA, Carson SS. Chronic critical illness. *Am J Respir Crit Care Med* 2010; **182**:446–54.

4. Carson SS, Bach PB. The epidemiology and costs of chronic critical illness. *Crit Care Clin* 2002; **18**:461–76.

5. MacIntyre NR, Epstein SK, Carson S, et al. National Association for Medical Direction of Respiratory C. Management of patients requiring prolonged mechanical ventilation: report of a namdrc consensus conference. *Chest.* 2005; **128**:3937–3954.

6. Kahn JM, Le T, Angus DC, et al. ProVent Study Group I. The epidemiology of chronic critical illness in the United States. *Crit Care Med* 2015; **43**:282–87.

7. Lamas D. Chronic critical illness. *N Engl J Med* 2014; **370**:175–77.

8. Unroe M, Kahn JM, Carson SS, et al. One-year trajectories of care and resource utilization for recipients of prolonged mechanical ventilation: a cohort study. *Ann Intern Med.* 2010; **153**:167–75.

9. Nomellini V, Kaplan LJ, Sims CA, Caldwell CC. Chronic critical illness and persistent inflammation: what can we learn from the elderly, injured, septic, and malnourished? *Shock* 2017.

10. Angus DC, Shorr AF, White A, et al. Critical care delivery in the United States: distribution of services and compliance

with leapfrog recommendations. *Crit Care Med* 2006; **34**:1016–24.

11. Seneff MG, Zimmerman JE, Knaus WA, Wagner DP, Draper EA. Predicting the duration of mechanical ventilation: the importance of disease and patient characteristics. *Chest* 1996; **110**:469–79.

12. Clark PA, Lettieri CJ. Clinical model for predicting prolonged mechanical ventilation. *J Crit Care* 2013; **28**(880): e881–87.

13. Estenssoro E, Gonzalez F, Laffaire E, et al. Shock on admission day is the best predictor of prolonged mechanical ventilation in the ICU. *Chest* 2005; **127**:598–603.

14. Sapijaszko MJ, Brant R, Sandham D, Berthiaume Y. Nonrespiratory predictor of mechanical ventilation dependency in intensive care unit patients. *Crit Care Med* 1996; **24**:601–7.

15. Troche G, Moine P. Is the duration of mechanical ventilation predictable? *Chest* 1997; **112**:745–51.

16. Clark PA, Inocencio RC, Lettieri CJ. I-trach: validating a tool for predicting prolonged mechanical ventilation. *J Intensive Care Med* 2016.

17. Anon JM, Gomez-Tello V, Gonzalez-Higueras E, et al. Prolonged mechanical ventilation probability model. *Med Intensiva* 2012; **36**:488–95.

18. Alves-Filho JC, de Freitas A, Spiller F, Souto FO, Cunha FQ. The role of neutrophils in severe sepsis. *Shock* 2008; **30** (Suppl 1):3–9.

19. Adams JM, Hauser CJ, Livingston DH, et al. Early trauma polymorphonuclear neutrophil responses to chemokines are associated with development of sepsis, pneumonia, and organ failure. *J Trauma* 2001; **51**:452–56; discussion 456–57.

20. Cummings CJ, Martin TR, Frevert CW, et al. Expression and function of the chemokine receptors cxcr1 and cxcr2 in sepsis. *J Immunol* 1999; **162**: 2341–46.

21. Gomez CR, Karavitis J, Palmer JL, et al. Interleukin-6 contributes to age-related

alteration of cytokine production by macrophages. *Mediators Inflamm* 2010; 2010:475139.

22. Asehnoune K, Roquilly A, Abraham E. Innate immune dysfunction in trauma patients: from pathophysiology to treatment. *Anesthesiology* 2012; **117**: 411–16.

23. Kovach MA, Standiford TJ. The function of neutrophils in sepsis. *Curr Opin Infect Dis* 2012; **25**:321–27.

24. Stortz JA, Murphy TJ, Raymond SL, et al. Evidence for persistent immune suppression in patients who develop chronic critical illness after sepsis. *Shock* 2017.

25. Slotwinski R, Sarnecka A, Dabrowska A, et al. Innate immunity gene expression changes in critically ill patients with sepsis and disease-related malnutrition. *Cent Eur J Immunol* 2015; **40**:311–24.

26. Wang H, Ye J. Regulation of energy balance by inflammation: common theme in physiology and pathology. *Rev Endocr Metab Disord* 2015; **16**:47–54.

27. Rosenthal MD, Moore FA. Persistent inflammatory, immunosuppressed, catabolic syndrome (PICS): a new phenotype of multiple organ failure. *J Adv Nutr Hum Metab* 2015; **1**.

28. Gentile LF, Cuenca AG, Efron PA, et al. Persistent inflammation and immunosuppression: a common syndrome and new horizon for surgical intensive care. *J Trauma Acute Care Surg* 2012; **72**: 1491–501.

29. Franceschi C, Bonafe M, Valensin S, et al. Inflamm-aging: an evolutionary perspective on immunosenescence. *Ann NY Acad Sci* 2000; **908**:244–54.

30. Fullerton JN, O'Brien AJ, Gilroy DW. Pathways mediating resolution of inflammation: when enough is too much. *J Pathol* 2013; **231**:8–20.

31. Castelo-Branco C, Soveral I. The immune system and aging: a review. *Gynecol Endocrinol* 2014; **30**:16–22.

32. van Duin D, Mohanty S, Thomas V, et al. Age-associated defect in human tlr-1/2 function. *J Immunol* 2007; **178**:970–75.

33. Villanueva JL, Solana R, Alonso MC, Pena J. Changes in the expression of HLA-class II antigens on peripheral blood monocytes from aged humans. *Dis Markers* 1990; **8**:85–91.

34. Simell B, Vuorela A, Ekstrom N, et al. Aging reduces the functionality of anti-pneumococcal antibodies and the killing of *Streptococcus pneumoniae* by neutrophil phagocytosis. *Vaccine* 2011; **29**: 1929–34.

35. Wenisch C, Patruta S, Daxbock F, Krause R, Horl W. Effect of age on human neutrophil function. *J Leukoc Biol* 2000; **67**:40–45.

36. Butcher SK, Chahal H, Nayak L, et al. Senescence in innate immune responses: reduced neutrophil phagocytic capacity and CD16 expression in elderly humans. *J Leukoc Biol* 2001; **70**:881–86.

37. Hazeldine J, Hampson P, Lord JM. Reduced release and binding of perforin at the immunological synapse underlies the age-related decline in natural killer cell cytotoxicity. *Aging Cell* 2012; **11**:751–59.

38. Grewe M. Chronological ageing and photoageing of dendritic cells. *Clin Exp Dermatol* 2001; **26**:608–12.

39. Nelson JE, Tandon N, Mercado AF, et al. Brain dysfunction: another burden for the chronically critically ill. *Arch Intern Med* 2006; **166**:1993–99.

40. Jackson JC, Girard TD, Gordon SM, et al. Long-term cognitive and psychological outcomes in the awakening and breathing controlled trial. *Am J Respir Crit Care Med* 2010; **182**:183–91.

41. Hope AA, Morrison RS, Du Q, Wallenstein S, Nelson JE. Risk factors for long-term brain dysfunction after chronic critical illness. *Ann Am Thorac Soc* 2013; **10**:315–23.

42. Girard TD, Jackson JC, Pandharipande PP, et al. Delirium as a predictor of long-term cognitive impairment in survivors of critical illness. *Crit Care Med* 2010; **38**: 1513–20.

43. Jubran A, Lawm G, Kelly J, et al. Depressive disorders during weaning from prolonged mechanical ventilation. *Intensive Care Med* 2010; **36**:828–35.

44. Chelluri L, Im KA, Belle SH, et al. Long-term mortality and quality of life after prolonged mechanical ventilation. *Crit Care Med* 2004; **32**:61–69.

45. Griffiths J, Fortune G, Barber V, Young JD. The prevalence of post traumatic stress disorder in survivors of ICU treatment: a systematic review. *Intensive Care Med* 2007; **33**:1506–18.

46. Jones C, Backman C, Capuzzo M, et al. Precipitants of post-traumatic stress disorder following intensive care: a hypothesis generating study of diversity in care. *Intensive Care Med* 2007; **33**: 978–85.

47. Twigg E, Humphris G, Jones C, Bramwell R, Griffiths RD. Use of a screening questionnaire for post-traumatic stress disorder (PTSD) on a sample of UK ICU patients. *Acta Anaesthesiol Scand* 2008; **52**:202–8.

48. Beishuizen A, Thijs LG. The immunoneuroendocrine axis in critical illness: beneficial adaptation or neuroendocrine exhaustion? *Curr Opin Crit Care* 2004; **10**:461–67.

49. Van den Berghe G, de Zegher F, Veldhuis JD, et al. The somatotropic axis in critical illness: effect of continuous growth hormone (GH)–releasing hormone and Gh-releasing peptide-2 infusion. *J Clin Endocrinol Metab* 1997; **82**: 590–99.

50. Van den Berghe G, de Zegher F, Veldhuis JD, et al. Thyrotrophin and prolactin release in prolonged critical illness: dynamics of spontaneous secretion and effects of growth hormone-secretagogues. *Clin Endocrinol (Oxf)* 1997; **47**:599–612.

51. Mechanick JI, Brett EM. Endocrine and metabolic issues in the management of the chronically critically ill patient. *Crit Care Clin* 2002; **18**:619–41, viii.

52. Boonen E, Vervenne H, Meersseman P, et al. Reduced cortisol metabolism during critical illness. *N Engl J Med* 2013; **368**: 1477–88.

53. Krinsley JS. Glycemic control in the critically ill: 3 domains and diabetic status means one size does not fit all! *Crit Care* 2013; **17**:131.

54. Spratt DI. Altered gonadal steroidogenesis in critical illness: is treatment with anabolic steroids indicated? *Best Pract Res Clin Endocrinol Metab* 2001; **15**:479–94.

55. Van den Berghe G, de Zegher F, Lauwers P, Veldhuis JD. Luteinizing hormone secretion and hypoandrogenaemia in critically ill men: effect of dopamine. *Clin Endocrinol (Oxf)* 1994; **41**:563–69.

56. Vanhorebeek I, Langouche L, Van den Berghe G. Endocrine aspects of acute and prolonged critical illness. *Nat Clin Pract Endocrinol Metab* 2006; **2**:20–31.

57. Arora NS, Rochester DF. Respiratory muscle strength and maximal voluntary ventilation in undernourished patients. *Am Rev Respir Dis* 1982; **126**:5–8.

58. Kelly SM, Rosa A, Field S, et al. Inspiratory muscle strength and body composition in patients receiving total parenteral nutrition therapy. *Am Rev Respir Dis* 1984; **130**:33–37.

59. Doekel RC, Jr, Zwillich CW, Scoggin CH, Kryger M, Weil JV. Clinical semi-starvation: depression of hypoxic ventilatory response. *N Engl J Med* 1976; **295**:358–61.

60. Fuhrman MP, Charney P, Mueller CM. Hepatic proteins and nutrition assessment. *J Am Diet Assoc* 2004; **104**:1258–64.

61. Schulman RC, Mechanick JI. Metabolic and nutrition support in the chronic critical illness syndrome. *Respir Care* 2012; **57**:958–77; discussion 977–58.

62. Nierman DM, Mechanick JI. Bone hyperresorption is prevalent in chronically critically ill patients. *Chest* 1998; **114**: 1122–28.

63. Van den Berghe G, Van Roosbroeck D, Vanhove P, et al. Bone turnover in prolonged critical illness: effect of vitamin D. *J Clin Endocrinol Metab* 2003; **88**: 4623–32.

64. Bonafe L, Berger MM, Que YA, Mechanick JI. Carnitine deficiency in chronic critical illness. *Curr Opin Clin Nutr Metab Care* 2014; **17**:200–9.

65. Aubier M, Murciano D, Lecocguic Y, et al. Effect of hypophosphatemia on diaphragmatic contractility in patients with acute respiratory failure. *N Engl J Med* 1985; **313**:420–24.

66. Loftus TJ, Moore FA, Moldawer LL. ICU-acquired weakness, chronic critical illness, and the persistent inflammation-immunosuppression and catabolism syndrome. *Crit Care Med* 2017; **45**: e1184.

67. Fan E, Dowdy DW, Colantuoni E, et al. Physical complications in acute lung injury survivors: a two-year longitudinal prospective study. *Crit Care Med* 2014; **42**: 849–59.

68. Schweickert WD, Hall J. ICU-acquired weakness. *Chest* 2007; **131**:1541–49.

69. Kress JP, Hall JB. ICU-acquired weakness and recovery from critical illness. *N Engl J Med* 2014; **370**:1626–35.

70. Latronico N, Shehu I, Seghelini E. Neuromuscular sequelae of critical illness. *Curr Opin Crit Care* 2005; **11**:381–90.

71. Batt J, dos Santos CC, Cameron JI, Herridge MS. Intensive care unit–acquired weakness: clinical phenotypes and molecular mechanisms. *Am J Respir Crit Care Med* 2013; **187**: 238–46.

72. Fenzi F, Latronico N, Refatti N, Rizzuto N. Enhanced expression of E-selectin on the vascular endothelium of peripheral nerve in critically ill patients with neuromuscular disorders *Acta Neuropathol* 2003; **106**:75–82.

73. Lacomis D. Electrophysiology of neuromuscular disorders in critical illness. *Muscle Nerve* 2013; **47**:452–63.

74. Lacomis D, Giuliani MJ, Van Cott A, Kramer DJ. Acute myopathy of intensive care: clinical, electromyographic, and pathological aspects. *Ann Neurol* 1996; **40**: 645–54.

75. Showalter CJ, Engel AG. Acute quadriplegic myopathy: analysis of myosin isoforms and

evidence for calpain-mediated proteolysis. *Muscle Nerve* 1997; **20**:316–22.

76. Crone C. Tetraparetic critically ill patients show electrophysiological signs of myopathy. *Muscle Nerve* 2017; **56**:433–40.

77. Goodman BP, Harper CM, Boon AJ. Prolonged compound muscle action potential duration in critical illness myopathy. *Muscle Nerve* 2009; **40**:1040–42.

78. Koch S, Spuler S, Deja M, et al. Critical illness myopathy is frequent: accompanying neuropathy protracts icu discharge. *J Neurol Neurosurg Psychiatry* 2011; **82**:287–93.

79. Latronico N. Neuromuscular alterations in the critically ill patient: critical illness myopathy, critical illness neuropathy, or both? *Intensive Care Med* 2003; **29**: 1411–13.

80. Intiso D, Amoruso L, Zarrelli M, et al. Long-term functional outcome and health status of patients with critical illness polyneuromyopathy. *Acta Neurol Scand* 2011; **123**:211–19.

81. Segredo V, Caldwell JE, Matthay MA, et al. Persistent paralysis in critically ill patients after long-term administration of vecuronium. *N Engl J Med* 1992; **327**: 524–28.

82. Cox CE, Martinu T, Sathy SJ, et al. Expectations and outcomes of prolonged mechanical ventilation. *Crit Care Med* 2009; **37**:2888–94; quiz 2904.

83. Carson SS, Bach PB, Brzozowski L, Leff A. Outcomes after long-term acute care: an analysis of 133 mechanically ventilated patients. *Am J Respir Crit Care Med* 1999; **159**:1568–73.

84. Scheinhorn DJ, Hassenpflug MS, Votto JJ, et al. Ventilation Outcomes Study G. Post-ICU mechanical ventilation at 23 long-term care hospitals: a multicenter outcomes study. *Chest* 2007; **131**:85–93.

85. Groves DS, Durbin CG, Jr. Tracheostomy in the critically ill: indications, timing and techniques. *Curr Opin Crit Care* 2007; **13**:90–97.

86. Levine S, Nguyen T, Taylor N, et al. Rapid disuse atrophy of diaphragm fibers in mechanically ventilated humans. *N Engl J Med* 2008; **358**:1327–35.

87. Jaber S, Petrof BJ, Jung B, et al. Rapidly progressive diaphragmatic weakness and injury during mechanical ventilation in humans. *Am J Respir Crit Care Med* 2011; **183**:364–71.

88. Scheinhorn DJ, Chao DC, Stearn-Hassenpflug M, Wallace WA. Outcomes in post-ICU mechanical ventilation: a therapist-implemented weaning protocol. *Chest* 2001; **119**:236–42.

89. Balas MC, Vasilevskis EE, Olsen KM, et al. Effectiveness and safety of the awakening and breathing coordination, delirium monitoring/management, and early exercise/mobility bundle. *Crit Care Med* 2014; **42**:1024–36.

90. Balas MC, Devlin JW, Verceles AC, Morris P, Ely EW. Adapting the abcdef bundle to meet the needs of patients requiring prolonged mechanical ventilation in the long-term acute care hospital setting: historical perspectives and practical implications. *Semin Respir Crit Care Med* 2016; **37**:119–35.

91. Chao DC, Scheinhorn DJ. Determining the best threshold of Rapid Shallow Breathing Index in a therapist-implemented patient-specific weaning protocol. *Respir Care* 2007; **52**:159–65.

92. Umbrello M, Formenti P. Ultrasonographic assessment of diaphragm function in critically ill subjects. *Respir Care* 2016; **61**:542–55.

93. Treggiari MM, Romand JA, Yanez ND, et al. Randomized trial of light versus deep sedation on mental health after critical illness. *Crit Care Med* 2009; **37**:2527–34.

94. Bioc JJ, Magee C, Cucchi J, et al. Cost effectiveness of a benzodiazepine vs a nonbenzodiazepine-based sedation regimen for mechanically ventilated, critically ill adults. *J Crit Care* 2014; **29**: 753–57.

95. Wei LA, Fearing MA, Sternberg EJ, Inouye SK. The confusion assessment method: a systematic review of current usage. *J Am Geriatr Soc* 2008; **56**: 823–30.

96. Mechanick JI, Brett EM. Nutrition and the chronically critically ill patient. *Curr Opin Clin Nutr Metab Care* 2005; **8**: 33–39.

97. Buzby GP, Knox LS, Crosby LO, et al. Study protocol: a randomized clinical trial of total parenteral nutrition in malnourished surgical patients. *Am J Clin Nutr* 1988; **47**:366–81.

98. Kondrup J, Rasmussen HH, Hamberg O, Stanga Z, Ad Hoc ESPEN Working Group. Nutritional risk screening (NRS 2002): a new method based on an analysis of controlled clinical trials. *Clin Nutr* 2003; **22**:321–36.

99. Anthony PS. Nutrition screening tools for hospitalized patients. *Nutr Clin Pract* 2008; **23**:373–82.

100. Artinian V, Krayem H, DiGiovine B. Effects of early enteral feeding on the outcome of critically ill mechanically ventilated medical patients. *Chest* 2006; **129**:960–67.

101. Barr J, Hecht M, Flavin KE, Khorana A, Gould MK. Outcomes in critically ill patients before and after the implementation of an evidence-based nutritional management protocol. *Chest* 2004; **125**:1446–57.

102. Grau T, Bonet A, Rubio M, et al. Liver dysfunction associated with artificial nutrition in critically ill patients. *Crit Care* 2007; **11**:R10.

103. Cerra FB, Benitez MR, Blackburn GL, et al. Applied nutrition in ICU patients: a consensus statement of the American College of Chest Physicians. *Chest* 1997; **111**:769–78.

104. Solomon SM, Kirby DF. The refeeding syndrome: a review. *JPEN J Parenter Enteral Nutr* 1990; **14**:90–97.

105. Loss SH, Nunes DSL, Franzosi OS, et al. Chronic critical illness: are we saving patients or creating victims? *Rev Bras Ter Intensiva* 2017; **29**:87–95.

106. Kattelmann KK, Hise M, Russell M, et al. Preliminary evidence for a medical nutrition therapy protocol: enteral feedings for critically ill patients. *J Am Diet Assoc* 2006; **106**:1226–41.

107. McClave SA, Taylor BE, Martindale RG, et al. Guidelines for the provision and assessment of nutrition support therapy in the adult critically ill patient: Society of Critical Care Medicine (SCCM) and American Society for Parenteral and Enteral Nutrition (ASPEN). *JPEN J Parenter Enteral Nutr* 2016; **40**:159–211.

108. Elke G, van Zanten AR, Lemieux M, et al. Enteral versus parenteral nutrition in critically ill patients: an updated systematic review and meta-analysis of randomized controlled trials. *Crit Care* 2016; **20**:117.

109. Kompan L, Kremzar B, Gadzijev E, Prosek M. Effects of early enteral nutrition on intestinal permeability and the development of multiple organ failure after multiple injury. *Intensive Care Med* 1999; **25**:157–61.

110. Oltermann MH. Nutrition support in the acutely ventilated patient. *Respir Care Clin North Am* 2006; **12**:533–45.

111. Doley J, Mallampalli A, Sandberg M. Nutrition management for the patient requiring prolonged mechanical ventilation. *Nutr Clin Pract* 2011; **26**: 232–41.

112. Schweickert WD, Pohlman MC, Pohlman AS, et al. Early physical and occupational therapy in mechanically ventilated, critically ill patients: a randomised controlled trial. *Lancet* 2009; **373**:1874–82.

113. Martin UJ, Hincapie L, Nimchuk M, Gaughan J, Criner GJ. Impact of whole-body rehabilitation in patients receiving chronic mechanical ventilation. *Crit Care Med* 2005; **33**:2259–65.

114. Clini EM, Crisafulli E, Antoni FD, et al. Functional recovery following physical training in tracheotomized and chronically ventilated patients. *Respir Care* 2011; **56**:306–13.

115. Chiang LL, Wang LY, Wu CP, Wu HD, Wu YT. Effects of physical training on functional status in patients with

prolonged mechanical ventilation. *Phys Ther* 2006; **86**:1271–81.

116. Shahin ES, Dassen T, Halfens RJ. Pressure ulcer prevention in intensive care patients: guidelines and practice. *J Eval Clin Pract* 2009; **15**:370–74.

117. de Laat EH, Pickkers P, Schoonhoven L, et al. Guideline implementation results in a decrease of pressure ulcer incidence in critically ill patients. *Crit Care Med* 2007; **35**:815–20.

118. Wintermann GB, Weidner K, Strauss B, Rosendahl J, Petrowski K. Predictors of posttraumatic stress and quality of life in family members of chronically critically ill patients after intensive care. *Ann Intensive Care* 2016; **6**:69.

119. Truog RD, Campbell ML, Curtis JR, et al. Recommendations for end-of-life care in the intensive care unit: a consensus statement by the American College of Critical Care Medicine. *Crit Care Med* 2008; **36**:953–63.

120. Carson SS, Cox CE, Wallenstein S, et al. Effect of palliative care-led meetings for families of patients with chronic critical illness: a randomized clinical trial. *JAMA* 2016; **316**:51–62.

Chapter 3

Principles of Geriatric Pharmacotherapy

John W. Devlin and Jeffrey F. Barletta

Key Points

- Older adults frequently experience adverse drug events in the intensive care unit (ICU), due to age-related pharmacokinetic and pharmacodynamic changes, polypharmacy, and frequent transitions of care.
- Adverse drug events can be reduced in the geriatric population by individualizing dosing, avoiding potentially inappropriate medications when possible, recognizing prescribing cascades, reconciling medications at ICU discharge, and incorporating a critical care pharmacist on the ICU team.
- The effects of age on drug absorption, volume of distribution, and drug metabolism and clearance must be considered when optimizing medication therapy in the ICU setting.
- Important dosing considerations must be employed when nonintravenous routes of administration are used in critically ill older adults.
- Extremes in body weight are common in older adults and should be considered when optimizing pharmacotherapy in this population.
- Kidney function and the use of strategies such as renal replacement therapy (RRT) to support this function must be carefully evaluated and considered when optimizing drug therapy in older ICU adults.
- Older adults usually require far lower doses of opioids and sedatives and experience more adverse events with their use.
- Nonpharmacologic interventions such as early mobilization and the avoidance of delirium-causing medications (e.g., benzodiazepines) are more effective strategies to reduce the burden of delirium in older adults than initiating antipsychotic therapy.
- A number of pharmacodynamic and pharmacokinetic factors should be considered when optimizing anti-infective regimens in critically ill older adults.
- Body weight, kidney function, and the availability of a reversal agent should be considered when implementing anticoagulant therapy in the geriatric ICU population.

Introduction

Older adults (≥65 years) comprise an ever-increasing proportion of patients admitted to the ICU [1]. Very old adults (≥80 years) now make up more than 25 percent of the patients admitted to most ICUs. An ever-increasing proportion of older adults is chronically critically ill and frequently move between the long-term acute care hospital (LTACHs) and ICU settings [2]. Drug therapy plays a key role in improving outcomes after critical illness. With the average older adult admitted to an ICU administered 30 different medications throughout their stay, critical care clinicians are faced with making multiple drug-related decisions on a daily basis [3]. A number of different age-related effects increase the risk for medication-associated adverse events and drug interactions. Polypharmacy is a common consequence of critical illness among older adults and is associated with deleterious outcomes and increased costs [4]. This chapter reviews key concepts regarding medication choice, dosing, and monitoring in critically ill older adults and provides ICU clinicians with a number of strategies to improve the medication-related outcomes of geriatric patients under their care.

Epidemiology and Outcomes of Drug Therapy

Many older adults have multiple chronic conditions that require multiple medications and, on average, are prescribed 12 different prescription medications [5]. Adverse drug events account for more than 30 percent of all hospital admissions among older adults, and a drug-related cause is a frequent reason for ICU admission [6,7]. Use of herbal and over-the-counter (OTC) medications has doubled among older adults in the past 10 years; 10 percent will experience a major herbal/OTC–prescription drug interaction each year [8]. Prescribing cascades (i.e., a new medication is initiated to treat the side effects of another) remain an important driver of polypharmacy in the ICU setting.

Safe and effective medication use is crucial to ensure optimal patient care and ICU outcome. Critical illness–associated acute organ dysfunction will affect drug absorption, clearance, and response and increase adverse events [3]. Data generated in non-ICU settings should not be extrapolated to elderly ICU patients, in whom acuity of illness is higher, goals of therapy are different and change frequently with patient pathophysiologic condition, the duration of medication use is generally short, and monitoring practices are more rigorous [9]. There is a dearth of rigorous data to guide prescribing decisions for critically ill patients, which results in "off label" use for nearly half the medications ultimately prescribed [10].

Several drugs often used to treat critical illness are listed in the Beers List of low-benefit and/or high-risk medications – a list of medication deemed by geriatricians as "preferably avoided" in older adults in chronic healthcare settings [11]. Potentially inappropriate medications (PIMs) are frequently prescribed in the ICU setting [12]; the number of PIMs prescribed directly correlates with the duration of ICU stay [13]. Factors shown to increase the risk for a PIM being continued at ICU discharge include the number of PIMs prescribed during the ICU admission, admission to a surgical (versus medical) service, and discharge to another facility rather than home [14].

Transitions of care are frequent among older adults given the high proportion of this cohort that reside in long-term care facilities. They undergo frequent periods of decompensation, or suffer a new acute illness that requires management in the ICU. The post–intensive care syndrome (PICS), a new or worsening decrement in mental, cognitive, or physical health following critical illness persisting beyond the acute hospitalization, occurs frequently in older adults who survive their ICU admission [15]. Medications that potentiate glucose dysregulation and delirium or worsen ICU-acquired weakness may worsen PICS [16].

Pharmacokinetic and Pharmacodynamic Alterations in Older Adults

Pharmacokinetics refers to the discipline that describes the absorption, distribution, metabolism, and elimination of drugs (i.e., what the *body* does to the drug). *Pharmacodynamics* is the study of the relationship between the concentration of a drug and the response obtained in a patient (i.e., what the *drug* does to the body). Several significant alterations develop in pharmacokinetic and pharmacodynamic parameters with aging and in the geriatric critically ill patient that must be considered in order to maximize outcomes and minimize drug toxicity and adverse effects.

Pharmacokinetics

Absorption

While splanchnic blood flow, gastric emptying time, and small intestine absorptive capacity are decreased in the elderly, drug absorption, for the most part, remains relatively unchanged in this population [17]. Nevertheless, a few key concepts should be considered. Delayed gastric emptying may be clinically significant for medications for which a rapid onset is desired (e.g., opioids). Because of reductions in liver mass and blood flow, the first-pass metabolism is lower in the elderly, and the bioavailability of medications that undergo extensive first-pass metabolism (e.g., labetalol, propranolol) may be higher.

Distribution

Volume of distribution is a mathematical concept that refers to the compartments into which a drug disperses. Significant age-related changes occur to body composition that have an impact on volume of distribution and hence drug concentration. Age-related reductions in total body water and increases in total body fat may lead to increased concentrations (due to a smaller volume of distribution) for hydrophilic drugs such as aminoglycosides and digoxin [18]. In contrast, lipophilic drugs (e.g., diazepam) will have a larger volume of distribution, and loading doses may need to be modified. However, clinicians should be cautious in increasing doses in elderly patients, given that age-related reductions in clearance may result in drug accumulation and prolonged effects.

Age-related changes in protein binding are of minimal clinical significance in most patients, but in the setting of critical illness, they can be profound. Acidic drugs bind to albumin, which is often decreased in patients with burns, liver disease, sepsis, uremia, and trauma. Low albumin levels lead to reductions in drug-protein binding, which cause an increase in the unbound fraction of pharmacologically active drugs such as phenytoin and warfarin. Basic drugs such as morphine bind to alpha-1-acid glycoprotein, which is an acute-phase reactant and is often increased in patients with renal failure, burns, infections, and myocardial infarction and in those who have undergone recent surgery. Protein binding in these settings is elevated, and unbound drug concentrations are decreased.

Metabolism

Drug metabolism depends on both the amount of blood flow to the liver and the liver's ability to extract the drug from the bloodstream. Both of these processes are affected by age. Hepatic blood flow decreases by 30 percent between the ages of 30 and 75; thus the metabolism of drugs that rely on flow-dependent hepatic clearance (i.e., high-extraction drugs) may be negatively affected (e.g., labetalol, morphine, verapamil) [18]. Drugs that depend on enzymatic function for clearance (as opposed to hepatic blood flow) are considered low-extraction drugs (e.g., haloperidol, diazepam, phenytoin). These agents undergo either phase I reactions (i.e., oxidation, reduction, hydrolysis) or phase II reactions (i.e., glucuronidation, acetylation, sulfation). Phase I reactions are much more sensitive to age, and the clearance of drugs that are metabolized via these mechanisms may be reduced (e.g., diazepam, midazolam). Phase II reactions, in contrast, are not impaired in older adults, and the clearance of these agents is not reduced in an age-dependent fashion.

A common clearance pathway for many drugs used in the ICU setting is the cytochrome P-450 (CYP-450) system. The efficiency of the CYP-450 system may be affected by both advanced age and critical illness. However, not all CYP isoforms are equally affected by aging. Although wide variability has been noted, clearance appears to be lower for substrates of CYP-1A2 and CYP-2C19, decreased or unchanged for substrates of CYP-3A4 and CYP-2C9, and unchanged for substrates of CYP-2D6 [19].

Elimination

Increasing age is associated with several structural and functional changes in the kidney that result in decreased glomerular function and altered renal elimination. After age 30, there is a linear decline in glomerular filtration by approximately 8 ml/min per decade of life [20]. By age 70, a 30 to 50 percent loss of functioning glomeruli is observed [21]. This is likely due to decreases in renal mass, loss of functional nephrons, and diminished renal artery perfusion.

Pharmacodynamics

Aging is associated with several pharmacodynamic changes that can alter the therapeutic response and lead to adverse drug reactions. These changes can be due to altered receptor density, receptor affinity, signal transduction (i.e., ability of the cells to respond to receptor occupation), or homeostatic mechanisms [22]. Examples describing the pharmacodynamic variability of commonly used drugs in the ICU are presented in Table 3.1 [23–25].

Adverse Drug Events

One in seven Medicare beneficiaries experienced an adverse event when hospitalized in 2008. Between 2007 and 2009, almost 100,000 emergency hospitalizations in the United States were due to adverse drug events (ADEs) in adults 65 years of age and older. Nearly half were age 80 and older [26]. ADEs increase mortality, length of hospitalization, and healthcare costs, yet only 50 percent are reported in US hospitals. Adverse drug reactions or medication errors are only considered ADEs if there is documented harm to the patient (Figure 3.1) [27]. The medication classes most frequently associated with the ADEs in the ICU are drugs with CNS activities (e.g., opioids, sedatives), antimicrobials, drugs with cardiovascular effects, and anticoagulants.

Table 3.1 Age-Related Pharmacodynamic Alterations with Commonly Administered ICU Medications

Drug class	Pharmacodynamic alteration
Benzodiazepines	Differences in sensitivity to cognitive and sedative effects occur that are not attributable to the differences in pharmacokinetic parameters. This could be due to differences in drug distribution to the CNS. If benzodiazepines must be used, smaller doses should be administered. Lorazepam is least likely to accumulate because it is cleared by glucuronidation and does not have active metabolites (unlike midazolam and diazepam).
Opioids	Opioid receptor density, affinity, and binding may change with aging. Smaller opioid doses should be used. Morphine has an active metabolite that can accumulate and cause adverse effects. Alternatives are suggested.
Diuretics	A decreased diuretic and natriuretic response may be due to the age-related decrease in albumin (which transports the drug to the active site), decrease in the pharmacodynamic interactions, altered physiologic response, or age-related decreases in renal function.
Beta-blockers	Pharmacodynamic sensitivity declines with age. This may be due to receptor downregulation or receptor conformation, but the most likely mechanism is impaired signal transduction of beta receptors.
Warfarin	Anticoagulant effect may be increased due to decreased vitamin K stores or greater inhibition of vitamin K–dependent clotting factors

(*Sources:* Refs. [23–25].)

Older adults with complex medical conditions, many of whom require an admission to the ICU during their hospitalization, are at particularly high risk for errors during care transitions and experiencing ADEs secondary to polypharmacy and drug-drug interactions [4] (Table 3.2). During these transitions, patients are most vulnerable to medication errors, either through medication additions or omissions, that may lead to ADEs. Strategies to improve continuity of care and minimize gaps in care, such as better communication between clinicians, can reduce medication errors and improve patient outcomes [28].

Drug Dosing Considerations in Older Adults

Routes of Administration

Medications are frequently administered to critically ill geriatric patients by nonintravenous routes (e.g., oral/enteral, subcutaneous, transdermal, inhalational) when an IV formulation is not available, to prolong the duration of effect, to decrease monitoring requirements, to facilitate ICU discharge, and to decrease drug costs [9]. In general, bioavailability is nearly always lower when drugs are administered by nonintravenous routes. In addition, there can be considerable variability with the rate and extent of absorption, time of onset, magnitude of effect, and duration of action. These differences can have a substantial impact on treatment effect and clinical outcome, so several important factors should be considered (Table 3.3).

Table 3.2 Factors Associated with Polypharmacy and ADEs in Critically Ill Older Adults

- Failure to account for age and critical care–related pharmacokinetic changes.
- Failure to avoid high-risk drugs where possible.
- Failure to screen for pain, sedation, and delirium.
- Initiation of a new medication to treat a side effect from another drug.
- Failure to down titrate or discontinue medications on a daily basis.
- Failure to recognize drug-associated adverse effects.
- Initiation of medications that a patient stopped taking prior to the ICU admission.
- Failure to consider pre-ICU OTC, herbal, alcohol, or recreational drug use.
- Failure to consider medication withdrawal reactions.
- Lack of involvement of a critical care pharmacist in daily ICU care.
- Lack of involvement of family and friends in daily ICU care.
- Lack of medication reconciliation at ICU discharge/transitions of care.

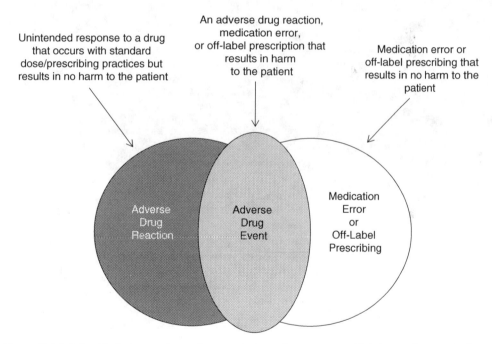

Figure 3.1 Relationship between adverse drug reactions, medication errors, off-label prescribing, and adverse events in older adults. (*Source:* Adapted from Nebeker, Barach, and Samore [27].)

Extremes in Body Mass

Obesity

An ever-increasing proportion of older adults is obese. Obesity is disproportionately present among patients in the ICU and may be associated with increased ICU mortality [29]. The pharmacokinetic parameters that are most important to consider when dosing medication in older, obese, critically ill patients are volume of distribution

Table 3.3 Dosing Considerations When Using Non-IV Routes of Administration

Oral/enteral:
- Numerous physiologic and end-organ changes are evident in critically ill geriatric patients that preclude extrapolation of data from pharmacokinetic studies evaluating bioavailability in healthy volunteers to the critically ill.
- Critically ill geriatric patients often have drug- or disease-induced decreases in gastric acid secretion. This may decrease the absorption of weak bases (e.g., ketoconazole, itraconazole) and alter the release characteristics of enteric-coated formulations (e.g., proton pump inhibitors).
- Delayed gastric emptying is common in geriatric patients, especially those with head injury or those who are mechanically ventilated. This is important for patients in whom the nasogastric tube is clamped after drug administration because if the drug has not emptied into the small intestine before nasogastric suction is reestablished, it will be removed and not absorbed.
- Administration of a medication through a gastric tube requires that a tablet be crushed, dissolved, and administered using an oral syringe. These added steps compound the risk that residual drug may be left behind in the receptacle where the tablet was crushed, in the syringe used for administration, or in the gastric tube itself.
- The bioavailability of several medications (e.g., phenytoin, ciprofloxacin) is substantially decreased when concomitantly administered with enteral nutrition. Enteral nutrition should therefore be held before and after drug administration. In these settings, tube feeding rate (if continuous) should be recalculated to account for the cessation in administration.

Subcutaneous:
- Subcutaneous administration is associated with erratic and/or incomplete absorption resulting in lower serum concentrations.
- This may be due to low cardiac output, peripheral edema, sepsis, and vasopressor-induced peripheral blood vessel vasoconstriction.
- For some medications, subcutaneous administration should be discouraged (e.g., vitamin K for warfarin reversal).

Transdermal:
- Transdermal drug absorption may be compromised in patients with alterations in blood flow to subcutaneous tissues (e.g., shock).
- With transdermal administration, the onset of effect is delayed (following application), and the duration is prolonged (following removal). This makes titration difficult and may present a safety concern should an adverse effect occur.
- For some medications, transdermal use has been associated with harm (e.g., fentanyl patch for acute pain).

Inhalational:
- Drugs administered by aerosol include beta-2 agonists, anticholinergics, mucolytics, corticosteroids, prostacyclins, and antibiotics.
- Drug doses administered to mechanically ventilated patients via metered-dose inhaler are typically twice that administered to patients not mechanically ventilated because of the ventilator circuit.
- Aerosolized antibiotics (e.g., aminoglycosides) have the advantage of enhanced penetration into the lung with minimal systemic exposure. One potential side effect is bronchospasm.

and clearance [30]. In general, drugs with a small volume of distribution are typically hydrophilic (e.g., aminoglycosides) with little distribution into adipose tissue [31]. In contrast, drugs with a larger volume of distribution are often more lipophilic, and thus distribution into adipose tissue and other body compartments is extensive. Studies describing the relationship between obesity and clearance have produced mixed results. Some studies demonstrate an increase in clearance (likely due to increased kidney size and blood flow in obesity), whereas others have shown no difference.

There are limited data describing how drugs should be dosed in the obese critically ill patient and even fewer that are specific to geriatrics. Nevertheless, when crafting a drug dosing regimen for the obese, critically ill geriatric patient, the clinician should first assess the degree of obesity present in the individual patient. With mild to moderate forms of obesity (e.g., body mass index [BMI] = 25–39 kg/m^2), published dosing recommendations are usually appropriate. With more extreme forms of obesity (e.g., BMI ≥ 40 kg/m^2), drug dosing becomes more complicated because these patients were often excluded from formal pharmacokinetic dosing studies [30,31]. In these settings, clinicians should seek clinical trials where dosing has been evaluated in morbid obesity. If these trials do not exist, then pharmacokinetic trials conducted in obese individuals should be sought, and the presence of dose proportionality should be evaluated. Dose proportionality suggests that as weight increases, pharmacokinetic parameters such as volume of distribution and clearance also increase by the same ratio. If dose proportionality exists, then the clinician must weigh the benefits versus risks of using total body weight (for weight-based dosing) or use a dose on the higher end of the dosing range (for non-weight-based dosing). If dose proportionality does not exist, then either lean or adjusted body weight should be used. Generally speaking, there are few drugs that are renally eliminated that display properties of dose proportionality. Other principles for drug dosing in obese, critically ill geriatric patients are listed in Table 3.4.

Table 3.4 Principles of Drug Dosing in Obese, Critically Ill Geriatric Patients

- All available weight measures (e.g., total body weight, ideal body weight, lean body weight) are limited by their inability to assess the ratio of fat mass to fat-free mass. This has implications for how hydrophilic versus lipophilic drugs may distribute.
- Seek consistency with the weight measure that is used for weight-based dosing and all dosing-related calculations.
- When consulting the literature, confirm that the weight of the specific patient in question is within the range of weights included in the clinical trial. This is especially important when dealing with extremes in body weight (e.g., BMI > 50 kg/m^2).
- The degree of variability in volume of distribution and clearance is greater in critically ill patients than in noncritically ill patients.
- The risk for an adverse effect associated with a higher dose of a medication must be balanced with the risk of treatment failure when using a lower dose.
- In some cases, it may be safer to use a series of smaller doses that can rapidly be titrated to effect versus a single large dose regardless of the weight measure that may be preferred for weight-based dosing.
- Therapeutic drug monitoring should be used whenever available.

Low Body Mass

At the other extreme, older adults may have a low body mass, particularly when patients have a chronic condition that has left them nutritionally depleted. Data describing drug dosing in patients with low body mass are limited. In general, standard drug doses or doses on the lower end of the dosing range should be appropriate. Caution should be exercised with fixed doses of anticoagulant medications (e.g., low-molecular-weight heparin) because standard doses commonly used for prophylaxis may actually achieve therapeutic anticoagulation levels.

Renal Insufficiency

Renal insufficiency is common in the critically ill older adults given the clear correlation between increasing age and reduced kidney function. One study identified an age of 65 years or older as an independent risk factor for acute kidney injury (odds ratio [OR] = 1.5; 95 percent confidence interval [CI] = 1.16–1.92) [32]. The most common method to estimate kidney function for the purposes of drug dosing in the ICU is the Cockcroft-Gault equation. However, the validity of this equation in the elderly ICU patient is poor, largely because it relies primarily on the serum creatinine concentration. Creatinine is not very sensitive to changes in the glomerular filtration rate, making the timely recognition of acute kidney insufficiency difficult. Moreover, the serum creatinine is heavily influenced by body muscle mass, which is usually diminished in most elderly patients. This can lead to false assumptions on creatinine clearance if traditional ranges of normal are used to interpret the serum creatinine concentration. To adjust for this issue, some institutions will round low serum creatinine values to an arbitrary value of 1 mg/dl. However, research has demonstrated that this practice will underestimate creatinine clearance and should be avoided because it may lead to subtherapeutic medication doses [33,34].

Many older ICU patients with renal insufficiency will require renal replacement therapy (RRT). Drug clearance with RRT depends on various factors, such as the drug's volume of distribution, degree of protein binding, molecular weight, and the duration and intensity of RRT. It is essential that clinicians understand local treatment practices, especially dialysis flow rates, because this will markedly affect drug removal. Discrepancies between local practices and published dosing recommendations may lead to either an over- or underestimation of extracorporeal drug removal and thus increase the likelihood for treatment failure or an adverse drug reaction.

Several resources exist to assist with drug dosing in RRT, but substantial variability exists in the dose recommended by each reference [35–37]. Many of these recommended doses are based on studies that used older dialyzer membranes that have poor permeability and lower effluent rates or were extrapolated from pharmacokinetic data in noncritically ill patients or those with chronic kidney disease. This is important because patients with chronic kidney disease also have compromised nonrenal clearance mechanisms, whereas in patients with acute kidney injury, nonrenal clearance mechanisms may be preserved. This has the potential to lead to the under dosing of medications that has been demonstrated with antibiotics such as imipenem, meropenem, and vancomycin [38]. In fact, several reports have demonstrated an inability to reach pharmacodynamic goals with doses commonly recommended for RRT [39]. Principles of drug dosing in elderly patients with acute kidney injury (AKI) or RRT are listed in Table 3.5.

Table 3.5 Principles of Drug Dosing in Geriatric Patients with AKI or Receiving RRT

- Serum creatinine values fail to increase with advanced age because creatinine production (which is directly proportional to muscle mass) decreases at nearly the same rate as the renal clearance of creatinine.
- Elderly patients are more vulnerable to dehydration because of a decrease in the capacity to concentrate urine. This and the use of diuretics may contribute to a higher propensity for drug toxicity.
- Many medications used in the ICU have active metabolites that can accumulate in renal failure (e.g., morphine, midazolam). These metabolites can contribute to the pharmacologic effect and lead to an adverse reaction.
- When making dosing adjustments in patients with AKI, the clinician should first consider what the starting dose would be if creatinine clearance were normal.
- Factors such as severity of illness, medication indication, adverse effect profile, and patient-specific pharmacokinetics (e.g., obesity) should be included in the strategy for drug dosing.
- When prescribing beta-lactam antibiotics in patients receiving continuous RRT, the use of loading doses and prolonged infusions should be considered to improve the likelihood that pharmacodynamic goals will be met.
- One of the most important factors influencing drug dosing in continuous RRT is the prescribed (and delivered) effluent rate, also referred to as the *continuous RRT dose*.
- Clinicians must review for stoppages in continuous RRT that may have resulted from filter clotting, circuit changes, or patient travel for procedures. These can result in meaningful reductions in extracorporeal drug clearance.

Hepatic Dysfunction

Drug dosing in hepatic dysfunction is challenging because of the general inability to estimate liver function. Although tests exist to detect hepatocellular changes (e.g., aspartate aminotransferase [AST], alanine aminotransferase [ALT]) and evaluate synthetic function (e.g., international normalized ration [INR]), none of these reflect the ability of the liver to metabolize drugs. Some medications can be adjusted based on the Child-Pugh score, but specific recommendations for commonly used-ICU medications using this strategy are limited. Nevertheless, dosing adjustments are not typically suggested until hepatic dysfunction becomes moderately (class B) or severely (class C) impaired [40].

Pharmacokinetic changes that occur with hepatic dysfunction are related to reductions in drug metabolism, plasma protein synthesis, and/or liver blood flow. Hepatic drug clearance is typically classified based on the dependence on hepatic blood flow (i.e., high-extraction drugs) or on the activity of drug-metabolizing enzymes (i.e., low-extraction drugs). Drugs that have a high degree of hepatic extraction are expected to have an increased bioavailability and decreased clearance in conditions associated with decreased hepatic blood flow. For medications that are administered orally, both the initial dose and maintenance doses should be reduced. For medications administered intravenously, only a reduction in the maintenance dose is necessary. For low-extraction drugs, metabolism is more so dependent on the degree of binding to albumin and the activity of metabolizing enzymes (e.g., CYP-450). This is further complicated by the fact that all CYP-450 enzymes do not uniformly decrease at the same severity of liver disease. Instead, a sequential progressive model has been described [41]. According to this model, patients with mild

Table 3.6 Principles of Drug Dosing in Geriatric Patients with Hepatic Failure

- Medications that are highly bound to albumin will have a higher free or unbound fraction in patients with hepatic failure.
- Hepatic failure is associated with larger volumes of distribution for water-soluble medications, resulting in lower peak concentrations. Higher loading doses may be necessary.
- Alterations in CYP-450 metabolism will vary based on the specific CYP subunit and the degree of hepatic insufficiency.
- Conjugation reactions such as glucuronidation are less affected by liver disease. As a result, clearance for benzodiazepines such as oxazepam, lorazepam, and temazepam is not reduced, whereas diazepam and midazolam (which undergo phase I reactions) clearance is decreased.
- Liver disease has been associated with a decreased pharmacodynamic response for drugs such as loop diuretics and beta-receptor antagonists. In contrast, an enhanced therapeutic effect can be expected for opioid analgesics, anxiolytics, and sedatives.
- Patients with liver cirrhosis are more sensitive to the adverse renal effects of nonsteroidal anti-inflammatory drugs (NSAIDs).
- The oral bioavailability of medications with a high-extraction ratio can be drastically increased in patients with chronic liver disease. Both initial and maintenance doses should be adjusted.
- For high-extraction drugs that are administered intravenously, clearance may be reduced in liver disease due to reduced hepatic blood flow. Maintenance doses should be adjusted.
- Clearance of low-extraction drugs will depend on the specific pathway, the degree of hepatic insufficiency, and the unbound fraction of drug.

hepatic dysfunction will experience a decrease in CYP-2C19 activity, but CYP-1A2, CYP-2D6, and CYP-2E1 will be sustained. As the level of hepatic dysfunction becomes more severe, a sequential reduction in CYP-1A2 activity, followed by CYP-2D6 activity, is noted. CYP-2E1 activity remains relatively preserved until hepatic decompensation or hepatorenal syndrome develops. Principles of drug dosing in hepatic dysfunction are listed in Table 3.6.

Drug/Disease-Specific Pharmacotherapy Issues

Analgesia and Sedation

Pain and discomfort are prevalent in critically ill older adults and thus require around-the-clock evaluation and treatment when they are present. Self-reporting of pain is considered the reference standard for pain assessment in this population. However, if a patient is nonverbal, the 2013 Pain, Agitation, and Delirium (PAD) Guidelines recommend the use of the Behavioral Pain Scale or the Critical Care Pain Observational Tool in the ICU [42]. Most ICU patients can be successfully treated with intermittent opioid therapy. Continuous opioid infusions may be required in some patients particularly when an analgesia-sedative approach to sedation management is being used. Older adults are at particularly high risk for developing sedative-associated coma and delirium particularly with benzodiazepine use. Increasing evidence suggests that using an opioid-first approach is safer and is associated with improved patient outcomes [42]. Despite strong evidence that patients who remain in a lightly sedated state have improved outcomes (e.g., less delirium, a shorter duration of mechanical ventilation, reduced posttraumatic stress disorder), over sedation remains a major concern in many ICUs. Deep sedation, particularly coma, should be avoided in all older adults unless it is a goal of therapy, given that even short periods spent in this state are associated with increased mortality [42,43].

The ABCDEF bundle (*a*ssess, prevent, and manage pain; *b*oth spontaneous awakening trials and spontaneous breathing trials; *c*hoice of drugs; *d*elirium: assess, prevent, and manage; *e*arly mobility and exercise; and *f*amily engagement and empowerment) has been shown to improve both short- and long-term outcome in older adults and help return patients back to their pre-ICU functional and cognitive status [2,42,44]. It should be emphasized that the appropriate choice of analgesic and sedative therapy (if needed) is only one factor affecting an older adult's cognitive and functional status after leaving the ICU.

Consideration of potential adverse events is the most important criterion when selecting opioid and sedative therapy in older adults given that these agents are usually administered at higher doses and for more prolonged periods than in non-ICU settings [45]. Adverse drug events with these agents are common in the ICU given that they are usually administered at far higher doses and for longer periods of time than outside the ICU. Furthermore, critically ill patients have a higher prevalence of end-organ dysfunction (e.g., renal, hepatic) that may result in higher drug concentrations than in patients on the floor [45]. Factors such as altered postreceptor binding, downregulation of receptors, and brain dysfunction may dramatically alter the response of ICU patients to these agents [45]. Cardiac dysfunction may increase the risk for dysrhythmias and hypotension. Adjuvants in the injectable formulations of sedatives (e.g., propylene glycol in parenteral lorazepam) may result in additional toxic effects.

Fentanyl is a synthetic opioid that is preferred over morphine given that it is associated with less hypotension and bronchospasm and its clearance is not affected by renal dysfunction [46]. Fentanyl has been reported to cause muscle rigidity and bradycardia. Fentanyl patches should be avoided for acute analgesia because the time to reach peak effect is delayed by up to 24 hours after patch application, and a prolonged drug effect is seen after patch removal. Hydromorphone has a half-life of 2 to 3 hours and also undergoes glucuronidation similar to morphine. However, the hydromorphone-3-glucuronide metabolite that is produced is inactive, making hydromorphone the opioid of choice for use in patients with end-stage renal disease. Ketamine and other opioid-sparing analgesics such as acetaminophen are being increasingly administered in the ICU to reduce opioid administration and the potential side effects associated with opioid use (e.g. constipation, respiratory depression, risk of future addiction) [42].

Compared with benzodiazepines (e.g., lorazepam and midazolam), propofol and dexmedetomidine are associated with faster neurologic recovery and a shorter duration of mechanical ventilation after discontinuation [47]. Moreover, given that benzodiazepine use is a well-established risk factor for delirium [48,49], the 2013 PAD Guidelines recommend that propofol or dexmedetomidine be used judiciously in older adults who require continuous sedation [42].

Propofol is an intravenous general anesthetic agent that has a rapid onset and offset of action and thus provides clinicians with a sedative option that is far more titratable than other sedative options. Propofol's duration of effect is longer in the very old elderly. The key safety concerns with propofol are bradycardia, hypotension, hypertriglyceridemia, and the propofol-associated infusion syndrome (PRIS). Propofol should not be bolused nor administered at a dose greater than 60 μg/kg per minute in the elderly. Serum triglyceride levels should be checked at least twice weekly. Propofol should be discontinued in a patient who exhibits sudden hypotension, metabolic acidosis, and cardiac failure given that these are the earlier and more common manifestations of PRIS.

Dexmedetomidine is a centrally acting alpha-2 agonist that has sedative and analgesic properties but no effect on respiratory drive [42]. Older adults are more likely to experience bradycardia and/or hypotension with its use, particularly patients with severe congestive heart failure, and thus it should be initiated at a dose of no more than 0.2 μg/kg per hour and titrated upward with care. Dexmedetomidine can be particularly effective in older adults with agitated delirium or in those who are admitted with severe alcohol withdrawal.

Delirium

Delirium is a syndrome characterized by the acute onset of cerebral dysfunction with a change or fluctuation in baseline mental status, inattention, and either disorganized thinking or an altered level of consciousness [50,51]. Age is one of the most important underlying risk factors for delirium. More than a third of older adults have delirium at the time of ICU admission. Older adults in the ICU should be evaluated for delirium at least once per shift with a validated screening tool [42]. Treatment options for delirium in the ICU remain limited [52,53]. Therefore, clinicians should focus on delirium-prevention and risk-reduction strategies [42]. Many precipitating factors, such as patient immobility, application of patient restraints, excessive ambient noise, and admission to an ICU room without windows, clocks, or other features conducive to the maintenance of orientation and circadian normalcy, are modifiable and are important for clinicians to consider [54].

A number of medications have been reported to cause delirium in the critically ill [43] (Table 3.7). This is not surprising given the large number of medications administered in the ICU setting and the frequent presence of end-organ dysfunction that may influence drug response. The presence of conditions such as sepsis or stroke that may impair blood-brain barrier integrity and the use of medications with psychoactive properties may mimic delirium frequently [43]. Home medications such as benzodiazepines and opioids that are stopped at the time of ICU admission may cause a withdrawal syndrome, the symptoms of which are similar to those of delirium.

An increasing number of time-dependent, multivariate analyses that incorporate Markov models to focus on the association between medication exposure (e.g., benzodiazepines, corticosteroids, and anticholinergics) and the daily odds of transitioning from an

Table 3.7 Strategies to Reduce Medication-Associated Delirium

- Avoid polypharmacy, and ensure that medication dosing is appropriate.
- Consider medication withdrawal effects (particularly benzodiazepines).
- Avoid anticholinergic medications when possible.
- Avoid benzodiazepines when possible (including sleep aids).
- Avoid use of nonbenzodiazepine sleep aids when possible.
- Use the lowest effective corticosteroid dose.
- Use the lowest effective opioid dose to control pain/optimize nonopioid analgesic.
- Avoid metoclopramide when possible.
- If delirium occurs with levetiracetam, consider other anticonvulsant options.
- Reassess the need for continued antibiotic therapy.
- Monitor diuretic therapy for signs of dehydration and/or electrolyte abnormalities.

awake and nondelirious state to delirium the next day have been published [48,49,55–57]. A landmark 2006 study of 198 mechanically ventilated adults found that lorazepam administration was an independent risk factor for a daily transition to delirium (OR = 1.2; 95% CI = 1.1–1.4, p = 0.003) [48]. A more recent analysis of 1,112 critically ill adults found that midazolam administration was an independent risk factor for a daily transition to delirium (OR = 1.04; 95% CI = 1.02–1.05, p < 0.001 per every 5 mg/day of midazolam administered) [49]. This latter study suggests that for every 5 mg of midazolam administered to a patient who is awake and without delirium, there is a 4 percent chance that this patient will develop delirium the next ICU day. Given that the risk for delirium with benzodiazepine use is dose dependent, clinicians should employ strategies known to reduce the daily amount of benzodiazepine. Administration of sedatives that are associated with less delirium such as dexmedetomidine or propofol is preferable [42].

One cohort analysis of 520 mechanically ventilated adults with acute lung injury (ALI) found that systemic corticosteroid use was significantly associated with transitioning to delirium from a nondelirious, noncomatose state [55]. However, in a larger analysis of 1,112 patients who received a corticosteroid 35 percent of their ICU days at a median prednisone equivalent dose of 50 (25–75) mg, corticosteroid administration was not associated with a daily transition to delirium (OR = 1.08; 95% CI = 0.89–1.32 per each 10-mg increase in prednisone equivalent administered) [56]. Regardless of the exact risk for delirium with corticosteroid exposure in older adults, ICU clinicians should continue to evaluate their patients daily to ensure that they are receiving the lowest effective dose.

Cholinergic deficiency has been traditionally described as an important mechanistic cause for delirium occurrence. However, in one prospective study of 1,112 critically ill adults, in which anticholinergic burden was calculated on a daily basis using the Anticholinergic Drug Scale (ADS) score, a 1-unit increase in the ADS score resulted in a nonsignificant increase in the probability of delirium occurring the next day (OR = 1.05; 95% CI = 0.99–1.10) [57]. While medications without strong anticholinergic properties are preferred in the critically ill, the results of this investigation suggest that the association between anticholinergic medication use and delirium in the critically ill may not be as significant as previously thought.

Despite the limited evidence to support their use [52,53], antipsychotic agents are given off label to more than 10 percent of ICU patients, often at high and excessive doses [58]. Continuation of newly initiated antipsychotics beyond the care setting and context for which they were prescribed is frequent [58,59]. Moreover, patients with delirium who are agitated may also be initiated on benzodiazepines, opioids, or sedating anticonvulsants such as phenobarbital. These factors make delirium an important contributor to polypharmacy in critically ill older adults. A short course of antipsychotics may be indicated to treat agitation, particularly in patients for whom respiratory depression is of concern. Recent studies demonstrate the benefit of low-dose haloperidol in reducing agitation in patients with delirium [60] or subsyndromal delirium [61]. In addition to the side effects of dexmedetomidine (i.e., bradycardia and hypotension), the high acquisition cost and a requirement that it be administered as a continuous infusion in a monitored setting often preclude its administration [62]. There may be a role for antipsychotics at night in patients who report insomnia, in whom nonpharmacologic sleep improvement interventions fail, since sleep architecture (an important determinant of outcome) is less disrupted with antipsychotics than with benzodiazepines or propofol [63].

Anticoagulation

The risk-benefit decision to initiate anticoagulation therapy for either the prevention or treatment of venous thrombosis is similar between younger and older adults. However, the increased risk for the adverse effects, coupled with the pharmacokinetic variability that exists in critical illness, makes the provision of safe and effective anticoagulation therapy challenging in older adults in the ICU setting. Older adults may be more sensitive to the effects of warfarin. This may be related to receptor sensitivity, hypoalbuminemia, malnourishment, or decreased dietary intake of vitamin K. Age-related declines in renal function may lead to drug accumulation and increased bleeding because a number of anticoagulants are renally cleared (e.g., low-molecular-weight heparins, fondaparinux, dabigatran) Fondaparinux is contraindicated in patients with a creatinine clearance of less than 30 ml/min [64]. Both dabigatran and rivaroxaban have been associated with an increased risk for gastrointestinal bleeding compared with warfarin in patients over 75 years of age [65,66]. Dabigatran capsules cannot be opened; thus administration can be difficult in patients who cannot swallow.

The importance of rapid anticoagulation reversal in the setting of trauma and/or falls has been described previously [67]. Guidelines suggest that 4-factor prothrombin complex concentrates for the reversal of antifactor Xa inhibitors (e.g., rivaroxaban, apixaban, edoxaban), but data supporting this practice are limited [68]. Idarucizumab has recently been shown to rapidly and completely reverse dabigatran in a cohort of patients with serious bleeding or need for an urgent procedure [69]. While this study was not exclusive to older adults, the median age was 77 years (range 48–93 years), and only 13 percent had a creatinine clearances of 30 ml/min or less. Future large-scale pharmacoepidemiologic studies are needed to determine the efficacy and bleeding risk of these agents in geriatric patients.

Gastrointestinal

Constipation occurs frequently in elderly ICU patients and is associated with substantial morbidity [70]. More than 50 percent of long-term care residents (mean age 88 years), a population that often transitions back to the ICU, take at least one laxative daily, and more than half of these users take more than 60 doses per month [71]. A careful medication history is therefore important when elderly patients present to the ICU because constipation is a frequent side effect of several medications that are routinely used (e.g., opioid analgesics, anticholinergic agents, calcium supplements, iron). Bulking agents (e.g., psyllium), osmotic laxatives (e.g., PEG 3350), and stimulant laxatives (e.g., bisacodyl, senna) are recommended when constipation does occur [72]. Preemptive laxative therapy is suggested in high-risk patients such as those receiving scheduled opioid therapy [73].

Acid suppressive therapy for the provision of stress ulcer prophylaxis is widely used in the critical care setting, and proton pump inhibitors (PPIs) are the agents most commonly selected [74]. Nevertheless, there are several adverse effects related to PPI use that can substantially compromise care in the geriatric patient. Several studies have demonstrated an increased risk for *Clostridium difficile* infection with PPI therapy [75]. This appears to be associated with both dose and duration of therapy [76]. Some reports have suggested that PPIs are also associated with an increased risk for pneumonia [77]. Finally, PPI use has been linked to fractures, osteoporosis, dementia, and chronic kidney disease [78,79]. While these adverse effects appear to be related to long-term use, this risk cannot be overlooked given that many patients are inadvertently discharged on acid suppressive therapy [4]. One study even reported higher 1-year mortality in elderly patients who were discharged from acute care hospitals on PPI therapy [80]. Critically ill geriatric patients should therefore be appropriately screened for their risk for gastrointestinal (GI) bleeding, and stress ulcer prophylaxis should be offered only to patients considered to be high risk [74].

Endocrine

Abnormalities in blood glucose are common in geriatric ICU patients and can be the result of physiologic stress, diabetes, unrecognized diabetes, or initiation of new medications (e.g., corticosteroids). Approximately 26 percent of people age 65 or older in the United States have diabetes, and in many, this diagnosis is unknown [81,82]. In the outpatient setting, most patients are managed with oral hypoglycemic medications, but in the ICU, insulin is the preferred therapy for glucose control [83,84]. For the unstable patient, continuous IV insulin infusion is the best method for achieving glycemic targets. Insulin infusions provide the ability to rapidly titrate insulin administration and respond to changes in clinical status (e.g., hypothermia, edema, shock), interruptions in dextrose intake, and the provision of enteral/parenteral nutrition. Subcutaneous insulin may be an alternative for some ICU patients, particularly those who are clinically stable or preparing for ICU transfer. For patients who are NPO or have poor oral intake, a basal plus correction insulin regimen (e.g., insulin glargine plus regular insulin as needed) is preferred [83]. For patients tolerating oral diet, a basal-bolus regimen consisting of long-acting insulin (e.g., insulin glargine) plus short-acting insulin based on nutritional intake is suggested. The sole use of sliding-scale insulin is strongly discouraged.

Recommendations for a target blood glucose range vary, but guidelines from the Society of Critical Care Medicine state that insulin therapy should be titrated to keep the glucose concentration at less than 150 mg/dL and absolutely less than 180 mg/dL [85]. Careful consideration should be given to preventing hypoglycemia because even a single episode of hypoglycemia has been associated with poor outcome [86]. Geriatric patients in particular are at increased risk for hypoglycemia because of insulin deficiency, progressive renal insufficiency, variability in insulin sensitivity, slowed hormonal regulation/counterregulation, and slowed intestinal absorption [81].

Infectious Disease

More than half of ICU patients receive antibiotic therapy, and the prevalence of use is higher in older adults [87]. Geriatric patients typically display several of the pharmacokinetic characteristics that warrant dosage adjustment (e.g., decreased clearance, decreased volume of distribution), but careful evaluation is necessary to ensure that adequate serum concentrations are achieved. Several studies have revealed that in critically ill adults, standard doses may not achieve concentrations high enough to reach established pharmacodynamic goals associated with a clinical cure [88–90]. In one study, vancomycin doses in patients that did not reach goal area under the curve (AUC): minimum inhibitory concentration (MIC) targets on day 1 were associated with increased risk for clinical failure [91]. These data highlight the importance of early, aggressive dosing in the critically ill, especially when administering drugs that are generally considered safe (e.g., penicillins, cephalosporins, etc.).

When crafting an antimicrobial regimen in the critically ill geriatric patient, dosing principles should be the same regardless of patient age [9]. When applicable (e.g., similar susceptibility based on local antibiograms, actual culture and susceptibility, etc.), drugs with a favorable safety profile should be prioritized over those having a narrower therapeutic window. A careful assessment of kidney function is necessary. The decision to lower doses based on renal insufficiency must include a careful evaluation of the overall risk-benefit of making such adjustments. Practitioners should recognize that renal function estimates are often inaccurate in the critically ill and that the sequelae of under dosing may be more severe than the potential side effects of administering an excessive dose. In clinical settings where doses fall close to the threshold for a dosing adjustment, a more aggressive approach (i.e., the higher dose) should be considered, especially for agents with a favorable safety index. Therapeutic drug monitoring should be used where appropriate.

Strategies to Improve Medication Outcomes

With clinical data for any critically ill older adult being extensive, complex, and rapidly changing, clinicians must adopt strategies to regularly review drug therapy that are practical, systematic, and organized. If the use of an "at risk" medication cannot be avoided, the lowest dose of that medication should be prescribed. The medication profile of all ICU patients should be reviewed daily to identify medications that may be causing an adverse event, drug-drug interactions, or may no longer be needed [92]. Professional organizations and their members, such as the Society of Critical Care Medicine (SCCM), devote substantial resources and efforts to developing high-quality clinical practice guidelines and quality-improvement efforts, and this guidance should be incorporated into the routine care of all older adults [42,85,92].

The critical care pharmacist is now an essential part of the multidisciplinary ICU team and plays an important role in optimizing drug therapy. The critical care pharmacist identifies medication-related safety concerns and advises on situations where medication therapy can be stopped for the older adult population [92,94]. Numerous studies demonstrate the positive impact that the dedicated critical care pharmacist, when directly involved in bedside care, can have on the outcomes of critically ill older adults [92,94]. Not only is the critical care pharmacist adept at reducing adverse drug events, medication errors, and drug cost, but their daily presence in the ICU will reduce patient mortality and shorten the duration of ICU stay.

During the course of an illness, transitions of care occur when older adults are at the greatest risk of experiencing adverse events. Sustaining and properly communicating correct medication information across healthcare settings are important national safety goals of the Joint Commission on Accreditation of Healthcare Organizations [95]. Patients with cognitive impairment and taking more than five medications a day (i.e., polypharmacy) represent a substantial proportion of older adults being discharged from the ICU. They are at a particularly high risk of experiencing adverse drug events during transitions of care [95]. Medication deprescribing and reconciliation should be mandatory at the time of the ICU admission and discharge and should involve nurses, pharmacists, and physicians [9,96–98]. Potentially inappropriate medications such as antipsychotics, opioids, anticholinergics, antidepressants, acid suppressive agents, and drugs causing orthostasis should be targeted during this process.

Conclusions

Older adults are increasingly being admitted to the ICU, and the way in which drug therapy is initiated, monitored, and discontinued in this setting will influence their outcome. Critically ill older adults are among the most complex patients to optimize medications, given their multiple comorbidities, new end-organ damage, and high frequency of invasive/surgical procedures. All these factors can profoundly influence the safety and efficacy of any pre-scribed medication regimen and must be understood and evaluated when optimizing phar-macotherapy-related outcome. Clinicians seeking to optimize pharmacotherapy in the geriatric critically ill patient must have knowledge of the pharmacology, pharmacokinetics, and comparative evidence for all medications that are used in the ICU. Adverse drug events are common in the ICU and will frequently result in increased patient morbidity and mortality and higher healthcare costs. Critical care pharmacists can play an important role in helping to optimize medication-related outcomes in this population. Formal strategies such as medication reconciliation should be employed to reduce unnecessary post-ICU drug use.

References

1. Fuchs L, Chronaki CE, Park S, et al. ICU admission characteristics and mortality rates among elderly and very elderly patients. *Intensive Care Med* 2012; **38**(10): 1654–61.

2. Balas MC, Devlin JW, Verceles AC, et al. Adapting the ABCDEF bundle to meet the needs of patients requiring prolonged mechanical ventilation in the long-term acute care hospital setting: historical perspectives and practical implications. *Semin Respir Crit Care Med* 2016; **37**(1): 119–35.

3. Cullen DJ, Sweitzer BJ, Bates DW, et al. Preventable adverse drug events in hospitalized patients: a comparative study of intensive care and general care units. *Crit Care Med* 1997; **25**:1289–97.

4. Scales DC, Fisher HD, Li P, et al. Unintentional continuation of medications intended for acute illness after hospital discharge: a population-based cohort study. *J Gen Intern Med* 2015; **31**:196–202.

5. Bell CM, Brener SS, Gunraj N, et al. Association of ICU or hospital admission with unintentional discontinuation of medications for chronic diseases. *JAMA* 2011; **306**:840–47.

6. Budnitz DS, Pollock DA, Weidenbach KN, et al. National surveillance of emergency department visits for outpatient adverse drug events. *JAMA* 2006; **296**(15):1858–66.

7. Jolivot PA, Hindlet P, Pichereau C, et al. A systematic review of adult admissions to ICUs related to adverse drug events. *Crit Care* 2014; **18**(6):643.

8. Qato DM, Wilder J, Schumm LP, et al. Changes in prescription and over-the-counter medication and dietary supplement use among older adults in the United States, 2005 vs. 2011. *JAMA Intern Med* 2016; **176** (4):473–82.

9. Devlin JW, Barletta JF. Principles of drug dosing in the critically ill. In JW Parillo, RP Dellinger, eds., *Critical Care Medicine: Principles of Diagnosis and Management in the Adult* (3rd edn). Philadelphia, PA: Mosby-Elsevier, 2008: 343–76.

10. Lat I, Micek S, Janzen J, et al. Off-label medication use in adult critical care patients. *J Crit Care* 2011; **26**:89–94.

11. American Geriatrics Society. Beers Criteria Update Expert Panel: American Geriatrics Society 2015 updated Beers Criteria for potentially inappropriate medication use in older adults. *J Am Geriatr Soc* 2015; **63**: 2227–46.

12. Morandi A, Vasilevskis EE, Pandharipande PP, et al. Inappropriate medications in elderly ICU survivors: where to intervene? *Arch Intern Med* 2011; **171**(11): 1032–34.

13. Floroff CK, Slattum PW, Harpe SE, et al. Potentially inappropriate medication use is associated with clinical outcomes in critically ill elderly patients with neurological injury. *Neurocrit Care* 2014; **21**(3):526–33.

14. Morandi A, Vasilevskis E, Pandharipande PP, et al. Inappropriate medication prescriptions in elderly adults surviving an intensive care unit hospitalizations. *J Am Geriatr Soc* 2013; **61**: 1128–34.

15. Needham DM, Davidson J, Cohen H, et al. Improving long-term outcomes after discharge from intensive care unit: report from a stakeholders' conference. *Crit Care Med* 2012; **40**(2):502–9.

16. Stollings JL, Bloom SL, Huggins EL, et al. Medication management to ameliorate post–intensive care syndrome. *AACN Adv Crit Care* 2016; **27**(2):133–40.

17. Klotz U. Pharmacokinetics and drug metabolism in the elderly. *Drug Metab Rev* 2009; **41**(2):67–76.

18. Pisani MA. Considerations in caring for the critically ill older patient. *J Intensive Care Med* 2009; **24**(2):83–95.

19. Cusack BJ. Pharmacokinetics in older persons. *Am J Geriatr Pharmacother* 2004; **2**(4):274–302.

20. Mühlberg W, Platt D. Age-dependent changes of the kidneys: pharmacological implications. *Gerontology* 1999; **45**(5): 243–53.

21. Oskvig RM. Special problems in the elderly. *Chest* 1999; **115**(Suppl 5): S158S–64.

22. Turnheim K. When drug therapy gets old: pharmacokinetics and pharmacodynamics in the elderly. *Exp Gerontol* 2003; **38**(8): 843–53.

23. Akhtar S, Ramani R. Geriatric pharmacology. *Anesthesiol Clin* 2015; **33** (3):457–69.

24. Bowie MW, Slattum PW. Pharmacodynamics in older adults: a review. *Am J Geriatr Pharmacother* 2007; **5** (3):263–303.

25. ElDesoky ES. Pharmacokinetic-pharmacodynamic crisis in the elderly. *Am J Ther* 2007; **14**(5):488–98.

26. Naples JG, Hanlon JT, Schmade KE, et al. Recent literature on medication errors and adverse events in older adults. *J Am Geriatr Soc* 2016; **64**(2):401–8.

27. Nebeker JR, Barach P, Samore MH. Clarifying adverse drug events: a clinician's guide to terminology, documentation, and reporting. *Ann Intern Med* 2004; **140** (10):795–801.

28. Cook RI, Render M, Woods DD. Gaps in the continuity of care and progress on patient safety. *BMJ* 2000; **320**:791–94.

29. Nasraway SA Jr, Albert M, Donnelly AM, et al. Morbid obesity is an independent determinant of death among surgical critically ill patients. *Crit Care Med* 2006; **34**(4):964–70.

30. Erstad BL. Dosing of medications in morbidly obese patients in the intensive care unit setting. *Intensive Care Med* 2004; **30**(1):18–32.

31. Alobaid AS, Hites M, Lipman J, et al. Effect of obesity on the pharmacokinetics of antimicrobials in critically ill patients: a structured review. *Int J Antimicrob Agents* 2016; **47**(4):259–68.

32. de Mendonça A, Vincent JL, Suter PM, et al. Acute renal failure in the ICU: risk factors and outcome evaluated by the SOFA score. *Intensive Care Med* 2000; **26** (7):915–21.

33. Winter MA, Guhr KN, Berg GM. Impact of various body weights and serum creatinine concentrations on the bias and accuracy of the Cockcroft-Gault equation. *Pharmacotherapy* 2012; **32**(7):604–12.

34. Wilhelm SM, Kale-Pradhan PB. Estimating creatinine clearance: a meta-analysis. *Pharmacotherapy* 2011; **31** (7):658–64.

35. Scoville BA, Mueller BA. Medication dosing in critically ill patients with acute kidney injury treated with renal replacement therapy. *Am J Kidney Dis* 2013; **61**(3):490–500.

36. Heintz BH, Matzke GR, Dager WE. Antimicrobial dosing concepts and recommendations for critically ill adult patients receiving continuous renal replacement therapy or intermittent hemodialysis. *Pharmacotherapy* 2009; **29**(5):562–77.

37. Aronoff GR, Bennett WM, Berns JS, et al. *Drug Prescribing in Renal Failure: Dosing Guidelines for Adults and Children* (5th edn). Philadelphia, PA: American College of Physicians, 2007.

38. Vilay AM, Churchwell MD, Mueller BA. Clinical review: drug metabolism and nonrenal clearance in acute kidney injury. *Crit Care* 2008; **12**(6):235.

39. Lewis SJ, Mueller BA. Antibiotic dosing in patients with acute kidney injury: "enough but not too much." *J Intensive Care Med* 2016; **31**(3):164–76.

40. Halilovic J, Heintz BH. Antibiotic dosing in cirrhosis. *Am J Health Syst Pharm* 2014; **71** (19):1621–34.

41. Verbeeck RK. Pharmacokinetics and dosage adjustment in patients with hepatic dysfunction. *Eur J Clin Pharmacol* 2008; **64** (12):1147–61.

42. Barr J, Fraser GL, Puntillo K, et al. Clinical practice guidelines for the management of pain, agitation and delirium in adult ICU patients. *Crit Care Med* 2013; **41**(1): 263–30.

43. Devlin JW, Fraser GL, Riker RR. Drug-induced coma and delirium. In J Papadopoulos, B Cooper, S Kane-Gill, S Mallow-Corbett, J Barletta, eds., *Drug-Induced Complications in the Critically Ill Patient: A Guide for Recognition and Treatment* (1st edn). Chicago, IL: Society of Critical Care Medicine, 2011.

44. Balas MC, Vasilevskis EE, Olsen KM, et al. Effectiveness and safety of the awakening and breathing coordination, delirium monitoring/management, and early exercise/mobility bundle. *Crit Care Med* 2014; **42**:1024–36.

45. Devlin JW, Mallow-Corbett S, Riker RR. Adverse drug events associated with the use of analgesics, sedatives, and antipsychotics in the intensive care unit. *Crit Care Med* 2010; **38**(Suppl 6):S231–43.

46. Devlin JW, Roberts RJ. Pharmacology of commonly used analgesics and sedatives in the ICU: benzodiazepines, propofol, and opioids. *Anesthesiol Clin* 2011; **29**(4): 567–85.

47. Fraser GL, Devlin JW, Worby CP, et al. Benzodiazepine versus nonbenzodiazepine-based sedation for mechanically ventilated, critically ill adults: a systematic review and meta-analysis of randomized trials. *Crit Care Med.* 2013; **41**(9; Suppl 1):S30–38.

48. Pandharipande PP, Shintani A, Peterson J, et al. Lorazepam is an independent risk factor for transitioning to delirium in intensive care unit patients. *Anesthesiology* 2006; **104**(1):21–26.

49. Zaal IJ, Devlin JW, Hazelbag M, et al. Benzodiazepine-associated delirium in critically ill adults. *Intensive Care Med* 2015; **41**:2130–37.

50. Ely EW, Shintani A, Truman B, et al. Delirium as a predictor of mortality in mechanically ventilated patients in the intensive care unit. *JAMA* 2004; **291**: 1753–62.

51. Salluh JI, Wang H, Scheider EB, et al. Outcome of delirium in critically ill patients: systematic review and meta-analysis. *BMJ* 2015; **350**: H2538.

52. Neufeld KJ, Yue J, Robinson TN, et al. Antipsychotic medication for prevention and treatment of delirium in hospitalized adults: a systematic review and meta-analysis. *J Am Geriatr Soc* 2016; **64** (4):705–14.

53. Serafim RB, Bozza FA, Soares M, et al. Pharmacologic prevention and treatment of delirium in intensive care patients: a systematic review. *J Crit Care* 2015; **30**:799–807.

54. Trogrlić Z, van der Jagt M, Bakker J, et al. A systematic review of implementation strategies for assessment, prevention, and management of ICU delirium and their effect on clinical outcomes. *Crit Care* 2015; **19**:157.

55. Schreiber MP, Colantuoni E, Bienvenu OJ, et al. Corticosteroids and transition to delirium in patients with acute lung injury. *Crit Care Med* 2014; **42**(6):1480–86.

56. Wolters AE, Veldhuizjzen DS, Zaal IJ, et al. Systemic corticosteroids and transition to delirium in critically ill patients. *Crit Care Med* 2015; **43**(12):e585–88.

57. Wolters AE, Zaal IJ, Veldhuijzen DS, et al. Anticholinergic medication use and transition to delirium in critically ill patients: a prospective cohort study. *Crit Care Med* 2015; **43**(9):1846–52.

58. Marshall J, Herzig SJ, Howell MD, et al. Antipsychotic utilization in the intensive care unit and in transitions of care. *J Crit Care* 2016; **33**:119–24.

59. Rowe AS, Hamilton LA, Curtis RA, et al. Risk factors for discharge on a new antipsychotic medication after admission to an intensive care unit. *J Crit Care* 2015; **30**:1283–86.

60. Page VJ, Ely EW, Gates S, et al. Effect of intravenous haloperidol on the duration of delirium and coma in critically ill patients (Hope-ICU): a randomised, double-blind, placebo-controlled trial. *Lancet Respir Med* 2013; **1**:515–23.

61. Al-Qadheeb NS, Skrobik Y, Schumaker G, et al. Preventing ICU subsyndromal delirium conversion to delirium with low-dose IV haloperidol: a double-blind, placebo-controlled, pilot study. *Crit Care Med* 2016; **583–91**.

62. Reade MC, Eastwood GM, Bellomo R, et al. Effect of dexmedetomidine added to standard care on ventilator-free time in patients with agitated delirium: a randomized clinical trial. *JAMA* 2016; **315**:1460–68.

63. Pisani MA, Friese RS, Gehlbach BK, et al. Sleep in the intensive care unit. *Am J Respir Crit Care Med* 2015; **191**:731–38.

64. Arixtra [package insert]. GlaxoSmithKline, Research Triangle Park, NC, August 2009.

65. Romanelli RJ, Nolting L, Dolginsky M, et al. Dabigatran versus warfarin for atrial fibrillation in real-world clinical practice: a systematic review and meta-analysis. *Circ Cardiovasc Qual Outcomes* 2016; **9**(2):126–34.

66. Abraham NS, Singh S, Alexander GC, et al. Comparative risk of gastrointestinal bleeding with dabigatran, rivaroxaban, and warfarin: population based cohort study. *BMJ* 2015; **350**:H1857.

67. Ivascu FA, Howells GA, Junn FS, et al. Rapid warfarin reversal in anticoagulated patients with traumatic intracranial hemorrhage reduces hemorrhage progression and mortality. *J Trauma* 2005; **59**(5):1131–37.

68. Frontera JA, Lewin JJ 3rd, Rabinstein AA, et al. Guideline for reversal of antithrombotics in intracranial hemorrhage: a statement for healthcare professionals from the Neurocritical Care Society and Society of Critical Care Medicine. *Neurocrit Care* 2016; **24**(1):6–46.

69. Pollack CV Jr, Reilly PA, Eikelboom J, et al. Idarucizumab for dabigatran reversal. *N Engl J Med* 2015; **373**(6):511–20.

70. Gallegos-Orozco JF, Foxx-Orenstein AE, Sterler SM, et al. Chronic constipation in the elderly. *Am J Gastroenterol* 2012; **107**(1):18–25.

71. Harari D, Gurwitz JH, Avorn J, et al. Constipation: assessment and management in an institutionalized elderly population. *J Am Geriatr Soc* 1994; **42**(9):947–52.

72. Wald A. Constipation: advances in diagnosis and treatment. *JAMA* 2016; **315**(2):185–91.

73. Patanwala AE, Abarca J, Huckleberry Y, et al. Pharmacologic management of constipation in the critically ill patient. *Pharmacotherapy* 2006; **26**(7):896–902.

74. Barletta JF, Kanji S, MacLaren R, et al. Pharmacoepidemiology of stress ulcer prophylaxis in the United States and Canada. *J Crit Care* 2014; **29**(6):955–60.

75. Barletta JF, Sclar DA. Use of proton pump inhibitors for the provision of stress ulcer prophylaxis: clinical and economic consequences. *Pharmacoeconomics* 2014; **32**(1):5–13

76. Barletta JF, El-Ibiary SY, Davis LE, et al. Proton pump inhibitors and the risk for

hospital-acquired *Clostridium difficile* infection. *Mayo Clin Proc* 2013; **88**(10): 1085–90.

77. MacLaren R, Reynolds PM, Allen RR. Histamine-2 receptor antagonists vs. proton pump inhibitors on gastrointestinal tract hemorrhage and infectious complications in the intensive care unit. *JAMA Intern Med* 2014; **174**(4): 564–74.

78. Gomm W, von Holt K, Thomé F, et al. Association of proton pump inhibitors with risk of dementia: a pharmacoepidemiological claims data analysis. *JAMA Neurol* 2016; **73**(4): 410–16.

79. Lazarus B, Chen Y, Wilson FP. Proton pump inhibitor use and the risk of chronic kidney disease. *JAMA Intern Med* 2016; **176** (2):238–46.

80. Maggio M, Corsonello A, Ceda GP, et al. Proton pump inhibitors and risk of 1-year mortality and rehospitalization in older patients discharged from acute care hospitals. *JAMA Intern Med* 2013; **173**(7): 518–23.

81. American Diabetes Association. Older Adults. *Diabetes Care* 2016; **39**(Suppl 1): S81–85.

82. Carpenter DL, Gregg SR, Xu K, et al. Prevalence and impact of unknown diabetes in the ICU. *Crit Care Med* 2015; **43** (12):e541–50.

83. American Diabetes Association. Diabetes care in the hospital. *Diabetes Care* 2016; **39** (Suppl 1):S99–104.

84. Moghissi ES, Korytkowski MT, DiNardo M, et al. American Association of Clinical Endocrinologists and American Diabetes Association consensus statement on inpatient glycemic control. *Diabetes Care* 2009; **32**(6):1119–31.

85. Jacobi J, Bircher N, Krinsley J, et al. Guidelines for the use of an insulin infusion for the management of hyperglycemia in critically ill patients. *Crit Care Med* 2012; **40**(12):3251–76.

86. Krinsley JS, Grover A. Severe hypoglycemia in critically ill patients: risk factors and outcomes. *Crit Care Med* 2007; **35**(10):2262–67.

87. Magill SS, Edwards JR, Beldavs ZG, et al. Prevalence of antimicrobial use in US acute care hospitals, May–September 2011. *JAMA* 2014; **312**(14):1438–46.

88. Roberts JA, Ulldemolins M, Roberts MS, et al. Therapeutic drug monitoring of beta-lactams in critically ill patients: proof of concept. *Int J Antimicrob Agents* 2010; **36** (4):332–39.

89. Roberts JA, Paul SK, Akova M, et al. DALI: defining antibiotic levels in intensive care unit patients. Are current β-lactam antibiotic doses sufficient for critically ill patients? *Clin Infect Dis* 2014; **58**(8): 1072–83.

90. Taccone FS, Laterre PF, Dugernier T, et al. Insufficient β-lactam concentrations in the early phase of severe sepsis and septic shock. *Crit Care* 2010; **14**(4): R126.

91. Lodise TP, Drusano GL, Zasowski E, et al. Vancomycin exposure in patients with methicillin-resistant *Staphylococcus aureus* bloodstream infections: how much is enough? *Clin Infect Dis* 2014; **59**(5): 666–75.

92. Lewin JJ, Devlin JW. Critical care pharmacy practice. In University of the Sciences in Philadelphia, ed., *Remington: The Science and Practice of Pharmacy* (22nd edn). Philadelphia, PA: University of the Sciences in Philadelphia, 2012.

93. Society of Critical Care Medicine. ICU liberation campaign, 2016, available at www.iculiberation.org (accessed May 28, 2016).

94. Preslaski CR, Lat I, MacLaren R, et al. Pharmacist contributions as members of the multidisciplinary ICU team. *Chest* 2013; **144**(5):1687–95.

95. Hume AL, Kirwin J, Bieber HL, et al., for the American College of Clinical Pharmacy. Improving care transitions: current practice and future opportunities for pharmacists. *Pharmacotherapy* 2012; **32** (11):e326–37.

96. Scott IA, Hilmer SN, Reeve E, et al. Reducing inappropriate polypharmacy: the process of deprescribing. *JAMA* 2015; **11**: 852–57.

97. Varkey P, Cunningham J, O'Meara J, et al. Multidisciplinary approach to inpatient medication reconciliation in an academic setting. *Am J Health Syst Pharm* 2007; **64**: 850–54.

98. Rodehover C, Fearing D. Medication reconciliation in acute care: ensuring an accurate drug regimen on admission and discharge. *Jt Comm J Qual Patient Saf* 2005; **31**:406–13.

4

Respiratory Critical Care in the Elderly

Jonathan M. Siner and Margaret A. Pisani

Key Points

- The incidence of acute respiratory distress syndrome rises with age and is likely related to the increased incidence of sepsis with increasing age.
- Age-related changes in pulmonary function include a decrease in forced vital capacity (FVC), forced expiratory volume in 1 second (FEV_1), and arterial partial pressure of oxygen (PaO_2) and an increase in the oxygen arterial-alveolar (A–a) gradient.
- Both the incidence of pulmonary embolism and the mortality from pulmonary embolism increase with age.
- There are no specific guidelines related to optimal ventilator modalities for older patients.
- For older patients with ventilator-associated pneumonia, aspiration or microaspiration often is a contributing factor.
- Local hospital antibiograms should be used when treating patients with ventilator-associated pneumonia.

Introduction

Respiratory diseases in older patients are a major reason for admission to the intensive care unit (ICU), and critical complications related to underlying respiratory disease have a major impact on patient outcomes. The incidence of acute respiratory failure increases dramatically with age [1]. Older adults (defined as age > 65 years) comprise nearly 50 percent of ICU admissions in the United States [2,3]. Among all ICU patients who receive mechanical ventilation, 125,000 survive to discharge. Half of these survivors are ultimately readmitted to the hospital, and 30 to 60 percent die within 6 months. Interestingly, there is also evidence that older adults are receiving more intense care in critical care unit settings, and this may be the cause of decreased mortality [2]. Therefore, understanding the issues related to older adults with respiratory problems is essential to delivering appropriate medical care and providing accurate prognostication for this population [4,5].

Background: Respiratory Physiology and Age

The respiratory system undergoes many changes with aging that reduce reserve and have substantial impact on an individual's capacity to tolerate the stresses of critical illness.

Table 4.1 Respiratory System Age-Related Changes

Decreased vital capacity (VC)

Decreased forced expiratory volume in 1 second (FEV$_1$)

Increased functional residual capacity (FRC)

Increased residual volume (RV)

Reduced elastic recoil of the lung

Reduced arterial partial pressure of oxygen (PaO$_2$)

Increased O$_2$ arterial-alveolar (A–a) gradient

Increased chest wall stiffness, kyphoscoliosis

Decreased respiratory muscle strength

Decreased respiratory center sensitivity to hypoxia and hypercarbia

Table 4.1 lists some of the age-related changes in respiratory physiology. Age-related changes in respiratory function are defined by decreased strength of the respiratory muscles, a decrease in the elastic recoil of the lung, and a decrease in chest wall compliance [6]. Ventilatory reserve decreases substantially with age as a result of multiple interrelated physiologic changes: osteoporosis, kyphosis, and decreased mobility of joints (e.g., rib-vertebral articulation). Together these changes lead to decreases in lung volume and combined lung and chest wall compliance [7]. Elastance decreases, leading to increased lung compliance, as a result of changes in elastin structure and elastin-collagen ratios [8,9]. The combination of increased lung compliance and decreased chest wall compliance leaves total lung capacity unchanged, but the resulting increase in residual volume means that the vital capacity is reduced, along with a concomitant reduction in expiratory flow rates, as measure by forced expiratory volume in 1 second (FEV$_1$) [8]. There is also an age-related decrease in FEV$_1$ of 10 to 30 ml per year and a concomitant decrease in diffusing capacity after the age of 40 [10,11] (Figure 4.1). These limitations mean that the requirement for increased minute ventilation during exercise or illness is met in large part by increases in respiratory rate. Additionally, because age-related decreased chest wall compliance is proportionally larger than the increased lung compliance, the net compliance of the respiratory system is decreased, and therefore, resting work of breathing is increased and the diaphragm and abdominal muscles contribute proportionally *more* to the work of breathing than the thoracic muscles when compared with younger patients [12].

Respiratory muscle performance is impaired by age-related changes in muscle and bone relationships and increased FRC from decreased elastic recoil of the lung [12]. Respiratory muscle status is related to nutritional status and lean body mass; therefore, malnutrition reduces muscle strength and maximal ventilation [13]. Age is significantly correlated with reduced respiratory muscle function and walking capacity [14]. There is a progressive decline in diaphragmatic strength (25 percent) in healthy elderly persons. An investigation into the response of the respiratory muscles to graded exercise demonstrated greater participation of diaphragmatic motion together with rapid shallow breathing during lower-graded exercise in the elderly compared with the young [15]. With regards to gas exchange, an increase in dead space and shunt fraction and a reduction in diffusing capacity have been associated with increasing age [16]. It is estimated that the arterial partial

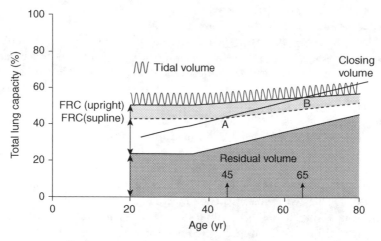

Figure 4.1 Changes in lung volumes and capacities with aging. Residual volume and functional residual capacity (FRC) increase with age, whereas total lung capacity remains the same. Closing volume increases with age and exceeds FRC in the supine position at about age 45 and exceeds FRC in the upright position at about age 65. (*Source:* Adapted from Corcoran TB, Hillyard S. Cardiopulmonary aspects of anaesthesia for the elderly. *Best Pract Res Clin Anaesthesiol* 2011; 25:329–54. Used with permission.)

pressure of oxygen (PaO_2) decreases by an average rate of 0.35 mmHg per year. Mean arterial oxygen tension on room air decreases from 95 mmHg at age 20 to less than 70 mmHg at age 80. These changes are caused by an increased degree of ventilation/perfusion (V/Q) mismatching and, to a lesser extent, pulmonary shunting. These changes would be expected to impair carbon dioxide elimination and oxygenation in the setting of a significant respiratory insult (e.g., acute respiratory distress syndrome [ARDS]). A study of airspace size relative to age found airspace enlargement in older subjects [17]. In addition to the physiologic changes in lung function, the neural sensing and modulating responses by the central nervous system (CNS) of the respiratory system also change with age. Older subjects have a significantly lower ventilatory response to both hypoxia and hypercapnia, and occlusion-pressure response to both hypercapnia and hypoxemia is reduced by a similar magnitude. The alteration in CNS efferent control is thought to be secondary to the lower augmentation of respiratory drive in older adults [18].

Older adults are more likely to have concomitant illnesses that have an impact on their respiratory system. Congestive heart failure has a significant negative effect on respiratory muscle strength and tension-time index, which is important given that cardiac disease and respiratory disease are commonly coincident [19]. In one study, the prevalence of inspiratory muscle weakness was as high as 76 percent in patients who were hospitalized because of acute heart failure [20]. Hypertension, lower extremity edema, and diabetes are independently associated with a lower level of lung function [21]. It is clear that concomitant diseases associated with aging taken together have a substantial impact on respiratory function.

Risk Factors for Respiratory Failure in Older Adults

Acute respiratory failure is a common complication of critical illness in older adults and is due in large part to the increase in prevalence of chronic illnesses, major organ dysfunction, and an increased risk of acquired causes of respiratory failure [22,23]. The incidences of pulmonary embolism, chronic obstructive pulmonary disease (COPD), congestive heart failure, and community-acquired pneumonia all rise with age [22,24]. Furthermore, as many as 47 percent of patients over age 65 who have acute respiratory failure have two diagnoses as the etiology of their respiratory decompensation. This is in large part due to the high incidence of congestive heart failure and COPD in this population. The increased incidence of major organ dysfunction combined with decreased pulmonary reserve is likely responsible for the exponential increase in respiratory failure from the third through the ninth decades of life [1,25,26]. Specifically, in the surgical population, an investigation regarding risk factors for postoperative intubation demonstrated that smoking status, presence of COPD, emergent intervention, and age were important determinants of risk [27]. A separate investigation had similar findings, confirming the role of age as a risk factor for unplanned postoperative intubations, and noted an 18-fold increase in mortality risk associated with unexpected requirement for mechanical ventilation [28]. In a review of surgical ICU admissions, it was noted that 48 percent of the readmissions were due to respiratory complications and that readmitted patients were older [29].

Acute Pulmonary Embolism

The occurrence of pulmonary embolism (PE) increases with age, and elderly patients have the highest risk of venous thromboembolic disease (VTE), with an incidence greater than 1 percent per year [30]. With regard to the clinical presentation of PE, older adults report less pleuritic chest pain and are more likely to present with syncope [31]. In an evaluation of older patients, it was noted that only 5 percent of those older than 80 years age have a negative D-dimer test compared with 50 percent of patients younger than 50 years of age [32]. A multicenter prospective management outcome study of patients with suspected PE demonstrated that an age-adjusted D-dimer cutoff was associated with a larger number of patients in whom PE could be ruled out [33].

Elderly patients with a PE have a high (>20 percent) 3-year mortality predominantly due to the high frequency of cancer and other comorbidities [34]. Risk assessment is generally performed based on echocardiography and measurement of circulating biomarkers associated with right ventricular strain. While echocardiographic evidence of right ventricular dysfunction is often used clinically to stratify risk, the extent of right ventricular dysfunction does not appear to be associated with mortality in older adults [35]. Cardiac biomarkers are more useful for identifying low-risk individuals with nonmassive PEs than echocardiography data, and these findings have been replicated in older adult populations [36,37].

New interventions for both massive and submassive PEs include ultrasound-assisted catheter-directed low-dose thrombolysis, which is still under investigation, but early studies have shown efficacy with possibly a lower risk of hemorrhage, although those studies may not be adequately powered to detect this complication [38,39]. Meta-analyses of prior investigations of thrombolysis for massive PEs have suggested that bleeding complications, including intracranial hemorrhage, are higher in those with advanced age, but whether is it is age or simply the concomitant risk factors, including malignancy, that increase risk is unknown [40,41]. While there are no specific independent guidelines for elderly adults who are critically ill with massive PEs, the current literature suggests that they be treated similar to the general population, but with recognition of the potential for increased risk of complications due to age and burden of comorbidities.

Pneumonia in Older Adults

Several studies have demonstrated that older patients have an increased incidence of pneumonia and greater mortality after pneumonia compared with younger patients. The physiologic changes discussed earlier and a reduced ability to expectorate and clear bacteria and decreased physiologic reserve are factors that increase this risk. In addition, oropharyngeal bacterial colonization with *Staphylococcus aureus, Klebsiella pneumonia,* and *Escherichia coli* are more common in elderly patients and serve as harbingers of subsequent pneumonia. Patients with severe community-acquired pneumonia who are older than 65 years of age have many preexisting diseases, including COPD (48 percent), heart disease (16 percent), diabetes (18 percent), and malignancy (12 percent) [42]. Elderly patients are more at risk for aspiration, including silent aspiration [43]. Factors supporting this include alterations in the swallowing mechanism that occur with age, cognitive impairment, medication use, malnutrition, poor oral health, and Parkinson's disease [44].

Frail older patients may not present with the typical fever, cough, and shortness of breath that characterize pneumonia in younger patients. Many older patients with pneumonia present with nonproductive cough, delirium, anorexia, falls and dizziness, or signs of sepsis. Older patients who present with hypothermia and sepsis from pneumonia have significant in-hospital mortality [45].

While older patients frequently have bacterial pneumonia and sepsis precipitating an ICU admission, they also are frequently critically ill secondary to viral respiratory infections. Patients older than 65 years have higher rates of hospitalization for laboratory-confirmed influenza. In the United States during the 2014–15 influenza season, the rates of hospitalization for patients older than 65 years was 258 per 100,000 population compared with 41 per 100,000 population for younger patients [46].

A recent systematic review examined current evidence on antibiotic treatment of older adults with community-acquired pneumonia (CAP), healthcare-associated pneumonia (HCAP), hospital-acquired pneumonia (HAP), and ventilator-associated pneumonia (VAP). This study demonstrated that patients older than age 65 are often excluded from clinical trials of bacterial pneumonia, and no data were found on the comparative efficacy of antibiotic treatment in elderly adults compared with younger patients [47]. What the study did note was increased treatment failure rates in participants who were aged 65 years and older.

Ventilator-associated pneumonia is a complication for older patients in the ICU who are mechanically ventilated. There are no studies examining the recognition or treatment of VAP in older patients, and general guidelines should be followed. The 2016 Infectious Disease Society of America guidelines on HCAP and VAP make recommendations regarding treatment, including using hospital-specific antibiograms to guide empirical antibiotic choices. There are no recommendations based on patient age [48]. One study using a molecular microbiology study of 44 patients age 60 years and older demonstrated that gastro-pulmonary aspiration is an important mechanism in the development of VAP, especially late-onset VAP [49]. Risk for aspiration should be recognized and evaluated in all older patients on mechanical ventilation and after extubation.

Acute Respiratory Distress Syndrome in Older Adults

Acute respiratory distress syndrome (ARDS) is a disease resulting in acute hypoxemic respiratory failure most commonly due to sepsis, pneumonia, aspiration, trauma,

Table 4.2 Acute Respiratory Distress Syndrome: The Berlin Definition

- Onset within 1 week of a known clinical insult or new/worsening respiratory symptoms.
- Chest imaging with bilateral opacities not fully explained by effusions, lobar/lung collapse, or nodules.
- Respiratory failure not fully explained by cardiac failure or fluid overload; objective assessment needed, such as echocardiography.
- Oxygenation:
  - Mild: 200 mmHg < PaO_2/FIO_2 ≤ 300 mmHg with PEEP or CPAP ≥ 5 cmH$_2$O
  - Moderate: 100 mmHg < PaO_2/FIO_2 ≤ 200 mmHg with PEEP or CPAP ≥ 5 cmH$_2$O
  - Severe: PaO_2/FIO_2 ≤ 100 mmHg with PEEP ≥ 5 cmH$_2$O

Abbreviations: PaO_2 = partial pressure of arterial oxygen; FIO_2 = fraction of inspired oxygen; PEEP = positive end-expiratory pressure; CPAP = continuous positive airway pressure.
(*Source:* From Ranier et al. [50].)

pancreatitis, and transfusion of allogeneic blood products. The injury of ARDS involves the alveolar epithelium and the lung capillary endothelium. The definition of ARDS was revised (Berlin definition) in 2012 and demonstrates better predictive validity for mortality compared with the 1994 American-European Consensus Conference definition. Table 4.2 lists the Berlin definition of ARDS [50]. The significantly increased incidence of ARDS associated with older age is partly due to the higher incidence of sepsis with aging, the primary risk factor for ARDS in adults [51,52]. An investigation of ARDS in the trauma population showed that the incidence of ARDS increases with age but plateaus in the 60- to 69-year-old population [53]. In a global incidence study, 10.4 percent patients with ICU admissions and 23.4 percent of patients requiring mechanical ventilation had ARDS. These results are similar to those of prior investigations, where clinical recognition of ARDS was only 51.3 percent for mild ARDS but increased to 78.5 percent for severe disease [54].

The first large randomized, controlled trial to evaluate a therapy for ARDS was published in 2000 and demonstrated that the ARDSnet approach to low-tidal-volume ventilation results in a substantial reduction in mortality [55]. The original ARDSnet investigation was notable for a young mean age and excluded patients with significant chronic lung disease, leaving open the question of whether this study is generalizable to the large population of older adults who develop sepsis and ARDS. Furthermore, because the low-tidal-volume strategy used tidal volumes and plateau pressures and older adults are known to have increased lung compliance and decreased chest wall compliance, it remains unknown whether the ARDSnet strategy would have the same effect in older adults with different pulmonary responses to similar volumes and pressures. A reanalysis of prior studies in ARDS found that while overall survival was high, older adults were twice as likely to die of acute lung injury and had greater difficulty achieving liberation from mechanical ventilation and being discharged from the ICU than younger adults [56]. In addition to low-tidal-volume ventilation, investigators have examined several other therapies for ARDS. A follow-up study by the ARDSnet investigators examined the role of corticosteroids as adjunctive therapy and showed that pulmonary parameters improved but that the increased rate of muscle weakness led to an increase in reintubations, and this would be of even greater concern in an older adult population [57]. Prone positioning has been investigated several times over the past decade, and the most definitive study of prone positioning for ARDS demonstrated improved outcomes, and importantly, the average age was approximately 60 years, but with large standard deviations consistent with the fact that a fair number of these patients were older adults. This trial showed significant reductions in mortality and ICU length of stay, and this approach has been adopted as a component of standard care for those with ARDS [58].

Additional supportive therapies that have received great attention in the past decade include a resurgent interest in the use of extracorporeal membrane oxygenation (ECMO). Most institutions and protocols have generally excluded the use of ECMO in older patients (age greater than 60 or 65 years). The authors of the CESAR trial recommended transferring patients with severe but potentially reversible hypoxemic respiratory failure, based on Murray score, to an ECMO center to improve survival without disability. The study itself started with 766 patients, of which 586 were excluded, and of those excluded, 10 percent of those referred for enrollment were excluded due to age (>65 or <18 years). These age-based exclusions are fairly standard for ECMO, and thus the implications of ECMO for older adults are unclear [59]. In a retrospective review of the Extracorporeal Life Support Organization (ELSO) registry from 1990 to 2013 for adults of age greater than 65 years, survival for older adults was 41 percent versus 55 percent for the entire population. Nonsurvivors were more likely to have hemorrhagic complications (cannulation site, pulmonary hemorrhage, disseminated intravascular coagulation, excessive hemolysis while on ECMO support). Death from withdrawal of life support occurred in 11 percent of patients. While the mortality rate in this review was certainly higher for older adults, the survival rate was still in a range that many clinicians would consider acceptable for a lethal disease when there are limited alternative options [60].

Mechanical Ventilation in Older Adults

There are no data to suggest that one mode of mechanical ventilation is better than any other mode of ventilation in older patients. As noted earlier in relation to ARDS, the study population used in the landmark study of low-tidal-volume ventilation did not include many older patients, and it also excluded many patients based on comorbidities, which are common in the elderly. Interestingly, a recent study using Medicare data demonstrated that among hospitalized nursing home residents with advanced dementia, there was an increase in the use of mechanical ventilation over time without substantial improvement in survival [61]. The use of mechanical ventilation increased from 39 per 1,000 hospitalizations in 2000 to 78 per 1,000 hospitalizations in 2013 [61]. As the number of ICU beds in a hospital increased over time, patients with advanced dementia were more likely to receive mechanical ventilation.

Discontinuation of Mechanical Ventilation and Prolonged Mechanical Ventilation

Expertise in liberation from mechanical ventilation has evolved over the past 20 years, yet it remains unclear specifically how the current knowledge applies to older adults. Because at baseline older adults have a respiratory exertional response that is similar to rapid shallow breathing, using this measure may be a less accurate marker of ongoing respiratory failure during weaning in the elderly [7,62]. Thus, physiologically, a patient may be judged to have failed a spontaneous breathing trial (SBT) when they have not. Yet this observation is further complicated by the fact that older adults also have a diminished response to hypoxia and hypercapnia, and therefore an older adult patient on a SBT may be more likely to appear comfortable despite having developed significant hypoxia or hypercapnia [18]. The most direct evidence regarding older adults and extubation comes from a study by Ely et al., who investigated outcomes of older patients in a large multicenter trial of ARDS [56]. Although older patients achieved physiologic recovery from acute lung injury in equal proportions to younger patients, their ICU length of stay and duration of mechanical ventilation were increased because of higher reintubation rates. In a medical ICU population, El Solh et al. observed that patients older than age 70, compared with a younger matched cohort, were more likely to fail extubation because of an inability to handle secretions [63]. While liberation from mechanical ventilation in older adults remains an area in which there are limited data, it is clear from an understanding of physiology and our limited data that the intensivist should carefully consider the impact of aging on respiratory function when making decisions on liberation from ventilation.

Prolonged mechanical ventilation (PMV) is defined as requiring mechanical ventilator support for longer than 21 days. Approximately 300,000 individuals annually in the United States require mechanical ventilation in the acute setting for more than 4 days [64]. Among these individuals, 3 to 7 percent will survive and remain ventilator dependent after 21 days [65]. Tracheostomy use in those requiring mechanical ventilation rose substantially from 1993 to 2008 (from 6.9 percent in 1993 to 9.8 percent) but then began a slow decline. This increase in the tracheostomy rate was driven primarily by patients in the surgical population and was associated with a decreased length of hospital stay [66]. A study of 437 admissions to a long-term acute care hospital (LTACH) for PMV between 2001 and 2006 investigated the impact of age on survival and discontinuation of mechanical ventilation. Increasing age was associated with more physiologic abnormalities and comorbidities, but after adjustment for these factors, the authors did not find an independent effect of age on ability to wean [67]. In the postacute settings, elderly adults were most likely to have successful discontinuation of mechanical ventilation if they had fewer comorbidities and less respiratory impairment, and interestingly, these factors were more important than physical function prior to the acute care hospitalization [68]. While the authors do not comment on this specifically, their data show that regardless of age, fewer than 10 percent of adults who failed to wean are alive at 24 months. While age alone was not associated with survival per se, for adults older than 84 years of age with PMV, those who were able to be weaned had a survival rate of only 20 percent at 24 months [68].

Conclusion

The respiratory system changes substantially with aging such that older adults have diminished ventilatory and oxygenation reserve and are at higher risk than younger adults of developing most common respiratory ailments, including pneumonia, ARDS, and respiratory failure. While much is known about these common respiratory ailments and there have been many controlled trials, age-specific knowledge is much more limited. Despite this, the evidence does suggest that while age increases the risk of developing certain adverse outcomes, it is important to keep in mind that it often the concomitant illness and comorbidities that drive the response to therapy and outcome more than simply the chronologic age.

References

1. Behrendt CE. Acute respiratory failure in the United States: incidence and 31-day survival. *Chest* 2000; **118**(4):1100–5.

2. Lerolle N, Trinquart L, Bornstain C, et al. Increased intensity of treatment and decreased mortality in elderly patients in an intensive care unit over a decade. *Crit Care Med* 2010; **38**(1):59–64.

3. Angus DC, Shorr AF, White A, et al. Critical care delivery in the United States: distribution of services and compliance with Leapfrog recommendations. *Crit Care Med* 2006; **34**(4):1016–24.

4. Wunsch H, Guerra C, Barnato AE, et al. Three-year outcomes for Medicare beneficiaries who survive intensive care. *JAMA* 2010; **303**(9):849–56.

5. Kahn JM, Benson NM, Appleby D, Carson SS, Iwashyna TJ. Long-term acute care hospital utilization after critical illness. *JAMA* 2010; **303**(22):2253–59.

6. Janssens JP. Aging of the respiratory system: impact on pulmonary function tests and adaptation to exertion. *Clin Chest Med* 2005; **26**(3):469–84, vi–vii.

7. Sprung J, Gajic O, Warner DO. Review article: age related alterations in respiratory function – anesthetic considerations. *Can J Anaesth* 2006; **53**(12):1244–57.

8. Knudson RJ, Burrows B, Lebowitz MD. The maximal expiratory flow-volume curve: its use in the detection of ventilatory abnormalities in a population study. *Am Rev Respir Dis* 1976; **114**(5):871–79.

9. Zeleznik J. Normative aging of the respiratory system. *Clin Geriatr Med* 2003; **19**(1):1–18.

10. Janssens JP, Pache JC, Nicod LP. Physiological changes in respiratory function associated with ageing. *Eur Respir J* 1999; **13**(1):197–205.

11. Knudson RJ, Kaltenborn WT, Knudson DE, Burrows B. The single-breath carbon monoxide diffusing capacity: reference equations derived from a healthy nonsmoking population and effects of hematocrit. *Am Rev Respir Dis* 1987; **135**(4):805–11.

12. Turner JM, Mead J, Wohl ME. Elasticity of human lungs in relation to age. *J Appl Physiol* 1968; **25**(6):664–71.

13. Arora NS, Rochester DF. Respiratory muscle strength and maximal voluntary ventilation in undernourished patients. *Am Rev Respir Dis* 1982; **126**(1):5–8.

14. Watsford ML, Murphy AJ, Pine MJ. The effects of ageing on respiratory muscle function and performance in older adults. *J Sci Med Sport* 2007; **10**(1):36–44.

15. Teramoto S, Fukuchi Y, Nagase T, Matsuse T, Orimo H. A comparison of ventilation components in young and elderly men during exercise. *J Gerontol A Biol Sci Med Sci* 1995; **50A**(1):B34–39.

16. Stam H, Hrachovina V, Stijnen T, Versprille A. Diffusing capacity dependent on lung volume and age in normal subjects. *J Appl Physiol* 1994; **76**(6):2356–63.

17. Gillooly M, Lamb D. Airspace size in lungs of lifelong non-smokers: effect of age and sex. *Thorax* 1993; **48**(1):39–43.

18. Peterson DD, Pack AI, Silage DA, Fishman AP. Effects of aging on ventilatory and occlusion pressure responses to hypoxia and hypercapnia. *Am Rev Respir Dis* 1981; **124**(4):387–91.

19. Mancini DM, Henson D, LaManca J, Levine S. Respiratory muscle function and dyspnea in patients with chronic congestive heart failure. *Circulation* 1992; **86**(3):909–18.

20. Verissimo P, Casalaspo TJ, Gonçalves LH, et al. High prevalence of respiratory muscle weakness in hospitalized acute heart failure elderly patients. *PLoS One* 2015; **10**(2): e0118218.

21. Enright PL, Kronmal RA, Higgins M, Schenker M, Haponik EF. Spirometry reference values for women and men 65 to 85 years of age: cardiovascular health study. *Am Rev Respir Dis* 1993; **147**(1): 125–33.

22. Marrie TJ, Lau CY, Wheeler SL, Wong CJ, Feagan BG. Predictors of symptom resolution in patients with community-acquired pneumonia. *Clin Infect Dis* 2000; **31**(6):1362–67.

23. Ray P, Birolleau S, Lefort Y, et al. Acute respiratory failure in the elderly: etiology, emergency diagnosis and prognosis. *Crit Care* 2006; **10**(3):R82.

24. Rich MW. Heart failure in the 21st century: a cardiogeriatric syndrome. *J Gerontol A Biol Sci Med Sci* 2001; **56**(2):M88–96.

25. Siner JM, Pisani MA. Mechanical ventilation and acute respiratory distress syndrome in older patients. *Clin Chest Med* 2007; **28**(4):783–91, vii.

26. El Solh AA, Ramadan FH. Overview of respiratory failure in older adults. *J Intensive Care Med* 2006; **21**(6):345–51.

27. Alvarez MP, Samayoa-Mendez AX, Naglak MC, Yuschak JV, Murayama KM. Risk factors for postoperative unplanned intubation: analysis of a national database. *Am Surg* 2015; **81**(8):820–25.

28. Nafiu OO, Ramachandran SK, Ackwerh R, et al. Factors associated with and consequences of unplanned post-operative intubation in elderly vascular and general surgery patients. *Eur J Anaesthesiol* 2011; **28**(3):220–24.

29. Timmers TK, Verhofstad MH, Moons KG, Leenen LP. Patients' characteristics associated with readmission to a surgical intensive care unit. *Am J Crit Care* 2012; **21**(6):e120–28.

30. Oger E. Incidence of venous thromboembolism: a community-based study in western France. EPI-GETBP Study Group. Groupe d'Etude de la Thrombose de Bretagne Occidentale. *Thromb Haemost* 2000; **83**(5):657–60.

31. Schouten HJ, Geersing GJ, Oudega R, et al. Accuracy of the Wells clinical prediction rule for pulmonary embolism in older ambulatory adults. *J Am Geriatr Soc* 2014; **62**(11):2136–41.

32. Righini M, Le Gal G, Bounameaux H. Venous thromboembolism diagnosis: unresolved issues. *Thromb Haemost* 2015; **113**(6):1184–92.

33. Righini M, Van Es J, Den Exter PL, et al. Age-adjusted D-dimer cutoff levels to rule out pulmonary embolism: the ADJUST-PE study. *JAMA* 2014; **311**(11):1117–24.

34. Faller N, Limacher A, Méan M, et al. Predictors and causes of long-term mortality in elderly patients with acute venous thromboembolism: a prospective cohort study. *Am J Med* 2016.

35. Hofmann E, Limacher A, Méan M, et al. Echocardiography does not predict mortality in hemodynamically stable elderly patients with acute pulmonary embolism. *Thromb Res* 2016; **145**:67–71.

36. Konstantinides S, Goldhaber SZ. Pulmonary embolism: risk assessment and management. *Eur Heart J* 2012; **33**(24): 3014–22.

37. Vuilleumier N, Simona A, Méan M, et al. Comparison of cardiac and non-cardiac biomarkers for risk stratification in elderly patients with non-massive pulmonary embolism. *PLoS One* 2016; **11**(5):e0155973.

38. Kucher N, Boekstegers P, Müller OJ, et al. Randomized, controlled trial of ultrasound-assisted catheter-directed thrombolysis for acute intermediate-risk pulmonary embolism. *Circulation* 2014; **129**(4):479–86.

39. Kuo WT, Banerjee A, Kim PS, et al. Pulmonary embolism response to fragmentation, embolectomy, and catheter thrombolysis (PERFECT): initial results from a prospective multicenter registry. *Chest* 2015; **148**(3):667–73.

40. Chatterjee S, Chakraborty A, Weinberg I, et al. Thrombolysis for pulmonary embolism and risk of all-cause mortality, major bleeding, and intracranial hemorrhage: a meta-analysis. *JAMA* 2014; **311**(23):2414–21.

41. Fiumara K, Kucher N, Fanikos J, Goldhaber SZ. Predictors of major hemorrhage following fibrinolysis for acute pulmonary embolism. *Am J Cardiol* 2006; **97**(1):127–29.

42. Rello J, Rodriguez R, Jubert P, Alvarez B. Severe community-acquired pneumonia in the elderly: epidemiology and prognosis. Study Group for Severe Community-Acquired Pneumonia. *Clin Infect Dis* 1996; **23**(4):723–28.

43. Kikuchi R, Watabe N, Konno T, et al. High incidence of silent aspiration in elderly

patients with community-acquired pneumonia. *Am J Respir Crit Care Med* 1994; **150**(1):251–53.

44. van der Maarel-Wierink CD, Vanobbergen JN, Bronkhorst EM, Schols JM, de Baat C. Risk factors for aspiration pneumonia in frail older people: a systematic literature review. *J Am Med Dir Assoc* 2011; **12**(5): 344–54.

45. Tiruvoipati R, Ong K, Gangopadhyay H, et al. Hypothermia predicts mortality in critically ill elderly patients with sepsis. *BMC Geriatr* 2010; **10**:70.

46. D'Mello T, Brammer L, Blanton L, et al. Update: influenza activity – United States, September 28, 2014–February 21, 2015. *MMWR Morb Mortal Wkly Rep* 2015; **64** (8):206–12.

47. Avni T, Shiver-Ofer S, Leibovici L, et al. Participation of elderly adults in randomized controlled trials addressing antibiotic treatment of pneumonia. *J Am Geriatr Soc* 2015; **63**(2):233–43.

48. Kalil AC, Metersky ML, Klompas M, et al. Management of adults with hospital-acquired and ventilator-associated pneumonia: 2016 Clinical Practice Guidelines by the Infectious Diseases Society of America and the American Thoracic Society. *Clin Infect Dis* 2016; **63**(5):e61–111.

49. Liu QH, Zhang J, Lin DJ, et al. Gastropulmonary route of infection and the prevalence of microaspiration in the elderly patients with ventilator-associated pneumonia verified by molecular microbiology-GM-PFGE. *Cell Biochem Biophys* 2015; **71**(3):1457–62.

50. Ranieri VM, Rubenfeld GD, Thompson BT, et al. Acute respiratory distress syndrome: the Berlin definition. *JAMA* 2012; **307**(23):2526–33.

51. Angus DC, Linde-Zwirble WT, Lidicker J, et al. Epidemiology of severe sepsis in the United States: analysis of incidence, outcome, and associated costs of care. *Crit Care Med* 2001; **29**(7):1303–10.

52. Manzano F, Yuste E, Colmenero M, et al. Incidence of acute respiratory distress

syndrome and its relation to age. *J Crit Care* 2005; **20**(3):274–80.

53. Hudson LD, Milberg JA, Anardi D, Maunder RJ. Clinical risks for development of the acute respiratory distress syndrome. *Am J Respir Crit Care Med* 1995; **151**(2 Pt 1):293–301.

54. Bellani G, Laffey JG, Pham T, et al. Epidemiology, patterns of care, and mortality for patients with acute respiratory distress syndrome in intensive care units in 50 countries. *JAMA* 2016; **315** (8):788–800.

55. Acute Respiratory Distress Syndrome Network. Ventilation with lower tidal volumes as compared with traditional tidal volumes for acute lung injury and the acute respiratory distress syndrome. *N Engl J Med* 2000; **342**(18):1301–8.

56. Ely EW, Wheeler AP, Thompson BT, et al. Recovery rate and prognosis in older persons who develop acute lung injury and the acute respiratory distress syndrome. *Ann Intern Med* 2002; **136**(1):25–36.

57. Steinberg KP, Hudson LD, Goodman RB, et al. Efficacy and safety of corticosteroids for persistent acute respiratory distress syndrome. *N Engl J Med* 2006; **354**(16): 1671–84.

58. Guérin C, Reignier J, Richard JC. Prone positioning in the acute respiratory distress syndrome. *N Engl J Med* 2013; **369**(10): 980–81.

59. Peek GJ, Mugford M, Tiruvoipati R, et al. Efficacy and economic assessment of conventional ventilatory support versus extracorporeal membrane oxygenation for severe adult respiratory failure (CESAR): a multicentre randomised controlled trial. *Lancet* 2009; **374**(9698):1351–63.

60. Mendiratta P, Tang X, Collins RT, et al. Extracorporeal membrane oxygenation for respiratory failure in the elderly: a review of the Extracorporeal Life Support Organization registry. *ASAIO J* 2014; **60**(4): 385–90.

61. Teno JM, Gozalo P, Khandelwal N, et al. Association of increasing use of mechanical ventilation among nursing home residents with advanced dementia

and intensive care unit beds. *JAMA Intern Med* 2016.

62. Zaugg M, Lucchinetti E. Respiratory function in the elderly. *Anesthesiol Clin North Am* 2000; **18**(1):47–58, vi.

63. El Solh AA, Bhat A, Gunen H, Berbary E. Extubation failure in the elderly. *Respir Med* 2004; **98**(7):661–68.

64. Zilberberg MD, Luippold RS, Sulsky S, Shorr AF. Prolonged acute mechanical ventilation, hospital resource utilization, and mortality in the United States. *Crit Care Med* 2008; **36**(3):724–30.

65. MacIntyre NR, Epstein SK, Carson S, et al. Management of patients requiring prolonged mechanical ventilation: report of a NAMDRC consensus conference. *Chest* 2005; **128**(6):3937–54.

66. Mehta AB, Syeda SN, Bajpayee L, et al. Trends in tracheostomy for mechanically ventilated patients in the United States, 1993–2012. *Am J Respir Crit Care Med* 2015; **192**(4):446–54.

67. Sansone GR, Frengley JD, Vecchione JJ, Manogaram MG, Kaner RJ. Relationship of the duration of ventilator support to successful weaning and other clinical outcomes in 437 prolonged mechanical ventilation patients. *J Intensive Care Med* 2016.

68. Dermot Frengley J, Sansone GR, Shakya K, Kaner RJ. Prolonged mechanical ventilation in 540 seriously ill older adults: effects of increasing age on clinical outcomes and survival. *J Am Geriatr Soc* 2014; **62**(1):1–9.

Chapter

Neurocognitive Dysfunction and Geriatric Neurocritical Care

Tracy J. McGrane, Pratik P. Pandharipande
and Christopher G. Hughes

Key Points

- Acute brain dysfunction is common among the elderly population and is often unrecognized, leading to long-term consequences.
- Increased hospital length of stay, increased hospital cost, increased morbidity and mortality, and reduced quality of life have all been attributed to acute brain dysfunction in elderly patients.
- The geriatric population tends to have a higher incidence of acute brain dysfunction due to an age-related increase in blood-brain barrier permeability to cytokines and a basal pro-inflammatory state.
- Changes in structure, function, metabolism, and blood flow in the aging brain lead to cognitive impairments, most frequently episodic memory changes, and an increased risk of delirium in the acute setting.
- The mechanism for delirium has not been fully elucidated, but current hypotheses support a multifactorial neuroinflammatory etiology.
- Education of healthcare professionals in diagnosing and managing delirium has been shown to reduce delirium rates and is a cost-effective delirium prevention strategy.
- Several risk factors for delirium are modifiable.
- Management of delirium is comprised of both pharmacologic and nonpharmacologic interventions.

Overview of Clinically Relevant Neurocognitive Changes with Aging

The population of septuagenarians, octogenarians, and even nonagenarians presenting for care in intensive care units (ICUs) has been increasing in recent years. Knowledge regarding physiologic changes that are specific to this patient population continues to evolve. Every major organ system has adaptive physiologic changes with increasing age, and the central nervous system (CNS) is no exception. Important neurophysiologic changes in the CNS include reduced brain volume, decreased neurotransmitters, reduced synaptic plasticity, increased blood-brain barrier permeability, and reduced microvascular blood flow [1]. Brain atrophy from neuronal cell death begins after 40 years of age and preferentially affects the prefrontal cortex, hippocampus, and cerebellum, with a greater loss of white matter compared with grey matter [2]. A decrease in neurotransmitter availability has been associated with declines in cognition, motor function, synaptic plasticity, and neurogenesis. Increased blood-brain barrier permeability results in an increased inflammatory response in the CNS, structural damage, and altered patterns of neuronal activity [3,4]. Finally, cerebral vascular resistance increases, capillary blood flow redistributes, and deformities in microvasculature increase with age, all contributing to altered microvascular blood flow in the brain [2].

The physiologic changes in the CNS of the elderly often manifest as changes in cognition. This typically includes a decline in memory, in particular episodic memory. Physiologic changes also play a role in the significant changes patients experience during and after critical illness, making elderly patients more susceptible to acute neurologic insults that cause further pathologic changes in the CNS (e.g., neurotransmitter imbalance, neuronal injury, neurodegeneration). The changes likely lead to the clinical presentation of acute brain dysfunction in the hospital and may contribute to changes in cognition after a critical illness.

Key Concepts with Evidence-Based Discussion

Acute Brain Dysfunction

Definition, Diagnosis, and Clinical Features

Acute brain dysfunction can occur when there is an imbalance of the brain's homeostatic reserve and acute stressors. The term *acute brain dysfunction* most commonly refers to delirium but may also include coma. Delirium is an acute disorder of attention and cognition [5]. A comprehensive psychiatric evaluation using criteria based on the *Diagnostic and Statistical Manual of Mental Disorders* (DSM), 5th edition, from the American Psychiatric Association [6], is considered the gold standard for diagnosing delirium. Important diagnostic features of DSM-5 delirium include sudden onset of altered consciousness, reduced capacity to maintain one's attention and awareness, and disorganized thought process, all of which cannot be better explained by another neurocognitive disorder or severely reduced arousal. Pragmatically, the DSM-5 definition may be challenging to apply in clinical settings, especially in geriatric critically ill patients who may have baseline cognitive impairment or neurologic injury [7]. The mental status therefore must be an acute change from baseline impairments and fluctuate throughout the day.

Clinically, delirium is often suspected when one has fluctuating attention and consciousness causing impaired awareness. One may also exhibit disorientation, episodic memory disorders, and delusions or hallucinations that lead to an abnormal perception of the environment. A number of well-validated approaches for diagnosing delirium in the critical care setting exist, with the most widely recognized methods being the Confusion Assessment Method for the Intensive Care Unit (CAM-ICU) [8] and the Intensive Care Delirium Screening Checklist (ICDSC) [9]. The CAM-ICU, originally described by Ely et al., is a four-element diagnostic algorithm that trained healthcare professionals can easily employ in less than 2 minutes [8]. It assesses for acute changes/fluctuations in mental status, inattention, disorganized thinking, and an altered level of consciousness (Table 5.1).

Table 5.1 Confusion Assessment Method–Intensive Care Unit (CAM-ICU)

Acute onset of mental status change *or* fluctuation course
AND
Inattention
AND
Disorganized thinking *or* altered level of consciousness

The ICDSC assesses eight diagnostic features of delirium over an entire nursing shift (altered level of consciousness, inattention, disorientation, psychosis, altered psychomotor activity, inappropriate speech/mood, sleep disturbance, and symptom fluctuation). Given the fluctuating nature of delirium, it is imperative that delirium assessments be performed serially. Of special challenge in geriatric critical care is delirium superimposed on dementia and delirium in those with primarily neurologic insult (i.e., stroke). The CAM-ICU has demonstrated high sensitivity and specificity, and the Richmond Agitation-Sedation Scale [10] has demonstrated moderate sensitivity and high specificity for delirium superimposed on dementia [11,12]. The CAM-ICU has also been validated for poststroke delirium assessment and should be employed for the detection of delirium in this subset of elderly patients [13].

Delirium can have varying clinical presentations, and three different motor subtypes of delirium (hypoactive, hyperactive, and mixed) have been described. Hypoactive delirium is characterized by symptoms of lethargy, decreased movement, and slowed mentation, whereas the hyperactive subtype manifests as agitation, heightened arousal, or aggression [14]. Additionally, a patient may have features of both subtypes, which is referred to as a *mixed delirium* [14]. Hypoactive delirium has been found to be the predominant subtype among elderly patients [15]. It is less clinically apparent than the hyperactive subtype, which may lead to a delayed diagnosis. In addition to diagnosing delirium and subtypes, the severity of the delirium may be rated using the Delirium Rating Scale–Revised-98 [16] or the Confusion Assessment Method–Severity (CAM-S) [17].

Postoperative delirium (POD), a commonly used clinical term, is recognized as a medical diagnosis code that is a subset of delirium in the tenth edition of the *International Statistical Classification of Diseases and Related Health Problems* (ICD-10) system. *Postoperative cognitive dysfunction* (POCD), another widely used term, is not recognized in the ICD-10 system. POCD typically refers to deficits that have a longer duration (weeks to years) than delirium (hours to days).

Outcomes Associated with Acute Brain Dysfunction

Previously, acute brain dysfunction was thought to be a transient, reversible, and self-limited process [18–22]. More recently, it has become clear that acute brain organ dysfunction in critically ill patients is a predictor of worse clinical outcomes and that delirium may have significant long-term consequences. Patients with delirium take longer to wean from mechanical ventilation and have longer ICU and hospital lengths of stay [23]. Furthermore, they are more likely to require institutionalization or to be readmitted after discharge [23,24]. Patients with delirium therefore have higher hospital costs [25,26].

In general, costs associated with delirium are estimated to be over $160 billion per year in the United States alone [5]. Delirium in the ICU has also been associated with increased risk of death, in particular when it persists for multiple days or after sedation has been discontinued [23,24,27,28]. Studies in surgical patients focusing on POD have found significant associations with increased length of stay, higher cost of care, readmission to the hospital, higher rates of institutionalization after discharge, and increased mortality [26,29,30]. Surgery combined with early postoperative neurologic dysfunction, including even minor reductions in performance (defined as a Mini Mental Status Exam score < 24), has recently been shown to be a negative prognostic factor among elderly patients with hip fractures with a nearly 15 percent mortality rate [31], which is double that of patients without delirium. Studies have now begun examining the association of subtype of delirium and severity of delirium with clinical outcome. In a study of elderly patients admitted to the ICU postoperatively after an elective surgery, patients suffering from hypoactive delirium had increased 6-month mortality compared with patients suffering from other subtypes [32]. Increased hospital length of stay and mortality have been associated with increased severity of delirium [17]. Poststroke delirium has been associated with increased hospital length of stay [13].

Although delirium represents acute brain dysfunction, it has additionally been linked to long-term cognitive impairment [33–36]. Recent observational studies of critically ill patients have shown that nearly three-fourths of survivors have cognitive impairment 1 year after the hospitalization [33] and that advancing age and duration of acute brain dysfunction were significant risk factors for worse global cognition [34]. Although the relationship has yet to be fully elucidated, POD appears to be associated with POCD [34–36] Furthermore, delirium has been shown to accelerate cognitive decline in patients with Alzheimer's disease [37,38] and be associated with worse cognitive decline in patients with and without dementia [39]. Thus long-term changes in cognition are a recognized complication associated with delirium in the geriatric population [33–36], but whether or not this reflects progression of the underlying pathology from delirium is unclear [40]. A better understanding of the disease process is needed prior to determining whether these are distinct entities or a single coherent syndrome. This is vitally important to patients because there is evidence that older adults with limited life expectancy may value preservation of cognitive status over survival [41]. Neither baseline nor post–critical illness cognitive status is routinely measured in a rigorous manner [42]; therefore, it has been difficult to determine which strategies are effective in preserving long-term brain function after critical illness, especially in the high-risk elderly patients.

Epidemiology

Incidence

The incidence of delirium in elderly patients has been reported as high as 50 to 80 percent, with the highest incidence among critically ill patients on mechanical ventilation [5,33]. Data demonstrate that most delirium in the ICU goes undiagnosed without a regular screening tool [43], and it is universally acknowledged that the incidence of delirium is likely to be underreported, with up to 50 percent of cases being undiagnosed [44]. Hypoactive delirium in particular is easily and frequently overlooked by healthcare professionals due to a lack of awareness of the importance of its recognition and lack of education on how to perform a formal delirium assessment [45,46]. Current critical care guidelines therefore recommend routine delirium screening, which is particularly important in elderly patients given their increased risk [47].

Risk Factors

Delirium diagnosis identifies the constellation of acute brain dysfunction signs but does not identify the etiology. It should therefore prompt further investigation into potential risk factors for delirium. Delirium risk factors are numerous and can be stratified into predisposing and precipitating factors (Table 5.2). Diminished preoperative cognitive status is probably the biggest risk factor for delirium in the elderly population [48]. Age greater than 75 years and cerebrovascular disease have also been identified as risk factors for delirium specific to the elderly [48]. Frailty, which is common in the elderly and refers to critically reduced or impaired functional reserves that may involve multiple organ systems, has been shown to be independently associated with a greater risk of developing delirium [49–51].

Other risk factors for delirium include lower levels of education, major comorbid disease, major surgery, acute renal failure, vision or auditory disturbances, alcoholism, infection, and electrolyte disorders [5,52]. Use of physical restraints, use of urinary catheters, malnutrition, and acute pain have also been reported as risk factors [53]. High and low mean arterial pressures, as well as overall blood pressure fluctuations, have been associated with increased risk of delirium in elderly individuals, but the optimal blood pressure target has not been determined with regard to delirium [54–56]. While transfusion and blood loss can be associated with delirium, liberal versus restrictive packed red blood cell transfusion targets found no difference in either delirium rates or severity in patients undergoing hip surgery [57,58].

Table 5.2 Delirium Risk Factors

Predisposing risk factors	Precipitating risk factors
Cognitive impairment	Medications (benzos, opioids, anticholinergics, steroids)
Functional impairment	Use of a urinary catheter
Visual impairment	Use of physical restraints
Hearing impairment	Infection
Dementia	Major surgery (cardiac, thoracic, vascular, orthopedic, abdominal)
Advanced age	Metabolic derangements
Alcohol abuse	Trauma
History of stroke	Coma
History of delirium	Poor pain control
Comorbid diseases	Sleep disturbances
Severity of illness	Hypotension
Malnutrition	Mechanical ventilation

A handful of sedative medications has been associated with delirium development, including benzodiazepines and opioids. Longer-acting benzodiazepines and opioids with active metabolites are more likely to be associated with increased risk of delirium. This is likely related to drug accumulation due to the normal physiologic changes that occur with aging, such as renal and hepatic insufficiency [59]. Benzodiazepine infusions to provide sedation for mechanically ventilated patients are strong contributors to delirium compared with other sedative regimens [60–62]. Deep levels of sedation also carry a higher risk of delirium [60]. General anesthetics have been hypothesized to contribute to both post-operative cognitive dysfunction and dementia, but the evidence is inconsistent, and clear causal association has yet to be established [63–66]. Furthermore, most recent studies have not demonstrated a link between general anesthesia and cognitive impairment [34,67–70].

Other medications hypothesized to precipitate delirium through altered neurotransmission include those with anticholinergic, serotonergic, or dopaminergic properties (commonly used hospital medications include classic antihistamines, cyclobenzaprine, meperidine, famotidine, scopolamine, benztropine, oxybutynin, and tricyclic antidepressants). Treatment with corticosteroids has also been linked to delirium, although it has not been fully elucidated as to whether this is due to the severity of illness and ensuing increased neuroinflammatory response or the known psychological side effects of steroid use [71].

Pathophysiology

The pathophysiology of delirium and its associated long-term cognitive impairment is presumed to be multifactorial due to the complex interactions between the aging brain, baseline comorbid conditions, acute insult, and decreased cognitive reserve. In general, elderly individuals are thought to have less physiologic reserve than their younger counterparts and therefore have less ability to maintain homeostasis to stressors, making them more susceptible to an exaggerated response [72]. Neuroinflammation, endothelial dysfunction leading to cerebral perfusion abnormalities and increased permeability of the blood-brain barrier, cholinergic deficiency and neurotransmitter imbalances, cerebral atrophy and global brain disorders, and modifiable clinical risk factors such as certain pharmacologic therapies have all been shown to play a role in the development of delirium. The majority of current studies investigating the pathophysiology of delirium have focused on the hypothesis that systemic insults lead to inflammatory signaling and increased permeability of the blood-brain barrier, resulting in neuroinflammation and neuronal injury or death [73–76].

The inflammatory response, resulting from a systemic insult such as major illness or major surgical procedure, leads to the widespread release of cytokines and mediators. These cytokines, which are a physiologic response to illness or surgery, then cross into other organs that are not inflamed such as the brain. In the brain, they likely cause an abnormal response such as microglial activation, neuronal apoptosis, and altered synaptic plasticity and long-term potentiation [77]. High baseline levels of interleukin 6 (IL-6) and tumor necrosis factor alpha (TNF-α), high oxidative stress, mitochondrial dysfunction, high free-radical production, cellular senescence, and dysregulation of the hypothalamic-pituitary-adrenal axis and sympathetic nervous system result in a deviant stress responses that leads to dysregulation of neuronal activity [78,79].

Endothelial cells lining the cerebral microvessels form a selective barrier known as the blood-brain barrier [80]. Blood-brain barrier permeability increases as a result of normal aging [1]. Infectious and inflammatory processes and pain stimulate the production of IL-6 and cause endothelial dysfunction, further increasing blood-brain barrier permeability [3].

Elevated plasma biomarkers of endothelial dysfunction such as plasminogen activator inhibitor-1, E-selectin, and S100B (which is a marker of disruption of the blood-brain barrier) have been shown to be elevated in critical illness, and higher levels have been associated with prolonged duration of delirium [73].

A significant number of disturbances in neurotransmitter function have been described as potential contributors to delirium. Normal aging is associated with a decrease in the synthesis of major brain neurotransmitters such as acetylcholine, dopamine, serotonin, and glutamate [81]. Central cholinergic deficiency has also been hypothesized to play a major role in delirium [14]. This hypothesis originated in the early 1980s when it was noted that delirium occurred with consumption of toxins and drugs that impair cholinergic function [82]. This has been further supported by neuroimaging showing areas of brain where cholinergic projections overlap with lesions associated with acute brain dysfunction [77]. Additionally, use of anticholinergic drugs in the perioperative period has been associated with an increased incidence of delirium in elderly patients. Human trials of cholinesterase inhibitors, however, have not demonstrated a benefit in prevention or management of delirium [82,83]. Dopamine, serotonin, and norepinephrine are integral to arousal and sleep-wake cycles and are mediated by cholinergic pathways. Increased levels of dopamine and serotonin have been associated with hyperactive delirium. Additionally, elevated CNS IL-6 levels are associated with delirium development and with degeneration of gamma-aminobutyric acid (GABA)ergic interneurons [84,85]. GABA is an inhibitory neurotransmitter, and GABA agonists such as benzodiazepines have been associated with increased incidence of delirium, which supports the theory that GABAergic dysregulation is a contributing factor for delirium [86]. It is the imbalance of these neurotransmitters that is believed to play a role in delirium, although the exact mechanism has been elusive [82].

Neuroimaging has consistently shown anatomic changes that occur as part of normal aging. Elderly persons experience a prominent loss of volume and thickness in the prefrontal cortex [87,88]. This area plays a prominent role in attention and executive function and is consistent with previous psychological experiments showing decreases in performance on tests of attention and executive function with aging [89,90]. Presumably these neuroanatomic changes that occur with normal aging predispose elderly individuals to the physiologic alterations that result from a systemic insult; application of before and after delirium multimodal neuroimaging, however, should be employed to further characterize this relationship. To date, neuroimaging studies have shown delirium to be associated with brain atrophy and decreased white matter integrity. A study of critically ill patients has shown that increasing duration of delirium in the hospital is associated with increased brain atrophy several months after discharge, including reductions in hippocampal and superior frontal lobe volume [91]. Additionally, increasing duration of delirium in the hospital is associated with increased white matter disruption several months after discharge, in particular in the anterior limb of the internal capsule and genu of the corpus callosum [92].

Strategies for Prevention and Management

Nonpharmacologic Interventions

First and foremost, delirium education programs for healthcare professionals have been found to consistently reduce hospital delirium rates [93,94]. These programs have focused on recognition of delirium, screening for delirium, risk factors for delirium, and approaches for prevention and management [94]. Despite initial costs and time, these programs have been shown to be cost-effective [95]. Reorientation, sleep enhancement using a nonpharmacologic sleep protocol and sleep hygiene, early mobility, adaptations for visual and hearing impairment, nutrition and fluid repletion, pain management, and prevention of constipation have all been strongly recommended by the American Geriatric Society as interventions for the prevention of delirium [96]. Inouye et al.'s Hospital Elder Life Program is an innovative model of care for the prevention of functional and cognitive decline of elderly hospitalized individuals. It employs trained staff and volunteers to help with nonpharmacologic prevention techniques such as those listed earlier, including reorientation, cognitive stimulation multiple times each day, assistance with ambulation or range-of-motion activities, visual and hearing aids when needed, feeding assistance, and sleep protocols, and is a potentially cost-effective model to improve outcomes in elderly hospitalized patients [97] (Table 5.3).

A coordinated approach to systematically lightening sedation, liberation from mechanical ventilation, avoidance of benzodiazepine sedation, routine delirium monitoring, and early mobility have consistently been shown to reduce delirium rates in ICU patients. The Awakening and Breathing Coordination, Delirium Monitoring/Management, and Early Exercise/Mobility (ABCDE) bundle was originally published in 2011 [98] and has been shown repeatedly to decrease delirium rates, mechanical ventilation duration, and hospital length of stay [99,100]. Additionally, widespread adoption of this type of bundle has been shown to improve survival and increase the number of days alive without delirium or coma [101].

Table 5.3 Strategies for Delirium Prevention

Nonpharmacologic	Pharmacologic
Education targeted to healthcare professionals	Pain management using nonopioid adjuncts
Serial evaluation for identification of delirium	Avoidance of benzodiazepines, anticholinergics, dopaminergics, and serotonergics
Cognitive reorientation	Targeted depth of anesthesia
Mobility	Regional anesthesia
Visual and hearing aids	Use of antipsychotics or alpha-2 agonists for hyperactive delirium
Sleep hygiene	Analgesia and sedation with fentanyl as first-line sedation in mechanically ventilated patients
Nutrition and hydration	Continuance of ongoing statin therapy
Prevention of constipation	
Faster liberation from mechanical ventilation	
Geriatric consultation	
Multidisciplinary coordination of care	

"Prehabilitation" (rehabilitation-like activities prior to the acute stressor), combining nutritional, physical, and cognitive support, may be a helpful preventive measure for elderly patients with planned surgical interventions who are at risk for delirium [48]. Physical exercise has been shown in experimental studies in rats to be associated with reduced inflammation of the microglia [102], and several human studies have shown the benefit of early mobility in critically ill patients, with interventions ranging from range-of-motion exercises to ambulation, in decreasing delirium [103,104].

Pharmacologic Interventions

In general, pharmacologic measures should be considered only after nonpharmacologic strategies have failed. As expected, pharmacologic strategies for delirium management have been targeted based on hypotheses of delirium pathogenesis. Avoidance of opioids, benzo-diazepines, and anticholinergics is a mainstay of delirium management [105]. While adequate pain control is paramount to delirium prevention, opioid-sparing techniques using multimodal analgesia pain regimens and regional anesthesia techniques should be employed to achieve adequate pain control while minimizing opioid use. Of the opioid options, meperidine has been shown to have a higher risk of delirium. A systematic review of postoperative analgesia in elderly patients found meperidine use to consistently be associated with higher rates of delirium [106]. The increased risk of delirium with meper-idine use in the elderly is presumably related to its anticholinergic effects and the seroto-nergic effects of its metabolite normeperidine.

Benzodiazepines, due to their GABAergic effect, have been shown in multiple studies to contribute to delirium in the acute setting, including multiple critically ill and operative cohorts [107–110]. The use of benzodiazepines for sedation has also been shown in large randomized, controlled trials to increase the risk of delirium. A study by Pandharipande et al. compared sedation with dexmedetomidine with lorazepam infusion in mechanically ventilated patients and found that patients receiving dexmedetomidine had 4 more delir-ium-free days than the lorazepam group and 30 percent less coma [60]. Subsequently, the increased risk of delirium with benzodiazepine infusion in critically ill patients was demon-strated by Riker et al. in a randomized, controlled trial comparing dexmedetomidine with midazolam, with a 20 percent reduction in the number patients developing delirium with the administration of dexmedetomidine [62]. Avoidance of benzodiazepines is therefore prudent when feasible.

Dexmedetomidine has also been shown to reduce delirium incidence and duration, ICU length of stay, and cost when compared with propofol when used in postoperative cardiac surgery patients [111]. Dexmedetomidine is widely used as an adjunct to antipsychotics in the management of delirium; the cost-benefit ratio of dexmedetomidine, however, has been questioned. Recently, dexmedetomidine has been shown to be a beneficial and cost-effective rescue drug compared with haloperidol in nonintubated critically ill patients [112]. Addition of dexmedetomidine in patients with agitated delirium on the ventilator reduced mechanical ventilation hours at 7 days in a nonelderly population [113]. A few recent trials have shown low doses of dexmedetomidine to prevent delirium compared with either placebo or propofol in subsets of postoperative patients [111,114,115]. The mechanism of dexmedetomidine beyond avoidance of the GABA receptor is unclear. It has been shown to suppress the serum inflammatory mediators IL-6, IL-8, and TNF-α, but further investigations are warranted. Recently, however, it has been recommended by the European Society of Anaesthesiology as an intraoperative adjunct for prevention of delirium in high-risk elderly patients [116].

Despite antipsychotics being a mainstay for delirium management in clinical practice, their administration in elderly patients has been controversial. In previous studies, haloperidol had been shown to worsen outcomes in elderly patients with delirium, specifically mortality, whereas other studies have shown no difference when compared with quetiapine for the treatment of delirium [117]. A more recent meta-analysis of 17 randomized, controlled trials assessing the mortality of conventional antipsychotics, and haloperidol in particular, did not show an increase in mortality risk in elderly patients [118]. Haloperidol has been investigated recently as a pharmacologic delirium prevention method in the perioperative setting and in critically ill, mechanically ventilated patients. Perioperative haloperidol prophylaxis in elderly hip surgery patients did not decrease the incidence of delirium but was associated with a shorter duration of delirium [119]. A low-dose haloperidol bolus and subsequent infusion in elderly critical care patients who underwent non-cardiac surgery decreased the incidence of delirium only after intra-abdominal surgeries [120]. A pre-post study of patients deemed at high risk for delirium found haloperidol prophylaxis to be associated with increased days alive and free of delirium and coma [121]. A randomized, double-blind, placebo-controlled trial conducted in medical and surgical ICUs, however, found that haloperidol reduced the hours patients spent with agitation but did not show a reduction in delirium incidence, delirium duration, days on mechanical ventilation, or ICU mortality [122].

With regard to delirium treatment, data on the efficacy of antipsychotic administration are also limited. In a study of critically ill patients at risk for delirium, placebo versus haloperidol versus ziprasidone for delirium treatment demonstrated no difference between the three groups in days alive and freedom from delirium [123]. A study of haloperidol versus olanzapine for delirium in the ICU found no difference in delirium duration, but patients who received haloperidol had more side effects [124]. Quetiapine in addition to haloperidol resulted in a faster resolution of delirium compared with placebo in addition to haloperidol [125].

Although cholinergic depletion is known to play a role in delirium development, acetylcholinesterase inhibitors such as rivastigmine and donezepil, which have been a mainstay in the treatment of Alzheimer's disease, have all had disappointing results in the prevention of delirium. They have not been established as an effective therapy in delirium management and actually may increase mortality [126–129].

Given the role of neuroinflammation in the pathogenesis of delirium, strategies targeting reduction of the inflammatory cascade seem prudent, but there are currently no studies showing this to be an effective measure. Prophylactic administration of dexamethasone to decrease systemic inflammatory response and neuroinflammation in patients undergoing cardiopulmonary bypass had no effect on either the incidence or the duration of delirium [130]. The pleiotropic anti-inflammatory effects of statin therapy have been hypothesized to play a role in the management of delirium. Continuation of ongoing statin therapy in critically ill patients has been associated with a decreased risk of delirium, whereas withholding statins in chronic users may increase the odds of developing delirium [131–133].

With regard to the role of anesthesia in the development of POD, studies monitoring the electroencephalogram (EEG) during general anesthesia have shown that current recommended doses of anesthetics for elderly patients may be placing them in a profound state of brain inactivation known as *burst suppression* [134,135]. Titration of anesthetic doses based on real-time EEG monitoring may help to reduce the incidence of postoperative cognitive disorders [134] and has been associated with reduced POD likely from reduced oversedation [136]. Monitoring of anesthetic depth and avoidance of deep anesthesia in the elderly are considered part of delirium prevention strategies [96].

Applications of Clinical Guidelines to Elderly Patients (>80 Years Old)

Increasing age is a known risk factor for delirium and cognitive impairment after acute illness or surgery. Investigations targeting this population are warranted, but unfortunately, at this time, no additional data exist regarding the application of clinical guidelines for the management of delirium in very elderly patients. Overall, the evidence does not support a single effective prevention or treatment approach in these patients. Although not targeted specifically for patients older than 80 years of age, the Society of Critical Care Medicine's ICU Liberation Collaborative with the ABCDEF bundle involving Assessment and management of pain, Both spontaneous awake trials (SATs) and spontaneous breathing trials (SBTs), Choosing sedation if required, Delirium monitoring and management, Early mobility, and Family involvement incorporates many aspects required to reduce delirium and improve patient outcomes related to delirium in the elderly [137]. Similarly, the American Geriatric Society has recommendations for the prevention of delirium in the elderly in the perioperative setting, including multicomponent nonpharmacologic intervention programs, optimization of pain control, avoidance of benzodiazepines and newly prescribed cholinesterase inhibitors, and use of antipsychotic medications only in patients who are agitated or of potential harm to self or others [96].

References

1. Farrall AJ, Wardlaw JM. Blood-brain barrier: ageing and microvascular disease–systematic review and meta-analysis. *Neurobiol Aging* 2009; **30**(3): 337–52.

2. Alvis BD, Hughes CG. Physiology considerations in geriatric patients. *Anesthesiol Clin* 2015; **33**(3): 447–56.

3. Abbott NJ, Ronnback L, Hansson E. Astrocyte-endothelial interactions at the blood-brain barrier. *Nat Rev Neurosci* 2006; **7**(1):41–53.

4. Sharshar T, Hopkinson NS, Orlikowski D, Annane D. Science review: the brain in sepsis – culprit and victim. *Crit Care* 2005; **9** (1):37–44.

5. Inouye SK, Westendorp RG, Saczynski JS. Delirium in elderly people. *Lancet* 2014; **383** (9920):911–22.

6. American Psychiatric Association. *Diagnostic and Statistical Manual of Mental Disorders* (5th edn). Washington, DC: APA, 2013.

7. Morandi A, Davis D, Bellelli G, et al. The diagnosis of delirium superimposed on dementia: an emerging challenge. *J Am Med Dir Assoc* 2017; **18**(1):12–18.

8. Ely EW, Inouye SK, Bernard GR, et al. Delirium in mechanically ventilated patients: validity and reliability of the Confusion Assessment Method for the Intensive Care Unit (CAM-ICU). *JAMA* 2001; **286**(21):2703–10.

9. Bergeron N, Dubois MJ, Dumont M, Dial S, Skrobik Y. Intensive care delirium screening checklist: evaluation of a new screening tool. *Intensive Care Med* 2001; **27** (5):859–64.

10. Sessler CN, Gosnell MS, Grap MJ, et al. The Richmond Agitation-Sedation Scale: validity and reliability in adult intensive

care unit patients. *Am J Respir Crit Care Med* 2002; **166**(10):1338–44.

11. Morandi A, Han JH, Meagher D, et al. Detecting delirium superimposed on dementia: evaluation of the diagnostic performance of the Richmond Agitation and Sedation Scale. *J Am Med Dir Assoc.* 2016; **17**(9):828–33.

12. Morandi A, McCurley J, Vasilevskis EE, et al. Tools to detect delirium superimposed on dementia: a systematic review. *J Am Geriatr Soc* 2012; **60**(11): 2005–13.

13. Mitasova A, Kostalova M, Bednarik J, et al. Poststroke delirium incidence and outcomes: validation of the Confusion Assessment Method for the Intensive Care Unit (CAM-ICU). *Crit Care Med* 2012; **40** (2):484–90.

14. American Geriatrics Society Expert Panel on Postoperative Delirium in Older Adults. American Geriatrics Society abstracted clinical practice guideline for postoperative delirium in older adults. *J Am Geriatr Soc* 2015; **63**(1):142–50.

15. Peterson JF, Pun BT, Dittus RS, et al. Delirium and its motoric subtypes: a study of 614 critically ill patients. *J Am Geriatr Soc* 2006; **54**(3):479–84.

16. Trzepacz PT, Mittal D, Torres R, et al. Validation of the Delirium Rating Scale–Revised-98: comparison with the delirium rating scale and the cognitive test for delirium. *J Neuropsychiatr Clin Neurosci* 2001; **13**(2):229–42.

17. Inouye SK, Kosar CM, Tommet D, et al. The CAM-S: development and validation of a new scoring system for delirium severity in 2 cohorts. *Ann Intern Med* 2014; **160**(8):526–33.

18. Abildstrom H, Rasmussen LS, Rentowl P, et al. Cognitive dysfunction 1–2 years after non-cardiac surgery in the elderly. ISPOCD group. International Study of Post-Operative Cognitive Dysfunction. *Acta Anaesthesiol Scand* 2000; **44**(10): 1246–51.

19. Bruce KM, Yelland GW, Smith JA, Robinson SR. Recovery of cognitive function after coronary artery bypass graft

operations. *Ann Thorac Surg* 2013; **95**(4): 1306–13.

20. Cormack F, Shipolini A, Awad WI, et al. A meta-analysis of cognitive outcome following coronary artery bypass graft surgery. *Neurosci Biobehav Rev* 2012; **36**(9): 2118–29.

21. Selnes OA, Gottesman RF, Grega MA, et al. Cognitive and neurologic outcomes after coronary-artery bypass surgery. *N Engl J Med* 2012; **366**(3):250–57.

22. Selnes OA, Grega MA, Bailey MM, et al. Neurocognitive outcomes 3 years after coronary artery bypass graft surgery: a controlled study. *Ann Thorac Surg* 2007; **84**(6):1885–96.

23. Salluh JI, Wang H, Schneider EB, et al. Outcome of delirium in critically ill patients: systematic review and meta-analysis. *BMJ* 2015; **350**:h2538.

24. Witlox J, Eurelings LS, de Jonghe JF, et al. Delirium in elderly patients and the risk of postdischarge mortality, institutionalization, and dementia: a meta-analysis. *JAMA* 2010; **304**(4):443–51.

25. Milbrandt EB, Deppen S, Harrison PL, et al. Costs associated with delirium in mechanically ventilated patients. *Crit Care Med* 2004; **32**(4):955–62.

26. Franco K, Litaker D, Locala J, Bronson D. The cost of delirium in the surgical patient. *Psychosomatics* 2001; **42**(1):68–73.

27. Klein Klouwenberg PM, Zaal IJ, Spitoni C, et al. The attributable mortality of delirium in critically ill patients: prospective cohort study. *BMJ* 2014; **349**:g6652.

28. Patel SB, Poston JT, Pohlman A, Hall JB, Kress JP. Rapidly reversible, sedation-related delirium versus persistent delirium in the intensive care unit. *Am J Respir Crit Care Med* 2014; **189**(6): 658–65.

29. Neufeld KJ, Leoutsakos JM, Sieber FE, et al. Outcomes of early delirium diagnosis after general anesthesia in the elderly. *Anesth Analg* 2013; **117**(2):471–78.

30. Lat I, McMillian W, Taylor S, et al. The impact of delirium on clinical outcomes in mechanically ventilated

surgical and trauma patients. *Crit Care Med* 2009; 37(6):1898–905.

31. Ruggiero C, Bonamassa L, Pelini L, et al. Early post-surgical cognitive dysfunction is a risk factor for mortality among hip fracture hospitalized older persons. *Osteoporos Int* 2017; 28(2):667–75.

32. Robinson TN, Raeburn CD, Tran ZV, Brenner LA, Moss M. Motor subtypes of postoperative delirium in older adults. *Arch Surg* 2011; 146(3):295–300.

33. Pandharipande PP, Girard TD, Jackson JC, et al. Long-term cognitive impairment after critical illness. *N Engl J Med* 2013; 369(14): 1306–16.

34. Hughes CG, Patel MB, Jackson JC, et al. Surgery and anesthesia exposure is not a risk factor for cognitive impairment after major noncardiac surgery and critical illness. *Ann Surg* 2016.

35. Saczynski JS, Marcantonio ER, Quach L, et al. Cognitive trajectories after postoperative delirium. *N Engl J Med* 2012; 367(1):30–39.

36. Inouye SK, Marcantonio ER, Kosar CM, et al. The short-term and long-term relationship between delirium and cognitive trajectory in older surgical patients. *Alzheimers Dement* 2016; 12(7): 766–75.

37. Fong TG, Jones RN, Marcantonio ER, et al. Adverse outcomes after hospitalization and delirium in persons with Alzheimer disease. *Ann Intern Med* 2012; 156(12): 848–56.

38. Fong TG, Jones RN, Shi P, et al. Delirium accelerates cognitive decline in Alzheimer disease. *Neurology* 2009; 72(18): 1570–75.

39. Davis DH, Muniz-Terrera G, Keage HA, et al. Association of delirium with cognitive decline in late life: a neuropathologic study of 3 population-based cohort studies. *JAMA Psychiatry* 2017; 74(3): 244–51.

40. MacLullich AM, Beaglehole A, Hall RJ, Meagher DJ. Delirium and long-term cognitive impairment. *Int Rev Psychiatry* 2009; 21(1):30–42.

41. Fried TR, Bradley EH, Towle VR, Allore H. Understanding the treatment preferences of seriously ill patients. *N Engl J Med* 2002; 346(14):1061–66.

42. Crosby G, Culley DJ, Hyman BT. Preoperative cognitive assessment of the elderly surgical patient: a call for action. *J Am Soc Anesthesiol* 2011; 114(6):1265–68.

43. van Eijk MM, van Marum RJ, Klijn IA, et al. Comparison of delirium assessment tools in a mixed intensive care unit. *Crit Care Med* 2009; 37(6):1881–85.

44. Spronk PE, Riekerk B, Hofhuis J, Rommes JH. Occurrence of delirium is severely underestimated in the ICU during daily care. *Intensive Care Med* 2009; 35(7): 1276–80.

45. Inouye SK, van Dyck CH, Alessi CA, et al. Clarifying confusion: the confusion assessment method – a new method for detection of delirium. *Ann Intern Med* 1990; 113(12):941–48.

46. Panitchote A, Tangvoraphonkchai K, Suebsoh N, et al. Under-recognition of delirium in older adults by nurses in the intensive care unit setting. *Aging Clin Exp Res* 2015; 27(5):735–40.

47. Barr J, Fraser G, Puntillo K, et al. American College of Critical Care Medicine clinical practice guidelines for the management of pain, agitation, and delirium in adult patients in the intensive care unit. *Crit Care Med* 2013; 41(1):263–306.

48. Benhamou D, Brouquet A. Postoperative cerebral dysfunction in the elderly: diagnosis and prophylaxis. *J Visc Surg* 2016; 153(Suppl 6):S27–32.

49. Kim S-w, Han H-S, Jung H-w, et al. Multidimensional frailty score for the prediction of postoperative mortality risk. *JAMA Surgery* 2014; 149(7): 633–40.

50. Leung JM, Tsai TL, Sands LP. Preoperative frailty in older surgical patients is associated with early postoperative delirium. *Anesth Analg* 2011; 112(5):1199.

51. Kelly AM, Batke JN, Dea N, et al. Prospective analysis of adverse events in surgical treatment of degenerative

spondylolisthesis. *Spine J* 2014; **14**(12): 2905–10.

52. Nadelson MR, Sanders RD, Avidan MS. Perioperative cognitive trajectory in adults. *Br J Anaesth* 2014; **112**(3):440–51.

53. Deiner S, Silverstein J. Postoperative delirium and cognitive dysfunction. *Br J Anaesth* 2009; **103**(Suppl 1):i41–46.

54. Wang NY, Hirao A, Sieber F. Association between intraoperative blood pressure and postoperative delirium in elderly hip fracture patients. *PLoS One* 2015; **10**(4): e0123892.

55. Bijker JB, van Klei WA, Kappen TH, et al. Incidence of intraoperative hypotension as a function of the chosen definition: literature definitions applied to a retrospective cohort using automated data collection. *Anesthesiology* 2007; **107** (2):213–20.

56. Hori D, Brown C, Ono M, et al. Arterial pressure above the upper cerebral autoregulation limit during cardiopulmonary bypass is associated with postoperative delirium. *Br J Anaesth* 2014; **113**(6):1009–17.

57. Carson JL, Terrin ML, Noveck H, et al. Liberal or restrictive transfusion in high-risk patients after hip surgery. *N Engl J Med* 2011; **365**(26):2453–62.

58. Gruber-Baldini AL, Marcantonio E, Orwig D, et al. Delirium outcomes in a randomized trial of blood transfusion thresholds in hospitalized older adults with hip fracture. *J Am Geriatr Soc* 2013; **61**(8): 1286–95.

59. Vasilevskis EE, Han JH, Hughes CG, Ely EW. Epidemiology and risk factors for delirium across hospital settings. *Best Pract Res Clin Anaesthesiol* 2012; **26**(3): 277–87.

60. Pandharipande PP, Pun BT, Herr DL, et al. Effect of sedation with dexmedetomidine vs lorazepam on acute brain dysfunction in mechanically ventilated patients: the MENDS randomized controlled trial. *JAMA* 2007; **298**(22):2644–53.

61. Kamdar BB, Niessen T, Colantuoni E, et al. Delirium transitions in the medical ICU:

exploring the role of sleep quality and other factors. *Crit Care Med* 2015; **43**(1):135.

62. Riker RR, Shehabi Y, Bokesch PM, et al. Dexmedetomidine vs midazolam for sedation of critically ill patients: a randomized trial. *JAMA* 2009; **301**(5): 489–99.

63. Sprung J, Jankowski CJ, Roberts RO, et al. Anesthesia and incident dementia: a population-based, nested, case-control study. *Mayo Clinic Proc* 2013; **88**(6): 552–61.

64. Chen C-W, Lin C-C, Chen K-B, et al. Increased risk of dementia in people with previous exposure to general anesthesia: a nationwide population-based case-control study. *Alzheimers Dement* 2014; **10**(2):196–204.

65. Hussain M, Berger M, Eckenhoff RG, Seitz DP. General anesthetic and the risk of dementia in elderly patients: current insights. *Clin Interv Aging* 2014; **9**:1619–28.

66. Liu Y, Pan N, Ma Y, et al. Inhaled sevoflurane may promote progression of amnestic mild cognitive impairment: a prospective, randomized parallel-group study. *Am J Med Sci* 2013; **345**(5):355–60.

67. Aiello Bowles EJ, Larson EB, Pong RP, et al. Anesthesia exposure and risk of dementia and Alzheimer's disease: a prospective study. *J Am Geriatr Soc* 2016; **64**(3):602–7.

68. Avidan MS, Searleman AC, Storandt M, et al. Long-term cognitive decline in older subjects was not attributable to noncardiac surgery or major illness. *Anesthesiology* 2009; **111**(5):964–70.

69. Dokkedal U, Hansen TG, Rasmussen LS, Mengel-From J, Christensen CK. Cognitive functioning after surgery in middle-aged and elderly Danish twins. *Anesthesiology* 2016; **124**(2):312–321.

70. Sprung J, Roberts RO, Knopman DS, et al. Mild cognitive impairment and exposure to general anesthesia for surgeries and procedures: a population-based case-control study. *Anesth Analg* 2017; **124** (4):1277–90.

71. Schreiber MP, Colantuoni E, Bienvenu OJ, et al. Corticosteroids and transition to

delirium in patients with acute lung injury. *Crit Care Med* 2014; **42**(6):1480.

72. Cunningham C, MacLullich AM. At the extreme end of the psychoneuroimmunological spectrum: delirium as a maladaptive sickness behaviour response. *Brain Behav Immun* 2013; **28**:1–13.

73. Hughes CG, Pandharipande PP, Thompson JL, et al. Endothelial activation and blood-brain barrier injury as risk factors for delirium in critically ill patients. *Crit Care Med* 2016; **44**(9):e809–17.

74. Cunningham C, Wilcockson DC, Campion S, Lunnon K, Perry VH. Central and systemic endotoxin challenges exacerbate the local inflammatory response and increase neuronal death during chronic neurodegeneration. *J Neurosci* 2005; **25**(40):9275–84.

75. Terrando N, Eriksson LI, Kyu Ryu J, et al. Resolving postoperative neuroinflammation and cognitive decline. *Ann Neurol* 2011; **70**(6):986–95.

76. Cerejeira J, Firmino H, Vaz-Serra A, Mukaetova-Ladinska EB. The neuroinflammatory hypothesis of delirium. *Acta Neuropathol* 2010; **119**(6): 737–54.

77. Hughes CG, Patel MB, Pandharipande PP. Pathophysiology of acute brain dysfunction: what's the cause of all this confusion? *Curr Opin Crit Care* 2012; **18** (5):518–26.

78. Walston J, Hadley EC, Ferrucci L, et al. Research agenda for frailty in older adults: toward a better understanding of physiology and etiology – summary from the American Geriatrics Society/National Institute on Aging Research Conference on Frailty in Older Adults. *J Am Geriatr Soc* 2006; **54**(6):991–1001.

79. Maldonado JR. Neuropathogenesis of delirium: review of current etiologic theories and common pathways. *Am J Geriatr Psychiatry* 2013; **21**(12):1190–222.

80. Abbott NJ. Astrocyte-endothelial interactions and blood-brain barrier permeability. *J Anat* 2002; **200**(5): 523–34.

81. Peters R. Ageing and the brain. *Postgrad Med J* 2006; **82**(964):84–88.

82. Hshieh TT, Fong TG, Marcantonio ER, Inouye SK. Cholinergic deficiency hypothesis in delirium: a synthesis of current evidence. *J Gerontol A: Biol Sci Med Sci* 2008; **63**(7):764–72.

83. Marcantonio ER. Postoperative delirium: a 76-year-old woman with delirium following surgery. *JAMA* 2012; **308** (1):73–81.

84. Westhoff D, Witlox J, Koenderman L, et al. Preoperative cerebrospinal fluid cytokine levels and the risk of postoperative delirium in elderly hip fracture patients. *J Neuroinflam* 2013; **10**(1):122.

85. Dugan LL, Ali SS, Shekhtman G, et al. IL-6 mediated degeneration of forebrain GABAergic interneurons and cognitive impairment in aged mice through activation of neuronal NADPH oxidase. *PLoS One* 2009; **4**(5):e5518.

86. Pandharipande PP, Ely E, Maze M. Dexmedetomidine for sedation and perioperative management of critically ill patients. *Semin Anesth Perioperat Med Pain* 2006.

87. Fjell AM, Westlye LT, Amlien I, et al. High consistency of regional cortical thinning in aging across multiple samples. *Cereb Cortex* 2009:bhn232.

88. Fjell AM, Westlye LT, Grydeland H, et al. Accelerating cortical thinning: unique to dementia or universal in aging? *Cereb Cortex* 2012:bhs379.

89. Kemps E, Newson R. Comparison of adult age differences in verbal and visuo-spatial memory: the importance of 'pure', parallel and validated measures. *J Clin Exp Neuropsychol* 2006; **28**(3):341–56.

90. West R, Schwarb H. The influence of aging and frontal function on the neural correlates of regulative and evaluative aspects of cognitive control. *Neuropsychology* 2006; **20**(4):468.

91. Gunther ML, Morandi A, Krauskopf E, et al. The association between brain volumes, delirium duration, and cognitive outcomes in intensive care unit survivors:

the VISIONS cohort magnetic resonance imaging study. *Crit Care Med* 2012; **40**(7): 2022–32.

92. Morandi A, Rogers BP, Gunther ML, et al. The relationship between delirium duration, white matter integrity, and cognitive impairment in intensive care unit survivors as determined by diffusion tensor imaging: the VISIONS prospective cohort magnetic resonance imaging study. *Crit Care Med* 2012; **40**(7): 2182–89.

93. Lundström M, Edlund A, Karlsson S, et al. A multifactorial intervention program reduces the duration of delirium, length of hospitalization, and mortality in delirious patients. *J Am Geriatr Soc* 2005; **53**(4): 622–28.

94. Robinson S, Rich C, Weitzel T, Vollmer C, Eden B. Delirium prevention for cognitive, sensory, and mobility impairments. *Res Theory Nurs Pract* 2008; **22**(2):103–13.

95. Rubin FH, Neal K, Fenlon K, Hassan S, Inouye SK. Sustainability and scalability of the hospital elder life program at a community hospital. *J Am Geriatr Soc* 2011; **59**(2):359–65.

96. American Geriatrics Society Expert Panel on Postoperative Delirium in Older Adults. Postoperative delirium in older adults: best practice statement from the American Geriatrics Society. *J Am Coll Surg* 2015; **220**(2):136–48.

97. Inouye SK, Bogardus ST Jr, Baker DI, Leo-Summers L, Cooney LM Jr. The Hospital Elder Life Program: a model of care to prevent cognitive and functional decline in older hospitalized patients. *J Am Geriatr Soc* 2000; **48**(12):1697–706.

98. Morandi A, Brummel NE, Ely EW. Sedation, delirium and mechanical ventilation: the "ABCDE" approach. *Curr Opin Crit Care* 2011; **17**(1):43–49.

99. Balas MC, Vasilevskis EE, Olsen KM, et al. Effectiveness and safety of the awakening and breathing coordination, delirium monitoring/management, and early exercise/mobility (ABCDE) bundle. *Crit Care Med* 2014; **42**(5):1024.

100. Dale CR, Kannas DA, Fan VS, et al. Improved analgesia, sedation, and delirium protocol associated with decreased duration of delirium and mechanical ventilation. *Ann Am Thorac Soc* 2014; **11**(3):367–74.

101. Barnes-Daly MA, Phillips G, Ely EW. Improving hospital survival and reducing brain dysfunction at seven California community hospitals: implementing PAD guidelines via the ABCDEF bundle in 6,064 patients. *Crit Care Med* 2017; **45**(2): 171–78.

102. Kohman RA, Bhattacharya TK, Wojcik E, Rhodes JS. Exercise reduces activation of microglia isolated from hippocampus and brain of aged mice. *J Neuroinflam* 2013; **10** (1):114.

103. Schaller SJ, Anstey M, Blobner M, et al. Early, goal-directed mobilisation in the surgical intensive care unit: a randomised controlled trial. *Lancet* 2016; **388**(10052): 1377–88.

104. Schweickert WD, Pohlman MC, Pohlman AS, et al. Early physical and occupational therapy in mechanically ventilated, critically ill patients: a randomised controlled trial. *Lancet* 2009; **373**(9678):1874–82.

105. American Geriatrics Society Beers Criteria Update Expert Panel. American Geriatrics Society updated Beers criteria for potentially inappropriate medication use in older adults. *J Am Geriatr Soc* 2012; **60**(4):616–31.

106. Fong HK, Sands LP, Leung JM. The role of postoperative analgesia in delirium and cognitive decline in elderly patients: a systematic review. *Anesth Analg* 2006; **102**(4):1255–66.

107. Lepouse C, Lautner CA, Liu L, Gomis P, Leon A. Emergence delirium in adults in the post-anaesthesia care unit. *Br J Anaesth* 2006; **96**(6):747–53.

108. McPherson JA, Wagner CE, Boehm LM, et al. Delirium in the cardiovascular ICU: exploring modifiable risk factors. *Crit Care Med* 2013; **41**(2):405–13.

109. Pandharipande PP, Shintani A, Peterson J, et al. Lorazepam is an independent risk

factor for transitioning to delirium in intensive care unit patients. *Anesthesiology* 2006; **104**(1):21–26.

110. Pandharipande PP, Cotton BA, Shintani A, et al. Prevalence and risk factors for development of delirium in surgical and trauma intensive care unit patients. *J Trauma* 2008; **65**(1):34–41.

111. Djaiani G, Silverton N, Fedorko L, et al. Dexmedetomidine versus propofol sedation reduces delirium after cardiac surgery: a randomized controlled trial. *Anesthesiology* 2016; **124**(2):362–68.

112. Carrasco G, Baeza N, Cabre L, et al. Dexmedetomidine for the treatment of hyperactive delirium refractory to haloperidol in nonintubated ICU patients: a nonrandomized controlled trial. *Crit Care Med* 2016; **44**(7):1295–306.

113. Reade MC, Eastwood GM, Bellomo R, et al. Effect of dexmedetomidine added to standard care on ventilator-free time in patients with agitated delirium: a randomized clinical trial. *JAMA* 2016; **315**(14):1460–68.

114. Su X, Meng ZT, Wu XH, et al. Dexmedetomidine for prevention of delirium in elderly patients after non-cardiac surgery: a randomised, double-blind, placebo-controlled trial. *Lancet* 2016.

115. Karren EA, King AB, Hughes CG. Dexmedetomidine for prevention of delirium in elderly patients after non-cardiac surgery. *J Thorac Dis* 2016; **8**(12):E1759–62.

116. Aldecoa C, Bettelli G, Bilotta F, et al. European Society of Anaesthesiology evidence-based and consensus-based guideline on postoperative delirium. *Eur J Anaesthesiol* 2017; **34**(4):192–214.

117. Grover S, Mahajan S, Chakrabarti S, Avasthi A. Comparative effectiveness of quetiapine and haloperidol in delirium: a single blind randomized controlled study. *World J Psychiatry* 2016; **6**(3):365–71.

118. Hulshof TA, Zuidema SU, Ostelo RW, Luijendijk HJ. The mortality risk of conventional antipsychotics in elderly patients: a systematic review and meta-analysis of randomized placebo-controlled trials. *J Am Med Dir Assoc* 2015; **16**(10):817–24.

119. Kalisvaart KJ, de Jonghe JF, Bogaards MJ, et al. Haloperidol prophylaxis for elderly hip-surgery patients at risk for delirium: a randomized placebo-controlled study. *J Am Geriatr Soc* 2005; **53**(10):1658–66.

120. Wang W, Li HL, Wang DX, et al. Haloperidol prophylaxis decreases delirium incidence in elderly patients after noncardiac surgery: a randomized controlled trial*. *Crit Care Med* 2012; **40**(3):731–39.

121. van den Boogaard M, Schoonhoven L, van Achterberg T, van der Hoeven JG, Pickkers P. Haloperidol prophylaxis in critically ill patients with a high risk for delirium. *Crit Care* 2013; **17**(1):R9.

122. Al-Qadheeb NS, Skrobik Y, Schumaker G, et al. Preventing ICU subsyndromal delirium conversion to delirium with low-dose IV haloperidol: a double-blind, placebo-controlled pilot study. *Crit Care Med* 2016; **44**(3):583–91.

123. Girard TD, Pandharipande PP, Carson SS, et al. Feasibility, efficacy, and safety of antipsychotics for intensive care unit delirium: the MIND randomized, placebo-controlled trial. *Crit Care Med* 2010; **38**(2):428–37.

124. Skrobik YK, Bergeron N, Dumont M, Gottfried SB. Olanzapine vs haloperidol: treating delirium in a critical care setting. *Intensive Care Med* 2004; **30**(3):444–49.

125. Devlin JW, Roberts RJ, Fong JJ, et al. Efficacy and safety of quetiapine in critically ill patients with delirium: a prospective, multicenter, randomized, double-blind, placebo-controlled pilot study. *Crit Care Med* 2010; **38**(2):419–27.

126. van Eijk MM, Roes KC, Honing ML, et al. Effect of rivastigmine as an adjunct to usual care with haloperidol on duration of delirium and mortality in critically ill patients: a multicentre, double-blind, placebo-controlled randomised trial. *Lancet* 2010; **376**(9755):1829–37.

127. Gamberini M, Bolliger D, Lurati Buse GA, et al. Rivastigmine for the prevention of postoperative delirium in elderly patients undergoing elective cardiac surgery: a randomized controlled trial. *Crit Care Med* 2009; 37(5):1762–68.

128. Liptzin B, Laki A, Garb JL, Fingeroth R, Krushell R. Donepezil in the prevention and treatment of post-surgical delirium. *Am J Geriatr Psychiatry* 2005; 13(12): 1100–6.

129. Marcantonio ER, Palihnich K, Appleton P, Davis RB. Pilot randomized trial of donepezil hydrochloride for delirium after hip fracture. *J Am Geriatr Soc* 2011; 59(Supple 2):S282–88.

130. Sauër A-MC, Slooter AJ, Veldhuijzen DS, et al. Intraoperative dexamethasone and delirium after cardiac surgery: a randomized clinical trial. *Anesth Analg* 2014; 119(5):1046–52.

131. Morandi A, Hughes CG, Girard TD, et al. Statins and brain dysfunction: a hypothesis to reduce the burden of cognitive impairment in patients who are critically ill. *CHEST Journal* 2011; 140(3):580–85.

132. Page VJ, Davis D, Zhao XB, et al. Statin use and risk of delirium in the critically ill. *Am J Respir Crit Care Med* 2014; 189(6): 666–73.

133. Morandi A, Hughes CG, Thompson JL, et al. Statins and delirium during critical illness: a multicenter, prospective cohort study. *Crit Care Med* 2014; 42(8):1899.

134. Chan MT, Cheng BC, Lee TM, Gin T, Group CT. BIS-guided anesthesia decreases postoperative delirium and cognitive decline. *J Neurosurg Anesthesiol* 2013; 25(1):33–42.

135. Purdon PL, Pierce ET, Mukamel EA, et al. Electroencephalogram signatures of loss and recovery of consciousness from propofol. *Proc Natl Acad Sci* 2013; 110 (12):E1142–51.

136. Radtke FM, Franck M, Lendner J, et al. Monitoring depth of anaesthesia in a randomized trial decreases the rate of postoperative delirium but not postoperative cognitive dysfunction. *Br J Anaesth* 2013; 110(Suppl 1):i98–105.

137. www.iculiberation.org.

Chapter

6 Geriatric Cardiovascular Critical Care

Ronald Pauldine

Key Points

- Aging is associated with an increased incidence of cardiovascular diseases, including ischemic heart disease, heart failure, atrial fibrillation, hypertension, valvular heart disease, pulmonary hypertension, and peripheral vascular disease.
- Progressive central aortic dilatation, increased thickness of the arterial wall, increased vascular stiffness, and altered nitric oxide–induced vasodilation occur with advancing age, leading to elevated mean arterial pressure and increased pulse pressure.
- Elderly patients are more likely to present with non-ST-segment-elevation myocardial infarction (NSTEMI) as opposed to ST-segment-elevation myocardial infarction (STEMI), and frequently present with nonspecific complaints including weakness, syncope, and increasing confusion.
- Overall 30-day mortality after coronary artery bypass grafting (CABG) in octogenarians is 6.8 versus 1.6 percent in the younger group.
- The elderly comprise the majority of patients with heart failure with preserved ejection fraction (HFpEF).
- The prevalence of moderate to severe aortic stenosis is estimated to be as high as 2.8 percent in patients older than 75 years of age, and complications associated with transcatheter aortic valve implantation (TAVI) appear to be greater in older patients.
- Age is the most important risk factor for the development of atrial fibrillation (AF). New-onset postoperative AF (POAF) is a common problem reported in 15 to 40 percent of patients following CABG, 40 percent following surgical valve replacement, 50 to 60 percent following combined CAGB-valve procedures, 20 to 25 percent of patients after esophagectomy, and 20 percent of patients following lung transplant.
- Meaningful outcome metrics in elderly patients who are admitted to the intensive care unit (ICU) and identifying those most likely to benefit from admission to the ICU still need to be delineated.

General Considerations

Practitioners of adult critical care medicine frequently encounter geriatric patients and by default are practitioners of geriatric critical care medicine. This may be even truer in the realm of cardiovascular medicine and cardiothoracic critical care. Aging is associated with an increased incidence of cardiovascular diseases, including ischemic heart disease, heart failure, atrial fibrillation, hypertension, valvular heart disease, pulmonary hypertension, and peripheral vascular disease [1] (Figure 6.1). Significant technological advances have resulted in an increasing array of minimally invasive interventions that can now be used in patients who may have insufficient physiologic reserve to tolerate more extensive procedures. This in particular includes the elderly. Minimally invasive valve replacement, valve repair, implantable electrical devices, and an expanding armamentarium of endovascular approaches to aortic disease are just a few examples. These technological realities, in combination with the significant rise in the elderly populations, place a large responsibility on all practitioners delivering cardiovascular critical care to meet the needs of this highly variable, dynamic, and often challenging patient population.

One may question what constitutes a working definition of geriatric cardiovascular critical care. In the simplest form, it is patient- and family-centered care that meets the needs of older adults. It includes a thorough and thoughtful consideration of age,

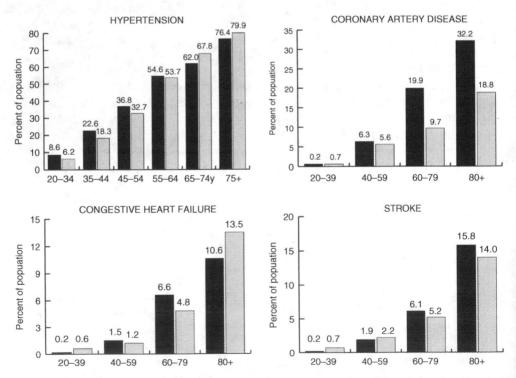

Figure 6.1 Prevalence of hypertension, coronary artery disease, congestive heart failure, and stroke with aging. (*Source:* Data from Mozaffarian et al. [1].)

comorbidities, and the available evidence to manage critical illness. Age alone should not be the deciding factor in determining therapeutic approach. Chronologic age and physiologic reserve can be incongruent. In many cases the presence of geriatric syndromes including frailty or dementia may influence outcome but do not necessarily correlate with patient age. Implicit in these considerations is a need to define the goals of care or intervention, including the expected outcome, patient values, and an understanding that aging is associated with an increase in the frequency and severity of iatrogenic complications and risk of harm from any treatment. Goals of care may differ widely depending on patient values and may change within a given period of care. Historically, outcome metrics have been largely preoccupied with mortality statistics, but an increasing emphasis is now been given to functional outcomes. In general, the therapeutic goal of most elderly patients should be to improve or maintain functional independence or alleviate pain. The complexity of medical decision making is increased by the potential effect of comorbidities and geriatric syndromes on the outcome of a specific therapy or intervention. In many situations, few data are available on which to base this estimate. Furthermore, these considerations take place in an environment of increasing cost containment and emphasis on value-based care. In considering value-based care, an understanding of expected outcomes is very important because the relationship of quality or outcome to cost is the defining principle of value-based care. Unfortunately, meaningful functional outcome data for cardiovascular therapies in critically ill elderly are sparse. However, some recent studies have sought to address these deficiencies. This chapter provides an overview of common cardiovascular problems that elderly patients encounter leading to admission to the ICU and their evidence-based management.

Cardiovascular Aging

Primary changes in cardiac function occur with advancing age. Morphologic changes include decreased myocyte number, increased collagen-to-elastin ratio, thickening of the left ventricular wall, and decreases in both conduction fiber density and the number of sinus node cells [1a]. Adrenergic activity and receptors also change with age [2]. These changes affect function, leading to decreased contractility, increased myocardial stiffness, increased ventricular filling pressures, and decreased β-adrenergic sensitivity.

Aging is associated with stiffening of the vasculature, or *arterial aging*, which leads to important secondary changes in the heart and other end organs, including the brain and kidney. Arterial aging is accelerated in the presence of cardiovascular comorbidities, including atherosclerosis, hypertension, diabetes, tobacco abuse, and obesity [2a–5].

Increased vascular stiffness leads to increased velocity of conduction of pulse waves down the vascular tree, resulting in earlier reflection of pulse waves from the periphery such that reflected pulse waves reach the heart during the latter phases of ejection leading to increased cardiac load [5]. This effect is evident on the arterial pressure tracing as late systolic peaking [6]. Increased left ventricular afterload leads to left ventricular wall thickening, hypertrophy, and impaired diastolic filling [7] (Figure 6.2). Cardiac contraction is prolonged to compensate for decreased ventricular compliance and increased afterload, resulting in decreased early diastolic filling time. With these changes, the atrial contribution to late ventricular filling becomes more important and explains in part the clinically

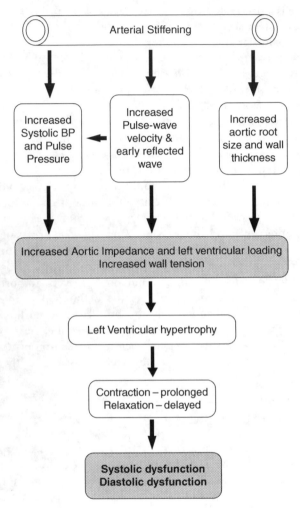

Figure 6.2 Effect of arterial stiffening on ventricular-vascular coupling, leading to increased left ventricular hypertrophy and systolic and diastolic dysfunction.

observed preload sensitivity and hemodynamic compromise often associated with failure to maintain sinus rhythm in elderly patients.

In the young, there is pulse pressure amplification as pulse waves travel down the vascular tree. This is observed as an increase in systolic pressure of 10 to 15 mmHg between the central aorta and the periphery with a slight decrease in diastolic and mean pressures. This a function of the cushioning effect of a compliant vasculature. With aging, this is lost resulting in an augmentation of central aortic pressure and increased impedance to left ventricular (LV) ejection [8]. Progressive central aortic dilatation, increased thickness of the arterial wall, increased vascular stiffness, and altered nitric oxide–induced vasodilation occur with advancing age, leading to elevated mean arterial pressure and increased pulse pressure [2–5] (Figure 6.2).

With aging there is a decrease in response to β-receptor stimulation and an increase in sympathetic nervous system activity [9]. This occurs as a result of both decreased receptor affinity and alterations in signal transduction [10]. With any physiologic stress, increased flow demands are placed on the heart. Attenuated β-receptor response in the elderly during stress is associated with decreased chronotropic and inotropic responses. In turn, the increased peripheral flow demand is met primarily by preload reserve, making the heart more susceptible to cardiac failure [1]. While β-receptor responsiveness is decreased, sympathetic nervous system activity increases with aging and may be another mechanism contributing to increased systemic vascular resistance [1]. Clinically, these autonomic changes lead to the heightened sensitivity of elderly patients to sympatholytic medications, with a greater likelihood of perioperative hemodynamic lability and a compromised ability to meet the metabolic demands of surgery.

Coronary Heart Disease: Acute Coronary Syndromes

Coronary heart disease (CHD) is a common problem in the elderly, with patients older than 65 and 75 years of age accounting for over half and over one-third of all patients, respectively, with a primary diagnosis of CHD at hospital discharge [11,12]. This same group experiences a considerably higher mortality rate, comprising approximately 82 percent of all deaths from CHD [13]. Modern cardiovascular care following acute myocardial infarction is associated with increased survival for the elderly, but survivors experience an increased incidence of heart failure [14]. The incidence of CHD and the burden of acute coronary syndromes (ACS) are expected to increase with projected growth in the population of older adults, increasing overall life expectancy, and a greater number of patients living longer with CHD due to improved therapies.

The elderly are underrepresented in previously published clinical trials of therapies for ischemic heart disease. In early studies, patients older than age 75 comprised only 2 percent of the patients enrolled. Over the past 20 years, this number has increased but falls short of reflecting the prevalence of CHD among the elderly [15]. While limited randomized, controlled trial data are available to offer clear treatment recommendations, current management is informed by existing clinical trial data, observational studies, and clinical guidelines. It has been well described, however, that treatment as recommended by clinical consensus guidelines is frequently underutilized in the elderly. Clinician concerns regarding patient safety are generally cited for this deficiency [16,17]. In 2007, the American Heart Association published a scientific statement on acute coronary syndromes in the elderly that includes discussions of considerations in ST-segment-elevation and non-ST-segment-elevation myocardial infarction [18,19] Recent updates to clinical guidelines for the management of ACS have recommended similar management for all, without age-specific differences. Nevertheless, it is important to appreciate that the elderly present with a different clinical profile with ACS. Older patients more frequently experience baseline functional limitations, compensated heart failure, past history of ischemic heart disease, and chronic kidney disease [20]. The elderly are more likely to have an unusual presentation with nonspecific complaints, including weakness, syncope, or increasing confusion [24]. This is important because atypical presentation can lead to delay in diagnosis and treatment. Evaluation may be further confounded by the presence of left bundle-branch block on electrocardiogram or elevated baseline levels of cardiac biomarkers in the aged [21,22]. Furthermore, elderly patients are more likely to present with non-ST-segment-elevation myocardial infarction (NSTEMI) as opposed to ST-segment-elevation myocardial infarction (STEMI) [23]. It has been well documented that delays in treatment and a greater frequency of triage decisions result in less intensive treatment in older patients presenting with ACS [19]. It is unclear whether this is the result of atypical presentation, frequency of concurrent illnesses, or clinical bias.

Increasing age is associated with an increasing incidence of heart failure as a complication of acute myocardial infarction with an incidence as high as 65 percent in patients older than 85 years of age [20]. As mentioned previously, multiple studies have suggested that more aggressive therapies are frequently withheld in the elderly [20,25,26]. While the elderly experience more heart failure following ACS than do their younger counterparts, including cardiogenic shock, bleeding, and in-hospital mortality, data suggest that with appropriate therapy a lower in-hospital mortality rate can be achieved [27,28]. Considerations for elders presenting with STEMI are similar to those for all patients with regard to route and timing of reperfusion interventions. Fibrinolysis is of known benefit in the elderly. Elderly patients have a greater absolute mortality benefit than patients younger than age 55. However, this mortality benefit comes at a greater risk of bleeding and stroke, with stroke rates as high as 2.9 percent in patients older than age 85 having been reported [29]. Overall outcomes with regard to stroke, recurrent myocardial infarction, and mortality tend to be better with percutaneous coronary intervention [13,18]. For this reason, fibrinolytic therapy generally should be considered only in clinical situations where there is confirmed STEMI presenting within 12 hours of symptom onset, no contraindications to treatments, and an expected time greater than 120 minutes to first-device activation for percutaneous coronary intervention (PCI) [21].

Initial NSTEMI management decisions include consideration for early invasive versus conservative therapy. Data support an early invasive approach for elderly patients meeting criteria because it has been associated with increased survival and decreased reinfarction rates [30]. An increasing number of patients older than age 75 and greater are presenting for open coronary artery revascularization [31]. For carefully selected patients with multivessel disease, surgery remains an option. One meta-analysis comparing PCI with CABG reported no significant difference in all-cause mortality at 30 days and 12 and 22 months. There was a higher rate of stroke in the CAGB patients but a greater need for repeat revascularization in the PCI group [32]. Off-pump CABG (OPCABG) has been proposed as a technique to limit complications associated with cardiopulmonary bypass and the associated aortic cannulation and cross-clamping. A trial of OPCABG specifically enrolling patients older than age 75 years failed to demonstrate benefit for OPCABG regarding death, myocardial infarction, stroke, need for renal replacement therapy, or need for repeat revascularization [33]. Consistent with other published OPCABG trials, the OPCABG group required fewer blood transfusions. Emergent open revascularization remains associated with increased mortality risk. As may be anticipated, elderly patients experience longer lengths of hospital stay following management of ACS or CABG [34,35]. Frailty also contributes to greater length of stay and higher rates of discharge to institutional care facilities [36,37]. Overall 30-day mortality after CABG in octogenarians is 6.8 percent versus 1.6 percent in the younger group [37a].

Heart Failure

Heart failure (HF) is common in the elderly, with the prevalence increasing exponentially with age. It is estimated that HF affects 6 to 10 percent of people older than 65 years of age. It is the leading cause of hospitalization in the elderly, with the majority of hospital inpatients between 70 and 75 years of age. Approximately 60 percent of elderly patients presenting with HF are women. A number of conditions are frequently present in patients presenting with HF, including atrial fibrillation, valvular heart disease, and dilated cardiomyopathy. Hospitalization for an episode of decompensated HF is associated with a high rate of readmission to the hospital and a 1-year mortality rate of nearly 30 percent. Patients may require ICU admission for acute decompensated heart failure (ADHF) or have chronic heart failure as a significant comorbidity in the setting of admission for another primary diagnosis. Clinical presentation of acute HF syndromes includes ADHF, acute pulmonary edema with normal blood pressure, acute pulmonary edema with hypertension, cardiogenic shock, high-output heart failure, and isolated right ventricular failure [38]. Heart failure can occur in the setting of reduced or preserved ejection fraction, although the elderly comprise the majority of patients with HF with preserved ejection fraction (HFpEF). The elderly may be less aggressively treated than younger patients with HF, and there is evidence of less use of diagnostic modalities and guideline-recommended therapeutic interventions [39]. The clinical presentation of HF is usually associated with congestion of the pulmonary and systemic vasculature and may include evidence of end-organ hypoperfusion. Therapeutic interventions may be directed at several targets to address these problems. Diuretics and vasodilators remain mainstays of therapy for HF. Heart failure with reduced ejection fraction (HFrEF) can be distinguished from diastolic dysfunction or HFpEF with echocardiography. Diastolic dysfunction is associated with decreased LV compliance and increased intracavitary pressures, which, in turn, result in increased pulmonary venous pressure. This can lead to frank HF and may be further exacerbated by conditions frequently encountered in ICU patients, such as volume overload, hypertension, and atrial fibrillation [40].

Patients with HF complicated by hypoxemia may require mechanical ventilation. Noninvasive positive-pressure ventilation (NIPPV) has demonstrated efficacy in the management of HF [41]. Elderly patients appear to benefit from this therapy as well, but patients should be carefully selected because contraindications to NIPPV, including altered mental status and an inability to clear secretions and protect the airway, may be present [42,43].

Long-term mechanical circulatory support (MCS) may be considered for subsets of elderly patients with end-stage HF. Ideally, selection criteria should include careful assessment of geriatric syndromes that may limit success or be incongruent with patient-centered values [44]. Clear guidelines for use of long-term MCS in elderly patients are not available but should be based on the demonstration of improved and cost-effective outcomes compared with standard medical therapy [45]. Studies have suggested safe implantation of continuous-flow devices in elderly patients, including those older than 70 years of age [46]. Age, however, is associated with a greater likelihood of discharge to care facilities and is not unexpectedly a predictor of increased mortality in the elderly population [46,47].

Patients with HF may experience ICU admission in the setting of noncardiac surgery, and up to 25 percent of these patients experience an acute exacerbation of HF in the perioperative period [48]. In this population, HF is strongly associated with increased perioperative mortality [49]. An increasing body of evidence suggests that routine use of inotropic medication is associated with harm [50,51]. A recent meta-analysis, however, provides a contrary viewpoint [52]. In light of the available evidence, it is prudent to consider limiting use of inotropic agents to patients with clinical evidence of low-cardiac-output states and impaired perfusion.

Valvular Heart Disease

Valvular heart disease, especially aortic stenosis (AS), is a frequently encountered problem in the elderly. The prevalence of moderate to severe aortic stenosis is estimated to be as high as 2.8 percent in patients over 75 years of age. As a comparison, the prevalence in the 18- to 45-year-old age group is 0.2 percent [53]. The only treatment that has been demonstrated to improve quality of life and increase survival is replacement of the valve. Historically, up to one-third of elderly patients with severe AS were not considered surgical candidates due to advanced age, LV dysfunction, or presence of significant comorbidities [54]. Mortality rate after surgical aortic valve replacement (AVR) in patients younger than 70 years of age is 1.3 percent, which increases to 5 percent in patients 80 to 95 years of age, with an increase to 10 percent in those older than 90 years of age.

Transcatheter aortic valve implantation (TAVI) techniques greatly expand treatment options for patients deemed to be at high surgical risk for open approaches. Overall, the available outcome data suggest symptomatic relief and survival advantage following TAVI in most, but not all, patients. Increasingly, emphasis has been placed on the attempt to determine which patients are most likely to benefit from intervention. This is a complex decision that does not currently have a clear answer because much remains to be learned concerning long-term outcomes in the elderly.

Technical aspects of TAVI include the type of valve implanted and the approach. The two most commonly used valves are the Edwards SAPIEN and the Core Valve, but technology is rapidly evolving, with newer generations of devices employing design features to decrease known complications. The Edwards SAPIEN is a balloon-expandable valve, and the Core Valve is self-expanding. Either valve can be placed via a retrograde approach through the femoral or axillary artery. For patients with significant peripheral vascular disease, transapical placement can be performed via a minithoracotomy. While early studies suggested no significant difference in mortality between transpical and transvascular approaches, it now appears that there is a survival advantage of transfemoral over transapical approaches [55–57]. During the valve deployment, rapid ventricular pacing to heart rates as high as 200 beats per minute is used to minimize cardiac ejection and cardiac motion so as to facilitate deployment of the valve. These periods may result in hemodynamic compromise, including the risk of myocardial ischemia with delayed recovery, especially affecting patients with poor ventricular function. This, in turn, may require inotropic or vasopressor support with obvious implications for postoperative management.

Several studies have examined outcomes of TAVI compared with open surgical AVR (SAVR). Most studies are observational in nature, but randomized, controlled trials have been conducted. The published data suggest better in-hospital recovery for TAVI with similar short- and long-term mortality. Much of the literature has been informed by various publications resulting from the Placement of AoRtic TraNscathetER Valves (PARTNER) trial. PARTNER trial was a multicenter, randomized trial comparing TAVI with SAVR and medical therapy in high-risk patients, with groups consisting of patients estimated to be at high surgical risk (group A) and a group not judged to be surgical candidates (group B).

These publications demonstrate noninferiority for TAVI versus SAVR in high-risk surgical patients with evidence of improved functional status and quality of life in some subgroups [58–62]. PARTNER trial data demonstrated similar rates of stroke, myocardial infarction, acute kidney injury, endocarditis, and permanent pacemaker placement at 1 and 2 years following TAVI or SAVR. TAVI was associated with a higher rate of vascular injury, and SAVR was associated with higher rates of major bleeding complications [63]. Other studies have reported higher rates of vascular injury, permanent atrioventricular (AV) block, and residual aortic valve regurgitation with TAVI [64].

Complications of TAVI appear to be greater in older patients. The most common complication after TAVI is vascular injury, including arterial dissection, perforation, and acute thrombosis. Patients undergoing TAVI are at risk for stroke. The incidence of stroke following TAVI has been reported to be from 2.5 percent to as high as 10 percent. Most strokes are ischemic in origin and are believed to be due to showering of emboli from the aorta during valve positioning and deployment. The majority of cerebral embolic events may be silent, as suggested by studies reporting new MRI findings in as many as 64 percent of patients following TAVI, with few patients manifesting any clinical signs of cerebral impairment [65]. The high-risk group from the PARTNER trial demonstrated a trend toward a greater incidence of stroke in TAVI versus SAVR that did not reach statistical significance [61]. TAVI is associated with a risk of conduction system injury that may require permanent pacemaker placement. The Core Valve appeared to have a greater risk of AV conduction problems compared with the Edwards SAPIEN valve. This may be explained by the self-expanding design of the valve structure, which includes a longer frame. Patients with underlying right bundle-branch block appear to be especially at risk to require permanent pacemaker placement owing to the relative risk of injury to the left bundle-branch pathway during valve deployment. Acute kidney injury (AKI) is observed following TAVI. In several studies that have evaluated risk factors for AKI following TAVI, patient age, quantity of intravenous contrast material delivered, and preexisting renal disease were not predictive of the development of AKI. Paravalvular leak can lead to aortic regurgitation (AR) and appears to be more common in TAVI than in SAVR. It is more likely to occur with self-expanding valves compared with balloon dilated devices. It is believed that central AR is the result of higher-grade paravalvular regurgitation after TAVI. Mild central AR appears to be well tolerated, but early severe AR is associated with increased mortality after TAVI [66,67]. In such cases, repeat valve replacement via valve-in-valve TAVI techniques can be considered. Valve malposition can occur and is usually noted at the time of valve deployment. Various complications can result, including embolization of the valve, blockage of the coronary ostia, paravalvular leak, interference with movement of the mitral valve leaflets, and dysrhythmias [68].

Postoperative considerations are largely the result of the physiologic consequences of valve replacement, underlying LV function, and the anticipated potential complications mentioned previously. Patients with severe AS often have impaired diastolic function related to long-standing increased in wall tension from the stenotic valve. Early after valve replacement, diastolic function has been observed to worsen in some cases [68]. Hemodynamic goals include avoidance of hypertension and maintenance of perfusion. Care should be taken to avoid pharmacologic agents that promote AV nodal blockade in patients with conduction system complications.

Much as TAVI has created treatment options for high-risk patients with severe AS, technological advances leading to techniques for transcatheter mitral valve repair have offered therapeutic considerations for high-risk patients with mitral regurgitation (MR) [69]. Degenerative MR in the elderly is a common problem, with significant MR demonstrated in over 10 percent of hospitalized patients older than 75 years of age [70]. Many of the same treatment dilemmas face elderly patients with MR as those with AS. Specifically, it is imperative to determine those most likely to benefit from treatment and align the available therapies with the goals of patients and their families. Realistic goals often address improvements in quality of life and functional status as opposed to prolonging survival [71]. As in other cardiac surgical populations, age is associated with risk in mitral valve surgery, with mortality rates reported to be 4.1 percent for those younger than age 50 and 17.0 percent for those older than age 80. Current data suggest that mitral valve repair is preferred to mitral valve replacement in the elderly. It is associated with decreased surgical mortality, lower risk of hemolysis and infection, avoidance of long-term anticoagulation, and improved long-term outcomes. However, open valve repair or replacement remains associated with poor functional recovery in the elderly [72]. The randomized multicenter EVEREST II trial compared percutaneous mitral valve repair to open surgery in low-risk patients with MR, concluding that percutaneous repair was not inferior to open surgery [73]. A high-risk cohort from the EVEREST II trial defined as estimated perioperative mortality of 12 percent or greater experienced a 30-day mortality of 6.7 percent, with survivors demonstrating improvement in New York Heart Association (NYHA) functional class and decreased hospital admission rates for heart failure [74].

Dysrhythmia

Through a variety of mechanisms, aging is associated with an increase in the prevalence of cardiac rhythm disturbances. Elderly patients may be admitted to the ICU for monitoring and management of primary dysrhythmic events or experience rhythm disturbances in the context of cardiac surgery, noncardiac surgery, or other acute critical illness. As is the case with many conditions in the aging population, presentation of disease may be atypical, and there is a risk of greater sensitivity to both therapeutic effects and adverse drug effects of medications frequently used to treat the underlying problem. Atrial fibrillation and bradydysrhythmias are particularly common in the elderly, and an increasing number of older patients have been considered for implantation of cardioverter-defibrillators for both primary and secondary management of malignant ventricular rhythms.

Bradydysrhythmias can be classified generally as abnormalities related to impulse generation or impulse conduction. Frequent underlying problems involve decreased automaticity of the sinus node or delay or blocked conduction in the sinus node or AV node or His-Purkinje system [75]. Aging has been associated with an increase in the prevalence of sinus node dysfunction, AV nodal block, and bundle-branch block. A wide variety of pathologic processes can contribute to conduction system disease, including age-related degeneration, ischemia, infection, infiltrative diseases, and trauma, including post–cardiac surgery effects. Secondary factors may also contribute to dysrhythmias and are frequently encountered in the ICU. These are electrolyte derangements, temperature imbalance, disorders of gas exchange, hypothyroidism, and adverse pharmacologic effects of medications. Treatment for symptomatic bradycardia frequently requires permanent pacemaker placement. Clinical trials suggest advantages for dual-chamber pacing over ventricular pacing alone and include a lower incidence of heart failure, reduction in the incidence of pacemaker syndrome, and a decreased incidence of the development of atrial fibrillation [76]. The observed advantages have been attributed to preservation of AV synchrony. However, long-term isolated right ventricular pacing may lead to an increased incidence of heart failure due to functional left bundle-branch block leading to ventricular dysynchrony [75].

Excluding a history of atrial fibrillation (AF), age is the most important risk factor for the development of AF [77]. Elderly patients may suffer from paroxysmal or persistent AF. New-onset AF is also frequently encountered in the ICU and is a well-described complication following cardiothoracic surgery, high-risk noncardiac surgery, trauma, or critical illness, including sepsis. The elderly are especially predisposed to developing AF due to structural and electrical changes observed with aging. Infiltrative processes and fibrosis lead to a reduction in atrial myocytes and nodal pacemaker cells, resulting in alterations in excitable tissue and conduction. These changes, along with age-related dilatation and remodeling of the left atrium and alterations in calcium conductance and potassium currents, create a milieu favoring AF [77]. Other risks factors commonly found in elderly patients that have been associated with AF include hypertension, diabetes mellitus, ischemic heart disease, valvular heart disease, heart failure, obesity, and chronic obstructive pulmonary disease (COPD).

New-onset postoperative AF (POAF) is a common problem reported in 15 to 40 percent of patients following CABG, 40 percent following surgical valve replacement, and 50 to 60 percent following combined CAGB-valve procedures [78]. Atrial fibrillation is also observed following noncardiac thoracic surgery, with a reported incidence of 12 to 30 percent in patients having pulmonary resection, 20 to 25 percent in patients undergoing esophagectomy, up to 50 percent of patients requiring extrapleural pneumonectomy, and 20 percent of patients following lung transplant [79–81]. A number of conditions exist following cardiothoracic procedures that strongly favor precipitation of AF. Operative trauma, myocardial ischemia, oxidative stress, ischemia-reperfusion injury, inflammation, increased atrial pressure, volume overload, alterations in autonomic tone, exogenous catecholamines, other inotropic agents, electrolyte disturbances, disordered acid-base homeostasis, altered gas exchange, and pain may interact with age-related changes in cardiac structure and conduction leading to slower conduction through normal pathways and shortened refractoriness that predispose to AF [82]. When AF occurs in the ICU setting, the severity of symptoms will influence the mode of therapy. Immediate synchronized electrical cardioversion is indicated for patients with acute instability including AF associated with hypotension, chest pain, shortness of breath, altered mental status, and acute congestive heart failure. Cardioversion enjoys high success rates, but when AF is not terminated, it is important to distinguish between conversion failure and early reinitiation of AF [83]. In conversion failure, cardioversion may be attempted at a higher energy level or after administration of an antiarrhythmic medication. If early reinitiation is the problem, repeated attempts at cardioversion are less likely to be effective until secondary factors have been addressed [84]. If AF is well tolerated hemodynamically, a decision must be made regarding rate versus rhythm control and timing and duration of anticoagulation. Institutional and individual practitioner preferences often affect this decision. A rate-control strategy appears to be safe and effective in elderly patients with normal LV function. Rhythm control is often an attractive therapeutic goal for patients who remain symptomatic with adequate rate control. Other potential advantages associated with rhythm control include decreased time to cardioversion, prolonged maintenance of normal sinus rhythm, and decreased hospital length of stay, but recent data do not support a long-term advantage for rhythm control in post–cardiac surgical patients [85]. Choice of antiarrhythmic agents is often dictated by the patient's underlying ventricular function because many agents exhibit negative inotropic effects and a greater risk of pro-arrhythmia in those with structural heart disease. For patients with permanent AF and poor tolerance of medical management, AF ablation or AV nodal ablation and permanent pacemaker placement may be considered [77].

Use of implantable cardioverter-defibrillators (ICDs) is common in the elderly, with an estimated 40 percent or more of ICDs and cardiac resynchronization therapy (CRT) devices implanted in those older than 70 years of age. The obvious questions regarding life expectancy and survival benefit are largely unanswered. The incidence of sudden cardiac death as a percentage of all-cause mortality decreases with age. Device implantation appears to be well tolerated [86].

Vascular Disease

An increasing array of options for the treatment of aortic and peripheral arterial disease has led to a rapid increase in the use of minimally invasive approaches to aortic aneurysm repair and treatment of carotid artery stenosis and critical limb ischemia. These interventions are attractive because they promise less physiologic stress, greater tolerance, and fewer periprocedure complications in patients with limited organ reserve. These procedures, however, have the potential to introduce new procedural risks and may not consistently produce better long-term outcomes congruent with the goals of patients because long-term data on functional outcomes are inconsistent or limited.

Endovascular repairs for both abdominal aortic aneurysms and thoracic aneurysms, as well as a variety of hybrid procedures for complex aortic disease, are now commonly performed. Endovascular approaches have been associated with a reduction in early morbidity and mortality compared with open approaches. Patients may be admitted to the ICU for hemodynamic and neurovascular monitoring, hemodynamic management, and management of lumbar drains for the prevention of spinal cord ischemia or for the management of associated complications. Associated complications may include AKI, postoperative bleeding, mesenteric ischemia, spinal cord ischemia, myocardial ischemia or infarction, distal embolization, AF, respiratory failure, and stroke. Technical issues with endovascular grafts may lead to different types of endoleaks. Age is not an absolute contraindication to endovascular aortic repair, and several reports suggest efficacy in octogenarians [87,88]. Nonagenarians have also been reported to tolerate endovascular aortic repair (EVAR) well but may not have the same mortality benefit compared with their younger counterparts [89]. This overall lack of benefit may be related to increased all-cause mortality after EVAR that compares with the high expected mortality of nonagenarians as a whole. Mortality data fail to consider quality of life, and there is evidence that physical performance remains impaired at 12 months in both open and endovascular aortic repair. These aspects of expected outcome should be considered in the treatment of the oldest old. While EVAR is associated with better early survival, the risk of late rupture appears greater than with open surgical repair [90].

Carotid disease is more prevalent in the elderly and often is present in patients with significant comorbidities. Following surgical procedures to treat symptomatic carotid stenosis, patients may be admitted to the ICU for hemodynamic monitoring and management and frequent serial neurologic assessments. Recent advancements in endovascular therapy have made carotid stenting an alternative approach to traditional carotid endarterectomy (CEA). Perioperative complications such as myocardial infarction, surgical site bleeding, and cranial nerve palsy occur less frequently with stenting. However, the risk of stroke is increased with stenting versus CEA [91–93]. A Cochrane Systematic Review reported the risk of procedural stroke or death with stenting to be 8.2 percent versus 5.0 percent for CEA (odds ratio [OR] 1.72, 95 percent confidence interval [CI] 1.29–2.31) [94]. A pooled analysis of several trials reporting an 8.9 percent incidence of stroke or death with stenting compared with 5.8 percent with CEA (relative risk [RR] 1.53, 95 percent CI 1.20–1.95). This difference, however, was strongly influenced by age, with an increased incidence of stroke and death only demonstrated in patients older than 70 years of age [95]. Both treatments are comparable in the long-term prevention of recurrent stroke [96].

Treatment of critical limb ischemia in the elderly is controversial. Patients often have severe comorbidities, poor functional status at baseline, and poor functional outcome [97]. Newer percutaneous approaches, including angioplasty, stenting, and atherectomy, may be better tolerated than traditional lower-extremity bypass, but outcome data are lacking [98]. Vogel et al. reported that endovascular procedures may not lead to better functional outcome as assessed by activities of daily living (ADLs) with critical limb ischemia compared with open approaches [99]. These results underscore the complexity of aligning treatment options with realistic goals where consistent outcome data are limited.

Other Considerations for Cardiovascular Critical Care of the Elderly

As noted previously, high-quality data to guide critical care of elderly cardiovascular patients are limited. Extrapolation of data from general ICU populations, with consideration of specific implications of the physiologic changes of aging affecting organ function, pharmacokinetics, and pharmacodynamics, along with baseline comorbidities, often drive the treatment approach in clinical practice. Other issues of concern for elderly patients in the ICU include delirium, postoperative cognitive dysfunction, and functional disability. The effects of the interaction of age, premorbid functional status, and geriatric syndromes on cardiovascular care are incompletely understood.

Delirium has an incidence of approximately 30 percent in cardiac surgical and cardiology patients [100,101]. Several risk factors have been identified in cardiac surgery patients, including a prior history of transient ischemic attack (TIA) or stroke, lower baseline Mini-Mental Status Examination scores, higher scores on screening for geriatric depression, and low serum albumin and low cardiac output states, including patients treated with intra-aortic balloon counterpulsation [101,102]. As in other ICU populations, it is prudent to screen for delirium in the cardiovascular ICU and employ nonpharmacologic strategies in an effort to decrease the incidence, including providing appropriate lighting condition to encourage diurnal variation, frequent reorientations, ensuring that patients are in possession of their visual or hearing aids, optimizing sleep hygiene, minimizing medical devices as possible, and avoiding the use of physical restraints. Early physical therapy and early mobilization may decrease duration of delirium [103]. Medications known to exacerbate delirium should be avoided. Antipsychotic medications, including haloperidol, and atypical agents, including quetiapine and risperidone, have been used in the pharmacologic management of delirium. Data on efficacy are mixed. One trial in cardiac surgical patients suggested therapeutic efficacy for risperidone in decreasing the incidence of delirium [104].

Postoperative cognitive decline has been widely reported in patients following cardiac surgery. Published studies have used various methods of testing and timing of test administration, making interpretation challenging [105]. A number of potential contributing etiologic factors have been explored, including cardiopulmonary bypass associated inflammation, cerebral ischemia, hypoxemia, and intraoperative blood pressure management. The data are conflicting, and it appears that patient factors, including preexisting cognitive dysfunction and educational status, may be more significant risk factors [106,107]. Duration of delirium has been correlated with cognitive decline but may be a marker for decreased cerebral reserve [108].

While a standardized definition has not been universally accepted, the concept of frailty may prove to be important in surgical decision making for cardiac surgical patients [109]. Frailty assessment has the potential to identify patients who are more likely to sustain lasting disability following surgical intervention [110]. In several studies of cardiac surgical patients, frailty as assessed by a variety of measures has been associated with increased perioperative morbidity and mortality [111–113]. Inclusion of frailty metrics in frequently employed surgical risk assessment tools appears to improve performance [114]. The implications of frailty on specific ICU-related therapies and interventions is unknown, but it is prudent to address evaluation of cognitive status, mobility, pain control, and nutrition. Use of geriatric consultation or inclusion of geriatric specialists as part of a multidisciplinary team in the ICU may be useful in defining goals of care that optimize patient-centered outcomes [115].

Areas of Uncertainty

Significant and rapid advances in technology have produced a growing array of therapies for cardiovascular diseases that have a variety of perceived advantages in the treatment of elderly patients. Minimally invasive modalities offer a lesser degree of physiologic stress that is frequently better tolerated by patients with decreased end-organ reserve. As with any progressive field, the available options may evolve faster than outcome data on which to base their implementation. Identifying patients most likely to benefit from aggressive intensive care and novel interventions is not an easy task. In patients with significant comorbidities, it may be difficult to clinically differentiate between the extent to which the cardiac disease is contributing to symptoms and functional limitation versus other coexisting conditions. Geriatric-specific syndromes and associated conditions including frailty, disability, impaired mobility, cognitive dysfunction, poor nutrition, polypharmacy, fall risk, mood disorders, and social isolation may influence prognosis in the elderly and may be more important determinants of outcome than traditional risk scoring systems [116]. In addition, individual therapy must carefully consider what outcomes are acceptable to patients and their families with an appreciation of the potential for goals of care to change over the course of an episode of care. In pursuing the best outcomes for elders with cardiovascular disease, much is yet to be learned. Rich et al. have proposed a research agenda for issues specific to the management of cardiovascular disorders [117]. Future research should include a patient-centered approach to delineating meaningful outcome metrics, defining and eliciting the impact of geriatric syndromes and commonly encountered comorbidities on outcome, and defining the patients most likely to benefit from admission to intensive care.

References

1. Mozaffarian D, Benjamin EJ, Go AS, et al. Heart disease and stroke statistics – 2016 update: a report from the American Heart Association. *Circulation* 2016; **133**(4): e38–360.

1a. Priebe HJ. The aged cardiovascular risk patient. *Br J Anaesth* 2000; **85**(5):763–78.

2. Brodde OE, Michel MC. Adrenergic and muscarinic receptors in the human heart. *Pharmacol Rev* 1999; **51**(4):651–90.

2a. O'Rourke MF, Adji A, Namasivayam M, Mok J. Arterial aging: a review of the pathophysiology and potential for pharmacological intervention. *Drugs Aging* 2011; **28**(10):779–95.

3. Brandes RP, Fleming I, Busse R. Endothelial aging. *Cardiovasc Res* 2005; **66** (2):286–94.

4. O'Rourke MF, ed. Function of conduit arteries. In MF O'Rourke, M Safar, VJ Dzau, eds., *Arterial Vasodilatation: Mechanisms and Therapy*. Philadelphia: Lea & Febiger, 1993: 1–9.

5. Steppan J, Barodka V, Berkowitz DE, Nyhan D. Vascular stiffness and increased pulse pressure in the aging cardiovascular system. *Cardiol Res Pract* 2011; **2011**: 263585.

6. O'Rourke MF, Kelly R, Avolio AP, eds. Factors determining normal pressure pulse contour. In MF O'Rourke, R Kelly, AP Avolio, eds., *The Arterial Pulse*. Philadelphia: Lea & Febiger, 1992: 47–72.

7. Frenneaux M, Williams L. Ventricular-arterial and ventricular-ventricular interactions and their relevance to diastolic filling. *Prog Cardiovasc Dis* 2007; **49** (4):252–62.

8. Barodka VM, Joshi BL, Berkowitz DE, Hogue CW Jr, Nyhan D. Review article:

implications of vascular aging. *Anesth Analg* 2011; **112**(5):1048–60.

9. Rooke GA. Cardiovascular aging and anesthetic implications. *J Cardiothorac Vasc Anesth* 2003; **17**(4):512–23.

10. Rooke GA. Autonomic and cardiovascular function in the geriatric patient. *Anesthesiol Clin North America* 2000; **18** (1):31, 46, v–vi.

11. Goldberg RJ, McCormick D, Gurwitz JH, et al. Age-related trends in short- and long-term survival after acute myocardial infarction: a 20-year population-based perspective (1975–1995). *Am J Cardiol* 1998; **82**(11):1311–17.

12. Roger VL, Jacobsen SJ, Weston SA, et al. Trends in the incidence and survival of patients with hospitalized myocardial infarction, Olmsted County, Minnesota, 1979 to 1994. *Ann Intern Med* 2002; **136** (5):341–48.

13. Ezekowitz JA, Kaul P. The epidemiology and management of elderly patients with myocardial infarction or heart failure. *Heart Fail Rev* 2010; **15**(5):407–13.

14. Ezekowitz JA, Kaul P, Bakal JA, et al. Declining in-hospital mortality and increasing heart failure incidence in elderly patients with first myocardial infarction. *J Am Coll Cardiol* 2009; **53**(1):13–20.

15. Saunderson CE, Brogan RA, Simms AD, et al. Acute coronary syndrome management in older adults: guidelines, temporal changes and challenges. *Age Ageing* 2014; **43**(4):450–55.

16. McCune C, McKavanagh P, Menown IB. A review of current diagnosis, investigation, and management of acute coronary syndromes in elderly patients. *Cardiol Ther* 2015; **4**(2):95–116.

17. Zaman MJ, Stirling S, Shepstone L, et al. The association between older age and

receipt of care and outcomes in patients with acute coronary syndromes: a cohort study of the myocardial ischaemia national audit project (MINAP). *Eur Heart J* 2014; **35**(23):1551–58.

18. Alexander KP, Newby LK, Armstrong PW, et al. Acute coronary care in the elderly: II. ST-segment-elevation myocardial infarction: a scientific statement for healthcare professionals from the American Heart Association Council on Clinical Cardiology in collaboration with the Society of Geriatric Cardiology. *Circulation* 2007; **115**(19):2570–89.

19. Alexander KP, Newby LK, Cannon CP, et al. Acute coronary care in the elderly: I. Non-ST-segment-elevation acute coronary syndromes: a scientific statement for healthcare professionals from the American Heart Association Council on Clinical Cardiology in collaboration with the Society of Geriatric Cardiology. *Circulation* 2007; **115**(19):2549–69.

20. Mehta RH, Rathore SS, Radford MJ, et al. Acute myocardial infarction in the elderly: differences by age. *J Am Coll Cardiol* 2001; **38**(3):736–41.

21. Dai X, Busby-Whitehead J, Alexander KP. Acute coronary syndrome in the older adults. *J Geriatr Cardiol* 2016; **13**(2):101–8.

22. Normann J, Mueller M, Biener M, et al. Effect of older age on diagnostic and prognostic performance of high-sensitivity troponin T in patients presenting to an emergency department. *Am Heart J* 2012; **164**(5):698, 705, e4.

23. Roger VL, Weston SA, Gerber Y, et al. Trends in incidence, severity, and outcome of hospitalized myocardial infarction. *Circulation* 2010; **121**(7):863–69.

24. Bayer AJ, Chadha JS, Farag RR, Pathy MS. Changing presentation of myocardial infarction with increasing old age. *J Am Geriatr Soc* 1986; **34**(4):263–66.

25. Paul SD, O'Gara PT, Mahjoub ZA, et al. Geriatric patients with acute myocardial infarction: cardiac risk factor profiles, presentation, thrombolysis, coronary interventions, and prognosis. *Am Heart J* 1996; **131**(4):710–15.

26. Stone PH, Thompson B, Anderson HV, et al. Influence of race, sex, and age on management of unstable angina and non-Q-wave myocardial infarction: the TIMI III registry. *JAMA* 1996; **275**(14):1104–12.

27. Alexander KP, Roe MT, Chen AY, et al. Evolution in cardiovascular care for elderly patients with non-ST-segment elevation acute coronary syndromes: results from the CRUSADE national quality improvement initiative. *J Am Coll Cardiol* 2005; **46**(8):1479–87.

28. Avezum A, Makdisse M, Spencer F, et al. Impact of age on management and outcome of acute coronary syndrome: observations from the global registry of acute coronary events (GRACE). *Am Heart J* 2005; **149**(1):67–73.

29. Gore JM, Granger CB, Simoons ML, et al. Stroke after thrombolysis. mortality and functional outcomes in the GUSTO-I trial: global use of strategies to open occluded coronary arteries. *Circulation* 1995; **92**(10):2811–18.

30. Bach RG, Cannon CP, Weintraub WS, et al. The effect of routine, early invasive management on outcome for elderly patients with non-ST-segment elevation acute coronary syndromes. *Ann Intern Med* 2004; **141**(3):186–95.

31. Seco M, Edelman JJ, Forrest P, et al. Geriatric cardiac surgery: chronology vs biology. *Heart Lung Circ* 2014; **23**(9):794–801.

32. Alam M, Virani SS, Shahzad SA, et al. Comparison by meta-analysis of percutaneous coronary intervention versus coronary artery bypass grafting in patients with a mean age of ≥70 years. *Am J Cardiol* 2013; **112**(5):615–22.

33. Diegeler A, Borgermann J, Kappert U, et al. Off-pump versus on-pump coronary-artery bypass grafting in elderly patients. *N Engl J Med* 2013; **368**(13):1189–98.

34. Alabas OA, Allan V, McLenachan JM, Feltbower R, Gale CP. Age-dependent improvements in survival after hospitalisation with acute myocardial infarction: an analysis of the myocardial

ischemia national audit project (MINAP). *Age Ageing* 2014; **43**(6):779–85.

35. Chee JH, Filion KB, Haider S, Pilote L, Eisenberg MJ. Impact of age on hospital course and cost of coronary artery bypass grafting. *Am J Cardiol* 2004; **93**(6): 768–71.

36. Ekerstad N, Swahn E, Janzon M, et al. Frailty is independently associated with short-term outcomes for elderly patients with non-ST-segment elevation myocardial infarction. *Circulation* 2011; **124**(22):2397–404.

37. Lee DH, Buth KJ, Martin BJ, Yip AM, Hirsch GM. Frail patients are at increased risk for mortality and prolonged institutional care after cardiac surgery. *Circulation* 2010; **121**(8):973–78.

37a. Sen B, Niemann B, Roth P, et al. Short- and long-term outcomes in octogenarians after coronary artery bypass surgery. *Eur J Cardiothorac Surg* 42(5):e102–7.

38. Gheorghiade M, Zannad F, Sopko G, et al. Acute heart failure syndromes: current state and framework for future research. *Circulation* 2005; **112**(25):3958–68.

39. Katsanos S, Bistola V, Parissis JT. Acute heart failure syndromes in the elderly: the European perspective. *Heart Fail Clin* 2015; **11**(4):637–45.

40. Vignon P. Ventricular diastolic abnormalities in the critically ill. *Curr Opin Crit Care* 2013; **19**(3):242–49.

41. Vital FM, Ladeira MT, Atallah AN. Non-invasive positive pressure ventilation (CPAP or bilevel NPPV) for cardiogenic pulmonary oedema. *Cochrane Database Syst Rev* 2013; 5:CD005351.

42. L'Her E, Duquesne F, Girou E, et al. Noninvasive continuous positive airway pressure in elderly cardiogenic pulmonary edema patients. *Intensive Care Med* 2004; **30**(5):882–88.

43. Ozsancak Ugurlu A, Sidhom SS, Khodabandeh A, et al. Use and outcomes of noninvasive ventilation for acute respiratory failure in different age groups. *Respir Care* 2016; **61**(1):36–43.

44. Vitale CA, Chandekar R, Rodgers PE, Pagani FD, Malani PN. A call for guidance in the use of left ventricular assist devices in older adults. *J Am Geriatr Soc* 2012; **60** (1):145–50.

45. Hiesinger W, Boyd JH, Woo YJ. Ventricular assist device implantation in the elderly. *Ann Cardiothorac Surg* 2014; **3** (6):570–72.

46. Kilic A, Sultan I, Yuh DD, et al. Ventricular assist device implantation in the elderly: nationwide outcomes in the united states. *J Card Surg* 2013; **28**(2):183–89.

47. Atluri P, Goldstone AB, Kobrin DM, et al. Ventricular assist device implant in the elderly is associated with increased, but respectable risk: a multi-institutional study. *Ann Thorac Surg* 2013; **96**(1):141–47.

48. Smit-Fun V, Buhre WF. The patient with chronic heart failure undergoing surgery. *Curr Opin Anaesthesiol* 2016.

49. van Diepen S, Bakal JA, McAlister FA, Ezekowitz JA. Mortality and readmission of patients with heart failure, atrial fibrillation, or coronary artery disease undergoing noncardiac surgery: an analysis of 38 047 patients. *Circulation* 2011; **124**(3):289–96.

50. Nielsen DV, Hansen MK, Johnsen SP, et al. Health outcomes with and without use of inotropic therapy in cardiac surgery: results of a propensity score-matched analysis. *Anesthesiology* 2014; **120** (5):1098–108.

51. Nielsen DV, Algotsson L. Outcome of inotropic therapy: is less always more? *Curr Opin Anaesthesiol* 2015; **28**(2):159–64.

52. Belletti A, Castro ML, Silvetti S, et al. The effect of inotropes and vasopressors on mortality: a meta-analysis of randomized clinical trials. *Br J Anaesth* 2015; **115** (5):656–75.

53. Nkomo VT, Gardin JM, Skelton TN, et al. Burden of valvular heart diseases: a population-based study. *Lancet* 2006; **368** (9540):1005–11.

54. Lindman BR, Alexander KP, O'Gara PT, Afilalo J. Futility, benefit, and transcatheter

aortic valve replacement. *JACC Cardiovasc Interv* 2014; 7(7):707–16.

55. Biancari F, Rosato S, D'Errigo P, et al. Immediate and intermediate outcome after transapical versus transfemoral transcatheter aortic valve replacement. *Am J Cardiol* 2016; 117(2):245–51.

56. Ewe SH, Delgado V, Ng AC, et al. Outcomes after transcatheter aortic valve implantation: transfemoral versus transapical approach. *Ann Thorac Surg* 2011; 92(4):1244–51.

57. Johansson M, Nozohoor S, Kimblad PO, et al. Transapical versus transfemoral aortic valve implantation: a comparison of survival and safety. *Ann Thorac Surg* 2011; 91(1):57–63.

58. Reynolds MR, Magnuson EA, Wang K, et al. Health-related quality of life after transcatheter or surgical aortic valve replacement in high-risk patients with severe aortic stenosis: results from the PARTNER (Placement of AoRTic TraNscathetER Valve) trial (cohort A). *J Am Coll Cardiol* 2012; 60(6):548–58.

59. Reynolds MR, Magnuson EA, Lei Y, et al. Health-related quality of life after transcatheter aortic valve replacement in inoperable patients with severe aortic stenosis. *Circulation* 2011; 124 (18):1964–72.

60. Leon MB, Smith CR, Mack MJ, et al. Transcatheter or surgical aortic-valve replacement in intermediate-risk patients. *N Engl J Med* 2016; 374(17):1609–20.

61. Smith CR, Leon MB, Mack MJ, et al. Transcatheter versus surgical aortic-valve replacement in high-risk patients. *N Engl J Med* 2011; 364(23):2187–98.

62. Makkar RR, Fontana GP, Jilaihawi H, et al. Transcatheter aortic-valve replacement for inoperable severe aortic stenosis. *N Engl J Med* 2012; 366(18):1696–704.

63. Kodali SK, Williams MR, Smith CR, et al. Two-year outcomes after transcatheter or surgical aortic-valve replacement. *N Engl J Med* 2012; 366(18):1686–95.

64. D'Errigo P, Barbanti M, Ranucci M, et al. Transcatheter aortic valve implantation versus surgical aortic valve replacement for severe aortic stenosis: results from an intermediate risk propensity-matched population of the Italian OBSERVANT study. *Int J Cardiol* 2013; 167(5): 1945–52.

65. Ghanem A, Kocurek J, Sinning JM, et al. Cognitive trajectory after transcatheter aortic valve implantation. *Circ Cardiovasc Interv* 2013; 6(6):615–24.

66. Tamburino C, Capodanno D, Ramondo A, et al. Incidence and predictors of early and late mortality after transcatheter aortic valve implantation in 663 patients with severe aortic stenosis. *Circulation* 2011; 123 (3):299–308.

67. Athappan G, Patvardhan E, Tuzcu EM, et al. Incidence, predictors, and outcomes of aortic regurgitation after transcatheter aortic valve replacement: meta-analysis and systematic review of literature. *J Am Coll Cardiol* 2013; 61(15):1585–95.

68. Huffmyer J, Tashjian J, Raphael J, Jaeger JM. Management of the patient for transcatheter aortic valve implantation in the perioperative period. *Semin Cardiothorac Vasc Anesth* 2012; 16 (1):25–40.

69. Taramasso M, Candreva A, Pozzoli A, et al. Current challenges in interventional mitral valve treatment. *J Thorac Dis* 2015; 7 (9):1536–42.

70. Taramasso M, Gaemperli O, Maisano F. Treatment of degenerative mitral regurgitation in elderly patients. *Nat Rev Cardiol* 2015; 12(3):177–83.

71. Mirabel M, Iung B, Baron G, et al. What are the characteristics of patients with severe, symptomatic, mitral regurgitation who are denied surgery? *Eur Heart J* 2007; 28 (11):1358–65.

72. Mehta RH, Eagle KA, Coombs LP, et al. Influence of age on outcomes in patients undergoing mitral valve replacement. *Ann Thorac Surg* 2002; 74(5):1459–67.

73. Mauri L, Foster E, Glower DD, et al. Four-year results of a randomized controlled trial of percutaneous repair versus surgery for mitral regurgitation. *J Am Coll Cardiol* 2013; 62(4):317–28.

74. Glower DD, Kar S, Trento A, et al. Percutaneous mitral valve repair for mitral regurgitation in high-risk patients: results of the EVEREST II study. *J Am Coll Cardiol* 2014; **64**(2):172–81.

75. Kumar P, Kusumoto FM, Goldschlager N. Bradyarrhythmias in the elderly. *Clin Geriatr Med* 2012; **28**(4):703–15.

76. Lamas GA, Lee K, Sweeney M, et al. The mode selection trial (MOST) in sinus node dysfunction: design, rationale, and baseline characteristics of the first 1000 patients. *Am Heart J* 2000; **140**(4):541–51.

77. Hakim FA, Shen WK. Atrial fibrillation in the elderly: a review. *Future Cardiol* 2014; **10**(6):745–58.

78. Hogue CW, Jr, Creswell LL, Gutterman DD, Fleisher LA, American College of Chest Physicians. Epidemiology, mechanisms, and risks: American College of Chest Physicians guidelines for the prevention and management of postoperative atrial fibrillation after cardiac surgery. *Chest* 2005; **128** (Suppl 2):9S–16S.

79. Vaporciyan AA, Correa AM, Rice DC, et al. Risk factors associated with atrial fibrillation after noncardiac thoracic surgery: analysis of 2,588 patients. *J Thorac Cardiovasc Surg* 2004; **127**(3):779–86.

80. Neragi-Miandoab S, Weiner S, Sugarbaker DJ. Incidence of atrial fibrillation after extrapleural pneumonectomy vs pleurectomy in patients with malignant pleural mesothelioma. *Interact Cardiovasc Thorac Surg* 2008; **7**(6):1039–42.

81. Mason DP, Marsh DH, Alster JM, et al. Atrial fibrillation after lung transplantation: timing, risk factors, and treatment. *Ann Thorac Surg* 2007; **84** (6):1878–84.

82. Echahidi N, Pibarot P, O'Hara G, Mathieu P. Mechanisms, prevention, and treatment of atrial fibrillation after cardiac surgery. *J Am Coll Cardiol* 2008; **51**(8):793–801.

83. Crawford TC, Oral H. Cardiac arrhythmias: management of atrial fibrillation in the critically ill patient. *Crit Care Clin* 2007; **23**(4):855, 72, vii.

84. Rho RW. The management of atrial fibrillation after cardiac surgery. *Heart* 2009; **95**(5):422–29.

85. Gillinov AM, Bagiella E, Moskowitz AJ, et al. Rate control versus rhythm control for atrial fibrillation after cardiac surgery. *N Engl J Med* 2016; **374**(20):1911–21.

86. Barra S, Providencia R, Paiva L, Heck P, Agarwal S. Implantable cardioverter-defibrillators in the elderly: rationale and specific age-related considerations. *Europace* 2015; **17**(2):174–86.

87. Lange C, Leurs LJ, Buth J, Myhre HO, EUROSTAR collaborators. Endovascular repair of abdominal aortic aneurysm in octogenarians: an analysis based on EUROSTAR data. *J Vasc Surg* 2005; **42** (4):624–30; discussion 630.

88. Henebiens M, Vahl A, Koelemay MJ. Elective surgery of abdominal aortic aneurysms in octogenarians: a systematic review. *J Vasc Surg* 2008; **47**(3):676–81.

89. Wigley J, Shantikumar S, Hameed W, et al. Endovascular aneurysm repair in nonagenarians: a systematic review. *Ann Vasc Surg* 2015; **29**(2):385–91.

90. Schermerhorn ML, Buck DB, O'Malley AJ, et al. Long-term outcomes of abdominal aortic aneurysm in the Medicare population. *N Engl J Med* 2015; **373** (4):328–38.

91. Blackshear JL, Cutlip DE, Roubin GS, et al. Myocardial infarction after carotid stenting and endarterectomy: results from the carotid revascularization endarterectomy versus stenting trial. *Circulation* 2011; **123** (22):2571–78.

92. Bonati L. Stenting or endarterectomy for patients with symptomatic carotid stenosis. *Neurol Clin* 2015; **33**(2):459–74.

93. Ouyang YA, Jiang Y, Yu M, Zhang Y, Huang H. Efficacy and safety of stenting for elderly patients with severe and symptomatic carotid artery stenosis: a critical meta-analysis of randomized controlled trials. *Clin Interv Aging* 2015; **10**:1733–42.

94. Bonati LH, Lyrer P, Ederle J, Featherstone R, Brown MM. Percutaneous transluminal

balloon angioplasty and stenting for carotid artery stenosis. *Cochrane Database Syst Rev* 2012; **9**:CD000515.

95. Carotid Stenting Trialists' Collaboration, Bonati LH, Dobson J, et al. Short-term outcome after stenting versus endarterectomy for symptomatic carotid stenosis: a preplanned meta-analysis of individual patient data. *Lancet* 2010; **376** (9746):1062–73.

96. Brott TG, Howard G, Roubin GS, et al. Long-term results of stenting versus endarterectomy for carotid-artery stenosis. *N Engl J Med* 2016; **374** (11):1021–31.

97. Duggan MM, Woodson J, Scott TE, Ortega AN, Menzoian JO. Functional outcomes in limb salvage vascular surgery. *Am J Surg* 1994; **168**(2):188–91.

98. Siracuse JJ, Menard MT, Eslami MH, et al. Comparison of open and endovascular treatment of patients with critical limb ischemia in the vascular quality initiative. *J Vasc Surg* 2016; **63** (4):958–65, e1.

99. Vogel TR, Petroski GF, Kruse RL. Functional status of elderly adults before and after interventions for critical limb ischemia. *J Vasc Surg* 2014; **59**(2): 350–58.

100. Cropsey C, Kennedy J, Han J, Pandharipande PP. Cognitive dysfunction, delirium, and stroke in cardiac surgery patients. *Semin Cardiothorac Vasc Anesth* 2015; **19** (4):309–17.

101. Rudolph JL, Jones RN, Levkoff SE, et al. Derivation and validation of a preoperative prediction rule for delirium after cardiac surgery. *Circulation* 2009; **119**(2):229–36.

102. Norkiene I, Ringaitiene D, Misiuriene I, et al. Incidence and precipitating factors of delirium after coronary artery bypass grafting. *Scand Cardiovasc J* 2007; **41** (3):180–85.

103. Collinsworth AW, Priest EL, Campbell CR, Vasilevskis EE, Masica AL. A review of multifaceted care approaches for the prevention and mitigation of delirium in intensive care units. *J Intensive Care Med* 2016; **31**(2):127–41.

104. Hakim SM, Othman AI, Naoum DO. Early treatment with risperidone for subsyndromal delirium after on-pump cardiac surgery in the elderly: a randomized trial. *Anesthesiology* 2012; **116**(5):987–97.

105. Bartels K, McDonagh DL, Newman MF, Mathew JP. Neurocognitive outcomes after cardiac surgery. *Curr Opin Anaesthesiol* 2013; **26**(1):91–97.

106. Selnes OA, Grega MA, Bailey MM, et al. Do management strategies for coronary artery disease influence 6-year cognitive outcomes? *Ann Thorac Surg* 2009; **88** (2):445–54.

107. Selnes OA, Gottesman RF, Grega MA, et al. Cognitive and neurologic outcomes after coronary-artery bypass surgery. *N Engl J Med* 2012; **366**(3):250–57.

108. Pandharipande PP, Girard TD, Jackson JC, et al. Long-term cognitive impairment after critical illness. *N Engl J Med* 2013; **369**(14):1306–16.

109. Morley JE, Vellas B, van Kan GA, et al. Frailty consensus: a call to action. *J Am Med Dir Assoc* 2013; **14**(6):392–97.

110. Graham A, Brown CH 4th. Frailty, aging, and cardiovascular surgery. *Anesth Analg* 2016.

111. Lee DH, Buth KJ, Martin BJ, Yip AM, Hirsch GM. Frail patients are at increased risk for mortality and prolonged institutional care after cardiac surgery. *Circulation* 2010; **121**(8):973–78.

112. Green P, Woglom AE, Genereux P, et al. The impact of frailty status on survival after transcatheter aortic valve replacement in older adults with severe aortic stenosis: a single-center experience. *JACC Cardiovasc Interv* 2012; **5**(9):974–81.

113. Sepehri A, Beggs T, Hassan A, et al. The impact of frailty on outcomes after cardiac surgery: a systematic review. *J Thorac Cardiovasc Surg* 2014; **148**(6):3110–17.

114. Afilalo J, Mottillo S, Eisenberg MJ, et al. Addition of frailty and disability to cardiac surgery risk scores identifies

elderly patients at high risk of mortality or major morbidity. *Circ Cardiovasc Qual Outcomes* 2012; **5**(2):222–28.

115. Mohanty S, Rosenthal RA, Russell MM, et al. Optimal perioperative management of the geriatric patient: a best practices guideline from the American College of Surgeons NSQIP and the American Geriatrics Society. *J Am Coll Surg* 2016; **222**(5):930–47.

116. Bell SP, Orr NM, Dodson JA, et al. What to expect from the evolving field of geriatric cardiology. *J Am Coll Cardiol* 2015; **66**(11):1286–99.

117. Rich MW, Chyun DA, Skolnick AH, et al. Knowledge gaps in cardiovascular care of older adults: a scientific statement from the American Heart Association, American College of Cardiology, and American Geriatrics Society: executive summary. *J Am Geriatr Soc* 2016; **64**(11): 2185–92.

Nutritional and Metabolic Derangements in the Critically Ill Elderly

Arturo G. Torres, Sasha Grek and Brenda G. Fahy

Key Points

- Aging nutritional physiology predisposes elderly individuals to malnutrition syndromes.
- Impaired intake and energy regulation and fuel metabolism derangements underscore the etiology of malnutrition in the elderly.
- The three main malnutrition syndromes are protein-energy malnutrition (or starvation), sarcopenia, and cachexia.
- Frailty is a reflection of the prolonged derangements from nutritional deficiencies and functional decline associated with the aging process.
- Malnourished elderly patients have a higher morbidity and mortality when hospitalized than their nourished counterparts.
- Protein-energy malnutrition is the only reversible condition responsive to nutritional interventions.
- A chronic inflammatory state exists in both sarcopenic and cachectic patients, leading to skeletal muscle mass loss and atrophy.
- Nutritional screening is necessary in all elderly hospitalized patients in order to identify those at higher nutritional risk.
- Feeding goals should be achieved within 48 hours in elderly intensive care unit patients with high nutritional risk factors.
- Enteral nutrition via gastric feeding should be the first-line choice for feeding. Consider small bowel feeding in those at high risk for aspiration or those who can have an enteral feeding tube placed in the small bowel.
- Obstacles that promote cessation of feeding must be identified and minimized on a daily basis.

Introduction

Nutritional and metabolic derangements are common in elderly patients in the intensive care unit (ICU) and are important to recognize due to the many complications that arise on admission and throughout the course of hospitalization. They are often present before ICU admission in many elderly patients. These nutritional and metabolic derangements are primary determinants of frailty. Medical, psychiatric, and socioeconomic factors influence

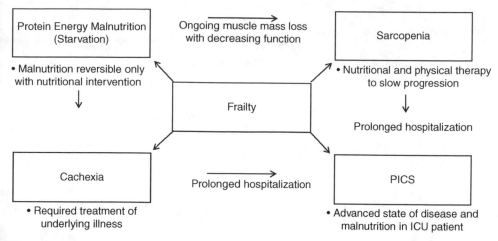

Figure 7.1 Overview of malnutrition syndrome (PICS = persistent inflammatory, immunosuppressed, catabolic syndrome).

the nutritional status of the elderly. Malnutrition is an independent factor for ICU morbidity and mortality [1]. This chapter explores the general malnutrition syndromes, including starvation, cachexia, and sarcopenia, that lead to frailty and its impact on the elderly ICU population (Figure 7.1). The physiologic derangements behind these processes, as well as assessments of their severity and potential interventions to treat them during ICU admission, will also be discussed. Current areas pertaining to specific nutritional interventions that may be helpful in critically ill patients will also be discussed. This chapter highlights the challenges of nutritional repletion in elderly ICU patients, which often falls below set goals and in and of itself is insufficient to reverse many of the nutritional and metabolic derangements that are present in the elderly.

Malnutrition Syndromes

Aging is associated with changes in nutritional physiology, promoting weight loss (Figure 7.2). The underlying mechanisms include impaired nutritional intake and alterations in energy expenditure and fuel processing. Decreased nutritional intake with aging has been attributed to reduced hunger and early satiety, as well as decreased senses of smell and taste. Delayed gastric emptying, insulin resistance, and decreased sensitivity to several digestive hormones are potentially responsible for these changes. Insulin resistance plays a central role in the overall process that leads to what has been termed the *anorexia of aging*, resulting in increasing satiation and promotion of skeletal muscle mass loss [2]. Longitudinal studies examining body composition and energy expenditures (including daily, activity, and basal), performed over the life span of healthy elderly subjects, have shown overall decreases in both body composition and energy expenditure with age. Of note, these studies also found that the greatest decline is in energy expenditure related to activity compared with the other components. The consequence of lower overall energy expenditure is associated with an increase in functional limitations, thus predisposing the

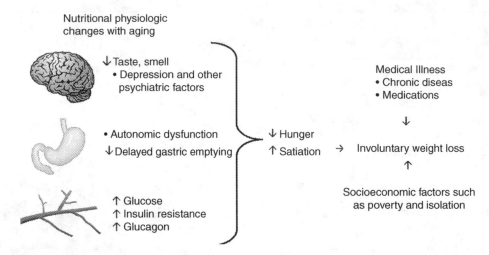

Figure 7.2 Factors contributing to involuntary weight loss in the elderly.

elderly to the increased risk of morbidities [3]. Based on these findings, the elderly are at an increased risk of malnutrition and frailty regardless of their current health status.

The term *frailty* is commonly used to describe the ailing elderly, and its definition continues to evolve as more studies are performed that improve our understanding. Currently, frailty describes a state of vulnerability that is responsible for an inability to maintain normal physiological balance and response to stress [3]. Frailty represents a physiologic trait that is independently associated with an increased risk of morbidity and mortality rather than a reflection of underlying comorbidities. The main signs heralding the presence of frailty are related to activity and nutrition. These include an unintentional weight loss of greater than 5 percent in a calendar year, decreased muscle strength, and a decrease in physical activity. Malnutrition, in combination with loss of muscle mass loss (sarcopenia), ultimately determines the degree of frailty present in a particular patient [4].

Sarcopenia represents a state involving muscle mass loss with its associated functional decline. The causes are multifactorial, including disuse, nutritional deficiencies, impaired response of skeletal muscle to nutrients, and endocrine dysregulation [4]. Hormonal imbalances are important because they lead to muscle catabolism; these hormonal imbalances include insulin resistance as well as decreases in both estrogen and testosterone, and they promote a disparity between muscle protein synthesis and muscle protein breakdown with resulting muscle catabolism [5]. As a person ages, there are associated alterations in muscle homeostasis and composition, including a decrease in muscle type II fibers, that are characterized by fast and powerful contractions with greater fatigue. The inability to generate power and the slowed rate of power development are hallmarks of both sarcopenia and frailty. These age-associated losses are further accelerated by malnutrition. Other derangements observed include an accumulation of damaged mitochondria and an increase in muscle apoptosis from excessive production of oxidative radicals. In sarcopenic patients, there exists some degree of chronic inflammation. This results in the presence of elevated protein markers, including tumor necrosis factor alpha (TNF-α), C-reactive protein, and interleukin 6 (IL-6). When TNF-α is elevated, an unregulated catabolic state is promoted that specifically targets skeletal muscle [5].

Starvation, more scientifically termed *protein-energy malnutrition* (PEM), is strictly caused by decreased intake. The prevalence of this state varies depending on the setting. For the community-dwelling elderly population, reported rates range from 5 to 10 percent, whereas in the elderly population in nursing homes and rehabilitation settings, the rates can be up to 70 percent. In the acute care setting, between 23 and 60 percent of elderly patients are malnourished [6]. Risk factors attributed to PEM are often referred to as the *nine d's* (dysphagia, dyspepsia, dementia, diarrhea, depression, disease, poor dentition, drugs, and dysfunction). These apply to all disorders of malnutrition and frailty, but the difference between PEM and the other disorders is that adequate feeding can reverse the negative effects of PEM.

Cachexia is defined as a "complex metabolic syndrome associated with underlying illness and characterized by loss of muscle, with or without loss of fat mass" [7]. Nutritional derangements include anorexia, insulin resistance, and increased muscle protein breakdown. In the elderly, there are multiple dysregulated nutritional pathways that lead to an imbalance between catabolism and anabolism, with the complications of this syndrome not responsive to nutritional interventions. Common disease processes responsible for cachexia are cancer, chronic obstructive pulmonary disease, end-stage renal disease, rheumatoid arthritis, and congestive heart failure. A key distinction between sarcopenia and cachexia is that most cachectic patients are sarcopenic, whereas the reverse is not true; that is, not all sarcopenic patients are cachectic. The difference relates to the malnutrition caused directly by the underlying illness in cachexia, although both sarcopenia and cachexia share a common pathway that leads to anabolism resistance mediated by chronic inflammatory processes [8].

One of the challenges in the elderly ICU patient population is that most elderly ICU patients will have an interplay of all three syndromes – starvation, cachexia, and sarcopenia. Clinical distinction is not always possible among the three because these states are not mutually exclusive. The key is to identify the patients who present with nutritional derangements in order to formulate a multidisciplinary approach to restore a degree of the nutritional status with the goal of improving patient outcomes.

Intersection of Frailty and Critical Illness

Many of the same mechanisms underlying malnutrition syndromes are present and amplified in the myopathy of critical illness. Sepsis, respiratory insufficiency, surgery, and trauma trigger a similar and common acute inflammatory pathway that leads to profound muscle wasting via TNF-α-mediated catabolism. One salient example is the effect of prolonged mechanical ventilation on sarcopenic elderly patients. The combination of decreased diaphragmatic muscular mass due to sarcopenia and disuse atrophy from mechanical ventilation leads to a vicious cycle of increased ventilator dependence. Emerging epidemiologic data suggest that frail elderly individuals have worse outcomes than their nonfrail counterparts. Even more alarming is that more than one-third of elderly patients meet the criteria for frailty. This figure will only continue to increase as the proportion of elderly population increases, with the effects of malnutrition superimposed on the high prevalence of chronic comorbidities. Interestingly, age alone is not consistently a predictor of mortality compared with frailty [9].

Furthermore, malnutrition syndromes are a major risk factor for persistent inflammatory immunosuppressed catabolic syndrome (PICS), a new phenotype of multiple-organ failure describing the underlying pathophysiology of chronic critical illness (defined as an ICU stay > 14 days) that is mostly associated with the elderly and has a high mortality rate. Similar to sarcopenia and cachexia, patients with PICS are refractory to nutritional supplementation. The underlying molecular pathophysiology shares a continuum with both sarcopenia and cachexia. The distinguishing features of PICS are the clinical setting and enhanced deterioration caused by the underlying illness and ensuing inflammatory insult [10].

Assessment

All patients admitted to the ICU require an immediate nutritional screening. Unlike the complexity of diagnosing sarcopenia and frailty, determining baseline nutritional risk is relatively simple. Current guidelines endorse the Nutritional Risk Screening (NRS) 2002 and the Nutrition Risk in Critically Ill (NUTRIC) scoring systems over others [11]. In contrast to other systems, both of these systems determine nutrition status and disease severity. Recent data support the use of assessment over screening tools in ICU patients because they indicate relevant outcomes (i.e., mortality, length of stay) independently. These assessments include Subjective Global Assessment and Mini Nutritional Assessment [12]. Regardless of the tool used for assessment, each has its shortcomings. The key is to have a standardized and consistent approach for identification of baseline nutritional status. Current data indicate that appropriate and early nutritional interventions for patients at higher risk can lead to improved outcomes, including reduced infection, total complications, and mortality, compared with patients at low nutritional risk [13].

Traditional serum protein markers, including albumin, prealbumin, and transferrin, among others, merely reflect the acute-phase response and do not accurately represent the nutrition status of the patient in the ICU (Table 7.1). Interestingly, the albumin levels of sarcopenic patients have been shown to correlate with all-cause mortality in the elderly [5]. Neither anthropometrics nor bioelectric impedance serves as a reliable assessment tool for sarcopenic status, nor do they assess the adequacy of nutritional therapy [14]. To date, markers of inflammation, including TNF-α, C-reactive protein, and others, are still being investigated and are discouraged from being used as surrogate markers [15]. Ultrasound and CT scan are emerging tools for muscle mass and body composition assessments. However, validation and reliability studies in ICU patients at the time of writing remain to be studied [16].

Nutritional experts opine that accurate estimation of energy expenditure is required to help guide an effective nutritional strategy. Indirect calorimetry remains the gold standard for determining energy requirements, yet there are no data suggesting that accurately measuring resting energy expenditure to determine nutritional requirements improves outcome [9]. A more practical recommendation is to use published predictive equations (e.g., Harris-Benedict, Penn State, etc.) or a simplistic weight-based equation (25–30 kcal/kg per day) to guide energy requirements. However, one of the shortcomings when using predictive equations is that they are less accurate in patients at the extremes of weight, that is, obese and underweight patients [18]. One advantage of using weight-based equations is the simplicity of their application. An important caveat when using weight-based calculations in the critically ill ICU patient is that with dynamic fluid shifts (e.g., fluid resuscitation,

Table 7.1 Serum Biomarkers Associated with Nutritional Status

Biomarker	Half-life	Comments
C-reactive protein	2 days	Acute-phase reactant.
		Levels influenced by underlying inflammation, infections, and cytokines.
Albumin	14–20 days	Long half-life limits usage in acute setting.
		Potential marker for long-term outcome in sarcopenic patients.
		Levels influenced by liver and renal disease, vascular permeability, and inflammation.
Prealbumin	12 hours	Negative acute-phase protein.
		Levels influenced by the inflammatory cascade, renal and liver disease.
Transferrin	8–9 days	Levels influenced by inflammation, iron content, malabsorption, and liver and renal disease.

edema), dry weight should be used instead of actual weight [11]. Regardless of the approach used, nutritional evaluations should be dynamic and ideally occur more than once per week.

Interventions

Once an elderly patient becomes frail, nutrition supplement in the form of feeding alone will not reverse the effects of the frailty. However, nutritional repletion is still necessary in the malnourished elderly patient [1]. A nutritional screen and/or further assessment should be performed, and if the patient is determined to be at high risk of malnourishment (Figure 7.3), early feeding is recommended whenever possible. Early feeding is preferred, provided that no active resuscitative efforts are taking place [18]. This recommendation is particularly relevant for sarcopenic elderly patients because they are already protein deficient. Even early starvation (<24 hours) should be avoided if possible due to the patient's underlying procatabolic state. In frail individuals, nearly 20 percent of resting energy expenditure during starvation is derived from protein stores. Importantly, type II muscle fibers, those that help prevent frailty, are the ones preferentially subjected to proteolysis [19]. Early initiation is paramount to decrease the ongoing PEM. The goal for these patients is to provide greater than 80 percent of estimated or calculated goal energy and protein requirements within at least the first 48 to 72 hours while monitoring for refeeding syndrome [20] (Table 7.2). Aggressive protein-driven diets (with a range of 1.2–2.0 g/kg of actual body weight per day) are the current recommendations, highlighting the importance of PEM and its deleterious effects. Protein requirements may be even higher in certain patient populations, which include patients with thermal injuries or elderly patients with polytrauma [11].

Current barriers exist that prevent optimal nutritional supplementation. These include both patient and institutional barriers (Table 7.3). In the current ICU setting, there is an

Table 7.2 Patients at Risk for Refeeding Syndrome

Elderly malnourished individuals

Postoperative patients

Patients with uncontrolled diabetes mellitus

Patients with alcoholism

Chronic users of antacids

Prolonged diuretic users

Table 7.3 Barriers Affecting Nutritional Supplementation in the ICU

Patient factors	Institutional factors
Uncertainty of feeding initiation due to resuscitation endpoint.	Perception that early feeding is not important
Degree of GI dysfunction	Relying on GRV
Intolerance to EN	Cessation due to scheduled tests or procedures
Change in patient status	Lack of specified nutrition bundles
Recommendations	
Prioritize early feeding.	
Define endpoints of resuscitation in order to begin feeds.	
GI dysfunction does not preclude feeding.	
Daily assessment of gastrointestinal function.	
Decrease reliance on GRV.	
Implement nurse-driven nutritional bundles.	

epidemic of underfeeding of patients [1]. On average, only about 50 percent of the recommended calories and proteins are administered to ICU patients. Several culprits have been identified, such as the reluctance of caregivers to initiate early feedings because of the concerns for the potential instability of the newly admitted patient, cessation of delivery for procedural reasons, nursing care, and other required tests. Perceived feeding intolerance is estimated to be inappropriate more than half the time. Intolerance misconceptions are speculative and include measurements of what is deemed high gastric volumes (GRVs) reliance, vasopressor therapy with stable blood pressure, and perceived gastric dysfunction [21]. Recent guidelines discourage the use of routinely measuring GRV because there is no evidence indicating higher rates of aspiration with high residuals. If GRV is still routinely used, then holding enteral nutrition (EN) for a GRV of less than 500 ml without signs of intolerance should be avoided. Daily assessments are crucial to identify true gastrointestinal intolerance from feedings (Figure 7.4). Recent surveys indicate that nurses

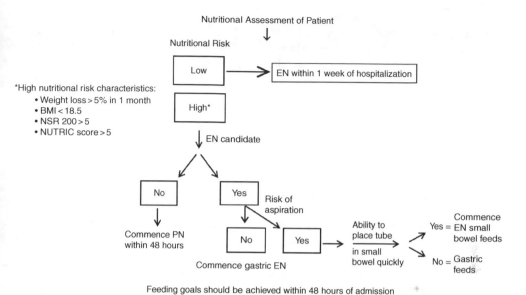

Figure 7.3 Feeding the ill elderly patient (EN = enteral nutrition).

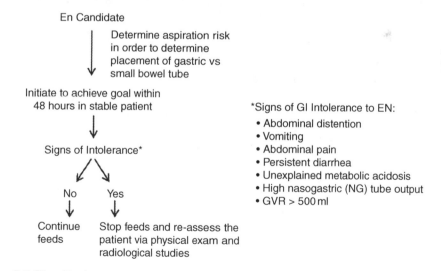

Figure 7.4 EN and intolerance assessment (EN = enteral nutrition; GRV = gastric residual volume).

solely used a GRV of greater than 200 ml as evidence of intolerance [22]. Hence a comprehensive approach using physical examination, signs and symptoms, and radiologic evaluations to determine true intolerance is required. For example, new onset of diarrhea is not a reason to discontinue EN; rather, EN should be continued while differentiating infectious versus osmotic diarrhea in a stable patient [11].

Enteral nutrition remains the standard of care for nutrition in the critically ill patient and continues to be preferred over parenteral nutrition (PN). For both practical and safety reasons, EN should be the primary mode of feeding. Accumulated evidence suggests that PN is not as deleterious as once thought [23]. Recent studies indicate that there is no difference in mortality, but EN is associated with a reduction in infectious morbidity [24]. The largest randomized, controlled trial to compare gastric versus small bowel EN found no difference in clinical outcomes [25]. Aggregated data from multiple randomized, controlled trials found a reduced risk of pneumonia with small bowel feeding, yet no difference in mortality or length of stay was seen [26]. Gastric EN to permit early feeding should be the initial approach unless the patient is deemed to be at high risk of aspiration or there is the ability for quick placement in the small bowel. Withholding EN before small bowel access is placed may be more harmful than commencing gastric EN in most patients [27].

Continuous EN of critically ill patients appears to be the global standard of care [11]. Although the alimentary tract in humans has evolved to digest intermittently, multiple animal studies suggest that a continuous approach inhibits skeletal muscle synthesis and promotes insulin resistance, which leads to muscle protein catabolism. Unfortunately, there are conflicting data regarding aspiration risk with intermittent bolus feeds [9,11]. At the time of writing, for any patient at risk for aspiration (Table 7.4), an intermittent approach to feeding cannot be recommended. Advanced age remains a risk factor for aspiration and thus makes the unstable elderly patient a nonviable candidate for bolus feeds. The potential for protein sparing and synthesis associated with intermittent bolus feeding needs further investigation and should not be cast aside without weighing the risks and benefits [28].

These recommendations apply to the general adult ICU population. Extrapolating them to the elderly ICU patient population should be done with careful consideration. Yet the general suggestions for early feeding with aggressive nutritional goal achievement (involving both calories and protein supplementation) with daily monitoring for intolerance are prudent.

Recommendations to proceed with PN depend on the nutritional status of the particular patient. For patients who are at low risk for complications related to malnutrition, withholding PN over the first 7 days of ICU admission is reasonable if EN is not possible. Yet, in a severely malnourished patient, immediate initiation of PN should be considered versus the standard therapy of withholding tube feeding for several days [28].

Some experts recommend a hybrid approach for severely malnourished elderly patients, that is, combining EN and PN to achieve nutritional goals. Guidelines caution that

Table 7.4 Factors Associated with a High Risk of Aspiration

Prolong mechanical ventilation
Age > 70 years
Neurologic deficits
Inadequate nurse-patient ratio
Supine positioning
Use of bolus intermittent EN
Severe gastroesophageal reflux

supplemental PN prior to a 7- to 10-day period in critically ill adult patients does not improve outcomes and may be detrimental [11,29,30]. Whether this approach is applicable to elderly ICU patients remains an area for investigation.

The goal for the volume of EN is to achieve greater than 80 percent of energy and protein needs within 48 hours regardless of the underlying illness. A randomized, single-center study compared trophic (i.e., low-volume EN) versus full EN supplementation during the first week of hospitalization in patients with acute respiratory distress syndrome. A lower incidence of gastrointestinal intolerance was seen in the trophic feeding group versus the full feeding group. Clinical outcomes in both groups were similar. The heterogeneity of the patient population and exclusion of malnourished patients from the design limit the conclusions and applicability of the study findings [28]. At this point, patients who present or develop acute respiratory distress syndrome or acute lung injury should not be subjected to trophic feeds unless clinically indicated by confirmed EN intolerance, especially ICU patients with underlying frailty.

The quality of evidence concerning EN formulation is sparse, especially for elderly ICU patients. The standard polymeric isotonic formula, at the moment, is one-size fit all. Other specially tailored formulas have not shown superiority over the standard polymeric isotonic formula. One exception would be the use of an immune-modulating formula in post-operative patients in the surgical ICU [11]. Emerging data suggest that targeted nutrient therapy may be beneficial in sarcopenic patients. In experimental observations, leucine supplementation promotes muscle synthesis [32]. Yet clinical observations are mixed, and such supplementation has not proven beneficial to date [33].

Muscle disuse or unloading is a common phenomenon in the critically ill elderly population. Within days, muscle unloading can lead to decrease muscle protein synthesis and skeletal mass in human models. Significant molecular changes involving decreased expression of amino acid cell membrane transports in a healthy elderly cohort after 7 days of bed rest has been observed. The obstacles of mobilizing critically ill elderly patients can be daunting due to myriad factors, yet the sequelae of prolonged bed rest and further muscle loss continue long after the patient survives the ICU [34]. Early aggressive mobilization is proven to be beneficial for ICU patients. Implementation protocols are feasible under the guidance of a multi-disciplinary team. In patients with significant disease burden (respiratory failure, shock, altered mental status), alternative nontraditional modalities should be considered, such as continuous passive motion devices and neuromuscular electrical stimulation [5].

Conclusion

The science behind nutritional support is in its infancy and continues to evolve. The current focus has revolved primarily around the adult ICU patient and has not specifically focused on the elderly ICU patient. Nutritional and metabolic derangements in the elderly stem from a predisposition for nutritional deficiencies due to physiologic changes, underlying illness, and an interplay of socioeconomic factors. These nutritional and metabolic derangements lead to frailty, further amplifying underlying comorbidities and nutritional derangements. Once a patient is admitted to the ICU, starvation is harmful, and efforts to aggressively feed these individuals are necessary. Daily assessments are mandatory to ensure that nutritional interventions are appropriate and advantageous. Ultimately, a multifaceted approach is required to address the underlying nutritional and medical derangements present because nutrition alone is insufficient.

References

1. Agarwal E, Miller M, Yaxley A, et al. Malnutrition in the elderly: a narrative review. *Maturitas* 2013; **76**:296–302.

2. Roberts S, Rosenberg I. Nutrition and aging: changes in the regulation of energy metabolism with aging. *Physiol Rev* 2006; **86**:651–67.

3. Boirie Y, Cano NJ, Caumon E, et al. Nutrition and protein energy homeostasis in elderly. *Mech Ageing Dev* 2014; **136–37**:76–84.

4. Guillet C, Prod'homme M, Balage M, et al. Impaired anabolic response of muscle protein synthesis is associated with S6K1 dysregulation in elderly humans. *FASEB J* 2004; **18**:1586–87.

5. Hanna JS. Sarcopenia and critical illness: a deadly combination in the elderly. *JPEN J Parenter Enteral Nutr* 2015; **39**:273–281.

6. Chapman I. Weight loss in older persons. *Med Clin North Am* 2011; **95**:579–93.

7. Evans W, Morley J, Argilés J, et al. Cachexia: a new definition. *Clin Nutr* 2008; **27**:793–799.

8. Muscaritoli M, Anker SD, Argilés J, et al. Consensus definition of sarcopenia, cachexia and pre-cachexia. *Clin Nutr* 2010; **29**:154.

9. Marik P. *Evidence-Based Critical Care*. New York, NY: Springer, 2015.

10. Rosenthal M, Moore F. Persistent inflammatory, immunosuppressed, catabolic syndrome (PICS): a new phenotype of multiple organ failure. *J Adv Nutr Hum Metab* 2015; **1**:1–9.

11. McClave S, Taylor B, Martindale R, et al. Guidelines for the provision and assessment of nutrition support therapy in the adult critically ill patient: Society of Critical Care Medicine (SCCM) and American Society for Parenteral and Enteral Nutrition (ASPEN). *JPEN J Parenter Enteral Nutr* 2016; **40**:159–211.

12. Lew CC, Yandell R, Fraser RJL, et al. Association between malnutrition and clinical outcomes in the intensive care unit: a systematic review. *JPEN J Parenter Enteral Nutr* 2017; **41**(5):744–58.

13. Doig G, Heighes P, Simpson F, et al. Early enteral nutrition, provided within 24 h of injury or intensive care unit admission, significantly reduces mortality in critically ill patients: a meta-analysis of randomised controlled trials. *Intensive Care Med* 2009; **35**:2018–202.

14. Raguso C, Dupertuis Y, Pichard C. The role of visceral proteins in the nutritional assessment of intensive care unit patients. *Curr Opin Clin Nutr Metab Care* 2003; **6**:211–16.

15. Davis C, Sowa D, Keim KS, et al. The use of prealbumin and C-reactive protein for monitoring nutrition support in adult patients receiving enteral nutrition in an urban medical center. *JPEN J Parenter Enteral Nutr* 2012; **36**:197–204.

16. Mourtzakis M, Wischmeyer P. Bedside ultrasound measurement of skeletal muscle. *Curr Opin Clin Nutr Metab Care* 2014; **17**:389–95.

17. Frankenfield D, Ashcraft C, Galvan D. Prediction of resting metabolic rate in critically ill patients at the extremes of body mass index *JPEN J Parenter Enteral Nutr* 2013; **37**:361–67.

18. Marik P, Zaloga G. Early enteral nutrition in acutely ill patients: a systematic review. *Crit Care Med* 2001; **29**:2264–70.

19. Abellan G. Epidemiology and consequences of sarcopenia. *J Nutr Health Aging* 2009; **13**:708–12.

20. Mehanna H, Nankivell P, Moledina J, et al. Refeeding syndrome: awareness, prevention and management. *Head Neck Oncol* 2009; **1**:4.

21. Khalid I, Doshi P, DiGiovine B. Early enteral nutrition and outcomes of critically ill patients treated with vasopressors and mechanical ventilation. *Am J Crit Care* 2010; **19**:261–68.

22. Metheny N, Stewart B, Mills A. Blind insertion of feeding tubes in intensive care units: a national survey. *Am J Crit Care* 2012; **21**:352–60.

23. Harvey S, Parrot F, Harrison DA, et al. Trial of the route of early nutritional support in critically ill adults. *N Engl J Med* 2014; **371**:1673–84.

24. Braunschweig C, Levy P, Sheean PM, et al. Enteral compared with parenteral nutrition: a meta-analysis. *Am J Clin Nutr* 2001; **74**:534–42.

25. Davies A, Morrison S, Bailey M, et al. A multicenter, randomized controlled trial comparing early nasojejunal with nasogastric nutrition in critical illness. *Crit Care Med* 2012; **40**:2342–48.

26. Kearns P, Chin D, Mueller L, et al. The incidence of ventilator-associated pneumonia and success in nutrient delivery with gastric versus small intestinal feeding: a randomized clinical trial. *Crit Care Med* 2000; **28**:1742–46.

27. Artinian V, Krayem H, DiGiovine B. Effects of early enteral feeding on the outcome of critically ill mechanically ventilated medical patients. *Chest* 2006; **129**:960–67.

28. Gazzaneo M, Suryawan A, Orellana R, et al. Intermittent bolus feeding has a greater stimulatory effect on protein synthesis in skeletal muscle than continuous feeding in neonatal pigs. *J Nutr* 2011; **141**:2152–58.

29. Heyland D, MacDonald S, Keefe L, et al. Total parenteral nutrition in the critically ill patient: a meta-analysis. *JAMA* 1998; **280**:2013–19.

30. Heidegger C, Berger M, Zingg W, et al. Optimisation of energy provision with supplemental parenteral nutrition in critically ill patients: a randomised controlled clinical trial. *Lancet* 2013; **381**:385–93.

31. Rice T, Wheeler A, Thompson BT, et al. Initial trophic vs full enteral feeding in patients with acute lung injury: the EDEN randomized trial. *JAMA* 2012; **307**:795–803.

32. Baptista I, Leal M, Artioli G, et al. Leucine attenuates skeletal muscle wasting via inhibition of ubiquitin ligases. *Muscle Nerve* 2010; **41**:800–8.

33. Bandt J, Cynober L. Therapeutic use of branched-chain amino acids in burn, trauma, and sepsis. *J Nutr* 2006; **136**:308–13.

34. Drummond M, Dickinson J, Fry CS, et al. Bed rest impairs skeletal muscle amino acid transporter expression, mTORC1 signaling, and protein synthesis in response to essential amino acids in older adults. *Am J Physiol Endocrinol Metab* 2012; **302**:1113–22.

Electrolyte and Renal Disorders in the Critically Ill Elderly

David S. Geller and Susan T. Crowley

Key Points

- There are well-described renal anatomic and physiologic adaptations associated with aging.
- While a loss of glomerular filtration rate (GFR) is not an absolute finding with aging, in general, GFR has an inverse relationship with age; estimation equations for GFR exist and should guide therapeutic decision making in the elderly with stable renal function.
- The typical renal functional changes of aging restrict the kidney's ability to maintain homeostasis in the face of physiologic challenges, resulting in an increased incidence of dysnatremias and other electrolyte disorders such as hypercalcemia and hyperkalemia.
- Acute kidney injury (AKI) is not exclusive to the elderly but is more common and is associated with an increased risk of nonrecovery of renal function in the aged compared with the young.
- A host of cellular mechanisms associated with senescence may collectively increase the risk of AKI and retard the regenerative capacity of the kidney, limiting renal recovery from AKI in the aged.
- The hazard of a renal biopsy is not increased by age itself, and specimen quality is not diminished; thus, in situations of diagnostic uncertainty of AKI, renal biopsy should not be withheld in the elderly because it may offer high diagnostic yield and effectively guide therapeutic treatment strategy.
- The mainstay of renal replacement therapy in the elderly is prevention of complications, particularly those related intradialytic hemodynamic instability and malnutrition.
- Current guidelines pertaining to the management of patients with AKI are age agnostic, yet elderly patients do have an increased risk of AKI and persistent renal dysfunction. This disconnect underscores the need for further research to establish evidenced-based critical care management strategies of the very elderly with AKI.

Introduction

Renal dysfunction is common in the critically ill elderly. In contrast, an understanding of the mechanisms contributing to this dysfunction is limited. Adopting a Bayesian approach, whereby available knowledge of normal renal senescence and acute kidney injury in the critically ill population are considered, the expected disruptions to renal homeostasis in the hospitalized elderly with life-threatening illness can be predicted and mitigated.

Renal Function and Aging: Epidemiology

A reduction in glomerular filtration rate (GFR) in the elderly compared with younger people was noted more than 60 years ago and has been confirmed by numerous subsequent studies [1]. In healthy adults, the average loss of GFR with increasing age is estimated to be approximately 0.75 ml/min per year [2]. Closer inspection, however, shows substantial heterogeneity in GFR loss across as well as within age strata. For example, a substantially higher rate of GFR decline is described in older healthy adults (40–80 years of age) compared with younger individuals (1.51 versus 0.26 ml/min, respectively) [2]. In addition, there is variation in the rate of decline within elderly cohorts, with over one-third of subjects manifesting no decrement in renal function with age [2,3], even when using GFR estimation equations in lieu of creatinine clearance [4] and among the "oldest old" [5]. Not surprisingly, the rate of decline of GFR in older populations that include subjects with comorbidities is substantially higher than the average reported for healthy cohorts, approximating 2.6 ml/min per year [6].

Thus, with aging, loss of GFR is not an absolute finding. Rather, there is variation in the decline in GFR with aging, with some healthy adults maintaining GFR, whereas in most adults the GFR declines at 1 ml/min per year and perhaps faster in the presence of additional comorbidities.

Estimating Renal Function in the Elderly

While serum creatinine (SCr) remains the most commonly used biomarker for estimating GFR, reduced dietary protein intake and changes in body composition with aging (e.g., sarcopenia) both reduce SCr. As a consequence, reliance on SCr alone leads to overestimation of GFR, and the presence of renal disease can be missed even when the SCr is within the laboratory reference range. This has led to a search for more reliable biomarkers of GFR as well as the development of equations with less variability in GFR estimation.

The Cockcroft-Gault (C-G) formula estimates creatinine clearance (eCrCl) using an equation derived from a small study of Caucasian men aged 18 to 92 years, with and without chronic kidney disease (CKD) [7]. As is true for measured urinary creatinine clearance, eCrCl typically overestimates GFR due to tubular secretion of creatinine.

Despite this limitation, for drug dosing, the eCrCl is the historical equation of choice for all ages, including the elderly. This is because eCrCl *underestimates* renal function [8] relative to the other commonly used GFR estimation equations (e.g., the Modification of Diet in Renal Disease [MDRD] formula, discussed below) [9]. GFR underestimation is especially preferred in the elderly because additional factors associated with aging may increase a drug's pharmacologic activity and toxicity (e.g., altered volume of distribution, reduced serum albumin concentration, changes in tubular handling). Because these latter factors are not considered when dosing a drug based on GFR alone, the more conservative GFR estimation approach to dosing is recommended.

The second SCr-based GFR estimation equation, widely adopted for laboratory core-porting of GFR along with SCr, is the Modification of Diet in Renal Disease (MDRD) formula. Generated from the Modification of Diet in Renal Disease study, it is derived from a population of predominantly Caucasian nondiabetic US adults from 18 to 70 years of age with an eGFR of less than 60 ml/min/1.73 m^2 [10]. While reportedly "suitable for use across populations with chronic kidney disease (CKD)" [11] and more accurate for estimating GFR in the elderly than eCrCl, in the absence of a study specifically validating its performance in the elderly, this claim remains debatable [8].

A third eGFR method, the Chronic Kidney Disease Epidemiology Collaboration (CKD-EPI) equation, is derived from the Chronic Kidney Disease Epidemiology Collaborative – a large (>10,000 subjects) racially and ethnically diverse population of men and women with and without CKD and diabetes [12]. In lieu of SCr, cystatin can be substituted as the serum biomarker. Regardless of the biomarker used, its relative precision as compared with the MDRD equation for estimating renal function in elderly patients with a GFR greater than 60 ml/min/1.73 m^2 remains to be determined.

Regardless of the formula used, all eGFR equations assume stability of SCr at the time of measurement, and thus laboratory-reported eGFR should be cautiously interpreted in patients with rapidly changing kidney function. Care is also warranted in the interpretation of GFR in the critically ill, where variable creatinine generation rates violate a second assumption of SCr-based equations. Further, SCr-based estimation of GFR may be inaccurate in patients with reduced muscle mass and those with irregular dietary intake, blood loss, or significant volume infusion, all of which are often seen in the elderly and/or critically ill [13].

Kidney Changes in Aging

The renal changes of aging are manifest throughout the nephron and are both structural and functional. Functionally, the aging renal vasculature demonstrates reduced endothelial cell capacity for nitric oxide production, as well as increased sensitivity to endothelin-1 and angiotensin II [14]. The elasticity of blood vessels also diminishes with age. The net result is a predictable rise in systolic arterial blood pressure (BP) with a widening of pulse pressure with progressive age [15]. Structurally, renal arteriolar hyalinosis accompanies the functional vascular changes of aging, with the relative contribution of hypertension versus aging as drivers of its development still under debate [15].

The restricted ability of the aging renal vasculature to effectively modulate blood flow in response to dynamic changes in arterial pressure results in increased glomerular capillary hydraulic pressure. Progressive glomerular sclerosis ensues, especially in the renal cortex, resulting in a loss of nearly 7,000 glomeruli per year after age 18 [16]. The involution of glomeruli results in atrophy of both afferent and efferent arterioles. As a consequence, the peritubular capillary density is eroded, and tubular atrophy and interstitial fibrosis become manifest. In juxtamedullary glomeruli, tuft sclerosis results in the development of direct arteriovenous shunts (*aglomerular arterioles*), accounting for the relative preservation of medullary blood flow in the senescent kidney [16]. Combined, the anatomic changes of aging result in reduced renal mass after the fourth decade, with cortical volume loss exceeding that of the medulla, and an average mass of less than 300 g by 80 years of age [16].

The tubular loss and interstitial fibrosis due to aging contribute to a variety of salt and water syndromes that are commonly manifest in the hospitalized as well community-dwelling elderly – notably the dysnatremias, hyperkalemia, and hypercalcemia.

Hypernatremia

Hypernatremia ($SNa^+ > 145$ mEq/liter) is relatively common in hospitalized patients with a reported incidence of roughly 1 percent in hospitalized patients as well as in long-term care facilities [17–19]. Hypernatremia is associated with substantial in-hospital mortality – up to 40 to 55 percent [17,18,20], although it should be noted that the mortality is typically related to the underlying disease process rather than the hypernatremia itself [19].

Hypernatremia is especially prevalent in the elderly; the mean age of patients admitted with this diagnosis is typically in the mid-70s [17,20]. Physiologic factors that predispose aging individuals to hypernatremia include the impaired renal concentration mechanisms that occur with age. Whereas young adults can achieve a urinary osmolality as high as 1,200 mOsm/kg, older individuals can achieve a maximum concentration of only 700 to 800 mOsm/kg [21]. Arginine vasopressin (AVP) levels are elevated in older individuals subjected to water deprivation, suggesting that the concentration deficit is due to renal tubular changes and not central deficiencies in osmoregulation. Studies in experimental animals suggest that this defect relates to decreased AVP-induced cyclic AMP generation and a consequent decrease in aquaporin expression [21–23]. In addition to these renal tubular epithelial (RTE) changes, healthy and cognitively intact elderly individuals do not have an adequate thirst response to water deprivation compared with younger subjects [22], and the risk is even greater in demented individuals [24].

Other clinical risk factors associated with hypernatremia in the elderly include female gender, age greater than 85 years, having more than four chronic conditions, limited mobility, infections, and altered mental status [19]. Additional contributing factors common in the elderly include febrile illness, diabetes, diarrhea, diuretics, gastrointestinal (GI) bleed, and intravenous (IV) solute [18], and a voluntary decrease in fluid intake due to concerns about urinary incontinence [19]. Increased water loss may be particularly problematic during the summer months [17]. Finally, hypernatremia may occur due to increased osmotic intake, whether via increased sodium/solute intake in patients with limited fluid intake or develop iatrogenically via the provision of hypertonic IV infusions, such as the use of IV bicarbonate in patients receiving cardiopulmonary resuscitation [19].

While the elderly are at particular risk of hypernatremia, the management of hypernatremia in the elderly does not differ substantially from that in any age group. The reader is thus referred to a general review of its management [25].

Hyponatremia

As with hypernatremia, renal functional changes leave elderly patients susceptible to hyponatremia. Hyponatremia is common in the elderly population, especially in institutionalized patients, in whom the prevalence is more than double that of age-matched ambulatory adults (18 versus 8 percent). Remarkably, 53 percent of nursing home denizens, particularly those with central nervous system or spinal cord lesions, experienced at least

Table 8.1 Pathophysiologic Mechanisms That Drive the Nonosmotic Release or Increased Effect of Vasopressin

- Release due to low effective circulating volume.
- Nonspecific stimuli, such as anxiety, stress, pain, and nausea.
- Drugs.
- Ectopic vasopressin (e.g., small cell lung cancer).
- Activating mutations in the vasopressin-2 receptor.
- Factors that increase the renal effects of vasopressin (e.g., cyclophosphamide).
- A reset Osmostat has been observed in certain types of dementia (e.g., multiple system atrophy, Lewy body dementia).

one episode of clinical hyponatremia in the preceding year [26], increasing the risk of hospitalization by 10 percent with a fourfold increased risk of an adverse outcome in hospitalized patients [27].

Clinically, the presentation of patients with hyponatremia depends not only on the severity of the hyponatremia but also on the rate at which it develops. Symptoms are often observed in cases of acute hyponatremia (i.e., the development of hyponatremia in < 48 hours). Patients with mild acute hyponatremia (SNa^+ = 130–134 mmol/liter) may be asymptomatic or may report anorexia, cramping, headache, or irritability. Moderate acute hyponatremia (SNa^+ = 125–129 mmol/liter) may lead to disorientation, confusion, weakness, or lethargy. Acute severe hyponatremia (SNa^+ < 125 mmol/liter) can lead to nausea, vomiting, seizures, coma, respiratory arrest, or permanent brain damage [21,28].

Previously believed to be inconsequential, hyponatremia is, to the contrary, associated with a significant increase in the risk of fracture in the elderly [29–32], independent of the presence of osteoporosis [32]. Likely contributors to this heightened fracture risk include increased gait instability, attention deficits, and falls [30]. The identification of such neurologic deficits raises the question of whether hyponatremia is truly benign in the elderly and whether more aggressive management of the hyponatremia should be considered [33].

Elevated vasopressin levels are overwhelmingly present in hospitalized patients with hyponatremia [34]. A number of pathophysiologic mechanisms drive the nonosmotic release or increased effect of vasopressin, many of which are more likely to be present in the elderly [21,35] (Table 8.1).

Management of Hyponatremia

The management of hyponatremia in the elderly patient is similar to that in other adults, and thus the reader is referred to recent guidelines for detailed recommendations [36]. Noteworthy is that the most dreaded complication of hyponatremia, brain herniation, typically occurs with the development of hyponatremia during rapid cerebral uptake of water. Because this more often occurs in settings of excessive water intake (e.g., marathon running, ecstasy use), it is less common in the elderly.

In contrast, the elderly more often present with chronic hyponatremia and are at risk of iatrogenic injury from overly rapid correction of hyponatremia. Patients with liver disease, alcoholism, hypokalemia, malnutrition, or a SNa$^+$ of less than 105 mEq/liter seem to be at particular risk of overly rapid correction. Current recommendations are that asymptomatic patients with chronic hyponatremia have their SNa$^+$ corrected by no more than 6 to 8 mEq/liter per day because rare cases of osmotic demyelination have been reported with correction rates as low as 10 mEq/liter per day [37]. A minimum correction of 4 to 8 mEq/liter per day has been advocated as well.

Patients who develop severe hyponatremia (SNa$^+$ < 120 mEq/liter) due to chronic thiazide use or hypovolemia are at particular risk of overly rapid correction. This is a consequence of a spontaneous aquaresis following volume-deficit correction. Also at high risk of overcorrection are patients whose hyponatremia develops as a result of cortisol deficiency or chronic desmopressin use. In such patients, therapeutic interventions to prevent rapid overcorrection are indicated. Serum Na$^+$ and urine volume should be monitored every 4 to 6 hours. If the daily target has been achieved, further correction of the serum Na$^+$ level via ongoing urinary water loss should be avoided by replacing it 1:1 with oral water or 5% dextrose or by parenteral desmopressin administration [36]. If the daily correction target has been exceeded, a relowering of the serum Na$^+$ level via water provision and use of desmopressin is recommended [36].

Hyperkalemia

Hyperkalemia is another frequent electrolyte disorder of the elderly due to renal functional changes with aging. The decline in GFR with age predisposes elderly patients to hyperkalemia but is typically not sufficient to cause hyperkalemia until the GFR is less than 30 ml/min, suggesting that disorders in tubular function contribute to the propensity to hyperkalemia as well. A number of mechanisms inhibit the distal nephron's ability to secrete potassium. Urinary tract obstruction, common among elderly males, triggers hyperkalemic renal tubular acidosis via a disruption of distal nephron potassium secretion [38]. Aldosterone is an important secretagogue of potassium in the distal nephron, but hyporeninemia, occurring as a by-product of the normal aging process or as a consequence of diabetes mellitus [39], may lead to hypoaldosteronemia. Certain medications, including nonsteroidal anti-inflammatory drugs, cyclooxygenase II inhibitors, and β-adrenergic blocking drugs, suppress renin secretion as well [40–43]. Selective hypoaldosteronism has also been described in association with amyloidosis, Sjögren syndrome, and cases of metastatic carcinoma to the adrenal gland [44–47] and is a well-known side effect of ketoconazole [39] and long-term heparin use [48]. Hyperkalemia is a common side effect of angiotensin-converting enzyme inhibitors, angiotensin-receptor blockers, and direct renin inhibitors. Amiloride and spironolactone directly antagonize the ability of the principal cell to secrete potassium, an activity shared by the antibacterial agent trimethoprim [43].

Potassium excretion in the distal nephron requires adequate sodium delivery and fluid flow [49]. Effective circulating volume depletion, either by hypovolemia (in the setting of diarrhea, sepsis, or liver disease or diuretic use) or hypervolemia (as seen with congestive heart failure) may lead to inadequate distal nephron sodium delivery, thus impairing the kidney's ability to secrete potassium. Similarly, flow-sensitive channels in the distal nephron secrete potassium in response to high urine flow – failure to maintain high flow due to hypovolemia or inadequate fluid intake will similarly compromise renal potassium excretion [43]. Elderly patients often avoid excess fluid intake either due to impaired thirst mechanisms or due to concerns about frequent urination or incontinence and thus may be at particular risk for hypovolemia, thus impairing the kidney's ability to secrete potassium.

Management of Hyperkalemia

Management of hyperkalemia in the elderly is similar to that in other adults, but with some important caveats. First, elderly patients with underlying cardiac disease or abnormal baseline electrocardiograms (ECGs) may experience a life-threatening conduction delay despite the absence of typical hyperkalemic ECG changes [50]. Second, nebulized β-agonists (10–20 mg) typically increase blood pressure and heart rate and thus are not recommended in elderly patients with coronary artery disease [50]. A combination of intravenous insulin (10–20 units) with 50 g of glucose is effective at inducing cellular uptake of potassium and is preferred in elderly patients. Sodium bicarbonate may also encourage cellular uptake of potassium, but its use should be reserved for patients with a severe metabolic acidosis who can tolerate a sodium load [50].

Ultimately, management of the hyperkalemia requires removal of excess potassium from the body. The use of potassium-binding resins such as sodium polystyrene sulfonate or patiromer may serve to facilitate colonic potassium excretion while waiting for dialysis to be initiated [39].

Hypercalcemia

The elderly are also at increased risk for is hypercalcemia. In the Netherlands, the overall incidence of hypercalcemia in elderly women is 3 percent, and severe hypercalcemia ($Ca^{2+} >$ 14 mg/dl) accounts for 3 percent of hospital admissions from the emergency department. Most cases are due to either primary hyperparathyroidism or malignancy, both of which occur with increasing incidence in the elderly [21]. In addition to these causes, the elderly are susceptible to hypercalcemia because of immobility, use of predisposing medications, and effective circulating volume depletion [21].

Hypercalcemia should be considered in any elderly patient presenting with decreased mental status. The diagnosis can be confirmed by measuring the ionized calcium level, important because a low serum albumin level may conceal the presence of hypercalcemia. If confirmed, a physical examination looking for evidence of volume depletion, neck masses, lymph nodes, or other signs of malignancy is essential. The evaluation and management of hypercalcemia are similar to those of other adults. Medications frequently prescribed to elderly individuals that predispose to hypercalcemia or potentiate its adverse effects include thiazides, vitamin D, vitamin A, calcium supplements, tamoxifen, and digoxin.

Severe hypercalcemia ($SCa^{2+} > 14$ mg/dl) or hypercalcemia with associated mental status changes requires urgent therapy. Because patients are often volume depleted due to the inhibitory effects of calcium on renal tubular sodium resorption, initial therapy for hypercalcemia normally involves volume repletion with IV normal saline at high rates (200–300 ml/h) [51]. Elderly patients are more likely to have a history of cardiovascular disease and thus need careful monitoring for signs of pulmonary congestion during fluid resuscitation. The reader is referred to further references for a detailed discussion of the use of loop diuretics, glucocorticoids, bisphosphonates and calcitonin in the management of hypercalcemia [51].

The Aging Kidney in Critical Illness: Epidemiology of Acute Kidney Injury in the Intensive Care Unit (ICU)

By far the most common renal manifestation described during critical illness is that of acute kidney injury (AKI). Defined as an abrupt increase in serum creatinine and/or onset of oliguria, AKI is identified disproportionately among the aged [52]. The most commonly reported cause of AKI in the critically ill is acute tubular necrosis (ATN), which may be secondary to absolute or relative renal parenchymal hypoperfusion, inflammation, and/or toxic injury [53,54].

Rodent models of ischemia-reperfusion AKI support an increased susceptibility of the aged animal to renal injury [55]. The human equivalent of an ischemia-reperfusion model occurs with renal transplantation. It is noteworthy that in this model, delayed graft function following renal transplantation is twofold higher in kidneys from older living donors compared with kidneys from younger donors, suggesting enhanced susceptibility of the aged kidney to injury and/or impaired recovery capability [55]. In addition, among hospitalized Medicare beneficiaries, the rate of AKI increases with age [56], with the most elderly (i.e., those 85 or more years of age) having nearly fourfold the rate of first hospitalization with AKI compared with the cohort of 66- to 69-year-olds [57]. Curiously, the rate of dialysis-requiring AKI is the same across all age-stratified Medicare cohorts, suggesting either a higher threshold for offering dialysis to the very elderly or a higher rate of declining dialysis to the very elderly with AKI. The substantially higher rate (~30 percent) of renal nonrecovery in older cohorts with AKI versus younger cohorts suggests greater injury and/or lower renal regenerative capacity in older subjects [55,57] Additionally, the risk of more severe and/or recurrent AKI is increased with age, lending further credence to the hypothesis that senescence is associated with increased risk of renal injury [52,57].

Kidney Adaptability in the Aged

The changes in renal tubular epithelial (RTE) cells that occur with senescence provide an explanation as to why there may be limited recovery from injury with advancing age. In response to stress, both non-telomerase- and telomerase-dependent pathways are activated in the aging RTE cell, resulting in an increased propensity for RTE cell cycle arrest. Aging kidney cells also demonstrate increased basal as well as stress-induced rates of apoptosis linked to alterations in the caspase cascade, which contributes to limited capability for RTE cellular repair. Diminished Klotho expression, associated with aberrations in Wnt signaling, is also linked to the reduced proliferative potential of the senescent cell. Lastly, age-related changes in macrophage-modulated RTE cell response to stress (*immunosenescence*) may also be an important determinant of recovery from AKI [55]. Collectively, these mechanisms of senescence interact to effectively retard the regenerative capacity of the RTE cell and hence limit renal recovery from AKI in the aged.

Management of AKI in Elderly with Critical Illness

Renal Biopsy and Renal Replacement Therapy (RRT)

Uncertainty about the cause of AKI is a common reason for pursuing a renal biopsy, particularly in the elderly, where AKI is the indication in nearly one-quarter of renal biopsies performed, in contrast to less than 10 percent in younger subjects [58]. The hazard of a renal biopsy is not increased by age itself, and the quality of the specimen obtained is not diminished [58]. In addition, the presumed clinical etiology of AKI in the elderly may be incorrect in the majority of the cases, making the diagnostic benefit of a biopsy substantial [59]. Therefore, renal biopsy should be considered in the elderly with AKI of unexplained origin or unrelenting duration [58]. Renal biopsy is also advisable if there is high potential for adverse effects related to empirical therapeutic treatment strategies and to exclude the possibility of an unanticipated superimposed cause of AKI such as drug-induced interstitial nephritis, which may require additional treatment [58,59].

Hemodialysis and hemofiltration therapies are the mainstay of RRT in the ICU. All forms of RRT incur risks for iatrogenic complications, the magnitude of which may be heightened in the elderly patient. First, each modality of RRT can result in hemodynamic instability and arrhythmia, particularly with intermittent hemodialysis (IHD) because of its shortened treatment time, high ultrafiltration rates, and rapid electrolyte flux. This is also especially true in the elderly with reduced cardiovascular reserve [60]. Second, because RRT incurs obligate nutrient loss, it can exacerbate existing nutritional deficiencies in the elderly. Further, because RRT itself is a catabolic process, it can fuel the excess catabolism of critical illness. Finally, all forms of RRT require central venous catheter (CVC) access, which in combination with the immunosuppression of uremia and perhaps advanced age incurs an increased risk of serious infection in the aged requiring acute RRT.

The mainstay of RRT in the elderly, then, is prevention of complications. Intradialytic hemodynamic instability is to be avoided by tempering ultrafiltration (UF) rates, establishing reasonable UF goals, and minimizing patient–dialysate electrolyte differentials. Careful attention to nutritional status and repletion of dialyzable essential vitamins and nutrients, as well as fastidious CVC care, are essential [60].

Conclusion

In summary, there are anatomic and functional renal changes that occur with aging, predisposing the elderly to detrimental electrolyte disorders and AKI, particularly in the critical care setting. The increased manifestation of renal dysfunction in the aged is a consequence of the progressive loss of renal resilience with senescence. The result is a constricted ability to maintain renal homeostasis in the face of critical illness. Enhanced awareness of the increased risk for AKI and electrolyte disorders in the elderly permits the implementation of preventative strategies to safeguard against their development in the ICU. The judicious use of eGFR equations and renal biopsy enhances the recognition of renal dysfunction in the elderly and may be useful in the early identification of potentially reversible causes of renal injury. The management of AKI requiring RRT centers on preventing hemodynamic instability, malnutrition, and infectious complications. Additional health services research targeting the clinical management of the elderly in the ICU is needed to define best practices for the prevention of adverse patient and renal outcomes.

References

1. Smith HW. *The Kidney: Structure and Function in Health and Disease* (Oxford Medical Publications). New York: Oxford University Press, 1951: xxii, 1049.

2. Lindeman RD, Tobin J, Shock NW. Longitudinal studies on the rate of decline

in renal function with age. *J Am Geriatr Soc* 1985; **33**(4):278–85.

3. Jiang S, et al. Age-related change in kidney function, its influencing factors, and association with asymptomatic carotid atherosclerosis in healthy individuals: a 5-year follow-up study. *Maturitas* 2012; **73** (3):230–38.

4. Wetzels JF, et al. Age- and gender-specific reference values of estimated GFR in Caucasians: the Nijmegen Biomedical Study. *Kidney Int* 2007; **72**(5):632–37.

5. Feinfeld DA, et al. Sequential changes in renal function tests in the old: results from the Bronx Longitudinal Aging Study. *J Am Geriatr Soc* 1995; **43**(4): 412–14.

6. Lauretani F, et al. Plasma polyunsaturated fatty acids and the decline of renal function. *Clin Chem* 2008; **54**(3):475–81.

7. Cockcroft DW, Gault MH. Prediction of creatinine clearance from serum creatinine. *Nephron* 1976; **16**(1):31–41.

8. Bolignano D, et al. The aging kidney revisited: a systematic review. *Ageing Res Rev* 2014; **14**:65–80.

9. Berman N, Hostetter TH. Comparing the Cockcroft-Gault and MDRD equations for calculation of GFR and drug doses in the elderly. *Natl Clin Pract Nephrol* 2007; **3** (12):644–45.

10. Levey AS, et al. A more accurate method to estimate glomerular filtration rate from serum creatinine: a new prediction equation. Modification of Diet in Renal Disease Study Group. *Ann Intern Med* 1999; **130**(6):461–70.

11. National Kidney Disease Education Program. *Estimation of Kidney Function for Prescription Medication Dosage in Adults*. Bethesda, MD: National Institute of Diabetes and Digestive and Kidney Diseases, 2015.

12. Levey AS, et al. A new equation to estimate glomerular filtration rate. *Ann Intern Med* 2009; **150**(9):604–12.

13. Poggio ED, et al. Performance of the Cockcroft-Gault and modification of diet in renal disease equations in estimating

GFR in ill hospitalized patients. *Am J Kidney Dis* 2005; **46**(2):242–52.

14. Yoon HE, Choi BS. The renin-angiotensin system and aging in the kidney. *Korean J Intern Med* 2014; **29**(3):291–95.

15. Del Giudice A, Pompa G, Aucella F. Hypertension in the elderly. *J Nephrol* 2010; **23**(Suppl 15):S61–71.

16. Schlanger L. *Online Curricula: Geriatric Nephrology*. American Association of Nephrology, 2009, available at www.asn-o nline.org/education/distancelearning/curri cula/geriatrics/.

17. Ates I, et al. Factors associated with mortality in patients presenting to the emergency department with severe hypernatremia. *Intern Emerg Med* 2015.

18. Snyder NA, Feigal DW, Arieff AI. Hypernatremia in elderly patients: a heterogeneous, morbid, and iatrogenic entity. *Ann Intern Med* 1987; **107** (3):309–19.

19. Adeleye O, et al. Hypernatremia in the elderly. *J Natl Med Assoc* 2002; **94**(8):701–5.

20. Long CA, et al. Hypernatraemia in an adult in-patient population. *Postgrad Med J* 1991; **67**(789):643–45.

21. AlZahrani A, Sinnert R, Gernsheimer J. Acute kidney injury, sodium disorders, and hypercalcemia in the aging kidney: diagnostic and therapeutic management strategies in emergency medicine. *Clin Geriatr Med* 2013; **29**(1):275–319.

22. Phillips PA, et al. Reduced thirst after water deprivation in healthy elderly men. *N Engl J Med* 1984; **311**(12):753–59.

23. Ledingham JG, et al. Effects of aging on vasopressin secretion, water excretion, and thirst in man. *Kidney Int Suppl* 1987; **21**: S90–92.

24. Shah, MK, Workeneh B, Taffet GE. Hypernatremia in the geriatric population. *Clin Interv Aging* 2014; **9**:1987–92.

25. Lindner G, Funk GC. Hypernatremia in critically ill patients. *J Crit Care* 2013; **28** (2):216, e11–20.

26. Miller M, Morley JE, Rubenstein LZ. Hyponatremia in a nursing home

population. *J Am Geriatr Soc* 1995; **43** (12):1410–13.

27. Choudhury M, et al. Hyponatremia in hospitalized nursing home residents and outcome: minimize hospitalization and keep the stay short! *J Am Med Dir Assoc* 2012; **13**(1):e8–9.

28. Nigro N, et al. Symptoms and characteristics of individuals with profound hyponatremia: a prospective multicenter observational study. *J Am Geriatr Soc* 2015; **63**(3):470–75.

29. Sandhu HS, et al. Hyponatremia associated with large-bone fracture in elderly patients. *Int Urol Nephrol* 2009; **41**(3):733–37.

30. Renneboog B, et al. Mild chronic hyponatremia is associated with falls, unsteadiness, and attention deficits. *Am J Med* 2006; **119**(1):71, e1–8.

31. Gankam Kengne F, et al. Mild hyponatremia and risk of fracture in the ambulatory elderly. *Q J Med* 2008; **101** (7):583–88.

32. Kinsella S, et al. Hyponatremia independent of osteoporosis is associated with fracture occurrence. *Clin J Am Soc Nephrol* 2010; **5**(2):275–80.

33. Decaux G. Is asymptomatic hyponatremia really asymptomatic? *Am J Med* 2006; **119** (7 Suppl 1):S79–82.

34. Anderson RJ, et al. Hyponatremia: a prospective analysis of its epidemiology and the pathogenetic role of vasopressin. *Ann Intern Med* 1985; **102**(2):164–68.

35. Hoorn EJ, et al. Hyponatremia due to reset osmostat in dementia with Lewy bodies. *J Am Geriatr Soc* 2008; **56**(3):567–69.

36. Verbalis JG, et al. Diagnosis, evaluation, and treatment of hyponatremia: expert panel recommendations. *Am J Med* 2013; **126**(10 Suppl 1):S1–42.

37. Ellis SJ. Severe hyponatraemia: complications and treatment. *Q J Med* 1995; **88**(12):905–9.

38. Batlle DC, Arruda JA, Kurtzman NA. Hyperkalemic distal renal tubular acidosis associated with obstructive uropathy. *N Engl J Med* 1981; **304**(7):373–80.

39. Palmer BF. Managing hyperkalemia caused by inhibitors of the renin-angiotensin-aldosterone system. *N Engl J Med* 2004; **351** (6):585–92.

40. Hay E, et al. Fatal hyperkalemia related to combined therapy with a COX-2 inhibitor, ACE inhibitor and potassium rich diet. *J Emerg Med* 2002; **22**(4):349–52.

41. Zimran A, et al. Incidence of hyperkalaemia induced by indomethacin in a hospital population. *Br Med J (Clin Res Ed)* 1985; **291**(6488):107–8.

42. Campbell WB, et al. Attenuation of angiotensin II- and III-induced aldosterone release by prostaglandin synthesis inhibitors. *J Clin Invest* 1979; **64**(6):1552–57.

43. Palmer BF, Clegg DJ. Hyperkalemia. *JAMA* 2015; **314**(22):2405–6.

44. Taylor HC, et al. Isolated hyperreninemic hypoaldosteronism due to carcinoma metastatic to the adrenal gland. *Am J Med* 1988; **85**(3):441–44.

45. Otabe S, et al. Selective hypoaldosteronism in a patient with Sjögren's syndrome: insensitivity to angiotensin II. *Nephron* 1991; **59**(3):466–70.

46. Zipser RD, et al. Hyperreninemic hypoaldosteronism in the critically ill: a new entity. *J Clin Endocrinol Metab* 1981; **53**(4):867–73.

47. Agmon D, et al. Isolated adrenal mineralocorticoid deficiency due to amyloidosis associated with familial Mediterranean fever. *Am J Med Sci* 1984; **288**(1):40–43.

48. Oster JR, Singer I, Fishman LM. Heparin-induced aldosterone suppression and hyperkalemia. *Am J Med* 1995; **98** (6):575–86.

49. Good DW, Wright FS. Luminal influences on potassium secretion: sodium concentration and fluid flow rate. *Am J Physiol* 1979; **236**(2):F192–205.

50. Perazella MA, Mahnensmith RL. Hyperkalemia in the elderly: drugs exacerbate impaired potassium homeostasis. *J Gen Intern Med* 1997; **12** (10):646–56.

51. Ariyan CE, Sosa JA. Assessment and management of patients with abnormal calcium. *Crit Care Med* 2004; **32**(Suppl 4): S146–54.

52. Wang X, Bonventre JV, Parrish AR. The aging kidney: increased susceptibility to nephrotoxicity. *Int J Mol Sci* 2014; **15** (9):15358–76.

53. Case J. et al. Epidemiology of acute kidney injury in the intensive care unit. *Crit Care Res Pract* 2013; **2013**:479730.

54. Anderson S, et al. Acute kidney injury in older adults. *J Am Soc Nephrol* 2011; **22**(1):28–38.

55. Schmitt R, Cantley LG. The impact of aging on kidney repair. *Am J Physiol Renal Physiol* 2008; **294**(6):F1265–72.

56. Xue JL, et al. Incidence and mortality of acute renal failure in Medicare beneficiaries, 1992 to 2001. *J Am Soc Nephrol* 2006; **17**(4):1135–42.

57. United States Renal Data System. *2015 USRDS Annual Data Report: Epidemiology of Kidney Disease in the United States.* Bethesda, MD: NIDDK, National Institutes of Health, 2015.

58. Di Palma AM, et al. Kidney biopsy in the elderly. *J Nephrol* 2010; **23**(Suppl 15): S55–60.

59. Haas M, et al. Etiologies and outcome of acute renal insufficiency in older adults: a renal biopsy study of 259 cases. *Am J Kidney Dis* 2000; **35**(3):433–47.

60. Santoro A, Mancini E. Hemodialysis and the elderly patient: complications and concerns. *J Nephrol* 2010; **23**(Suppl 15): S80–89.

Trauma and Musculoskeletal System Dysfunction in the Critically Ill Elderly

Felix Y. Lui and Kimberly A. Davis

Key Points

- Unintentional injury was the seventh leading cause of death in the population aged 65 years and older, and geriatric trauma patients consume a disproportionate share of healthcare costs.
- Patterns of injury differ between younger and older populations, as well as outcomes after traumatic injury.
- Alterations in cognition, vision, reflexes, muscular strength, and proprioception lead to increased rates of gait instability and subsequent falls, which contribute to an increased propensity for injury.
- Falls are the leading cause of injury and injury-related mortality for individuals older than age 75 and second only to motor vehicle collisions in those aged 65 to 74.
- Osteoporosis increases the risk of fractures and subsequent disability.
- Traumatic brain injuries (TBIs) are a significant contributor of morbidity and mortality in the elderly.
- Cervical spinal fractures are among the top five fractures in elderly patients.
- Elderly patients who sustain rib fractures have increased ventilator days, intensive care unit (ICU) and hospital lengths of stay, and rates of pneumonia and twice the mortality and thoracic morbidity than their younger counterparts.
- The annual mortality of patients older than age 80 with hip fractures is up to three times that of those without hip fractures.
- Older trauma patients have higher rates of functional impairment because of injury, requiring rehabilitation or placement in skilled care facilities.

Introduction

The aging population of the United States, coupled with increased independence and mobility of these individuals, makes traumatic injury of the elderly a challenging and growing problem in healthcare. The population aged 65 and older comprised 14.5 percent of the overall population in 2014, up from 13.0 percent in 2010, and it represents the fastest-growing segment of the population [1,2]. Accordingly, in 2014, unintentional injury was the seventh leading cause of death in the population aged 65 years and older and resulted in almost 4 million injuries and more than 865,000 hospitalizations [3].

Compared with younger patients, these elderly trauma patients tend to have longer hospital stays, greater medical expenditures, and higher mortality rates [4–6]. While accounting for one-tenth of the population, geriatric trauma patients consume a disproportionate share of healthcare costs. One-third of healthcare expenditures for trauma went toward trauma in the elderly [7]. Patterns of injury also differ between younger and older populations, as well as outcomes after traumatic injury, due to changes in function and the physiologic consequences of aging. While survival to discharge remains high, older trauma patients have higher rates of functional impairment because of injury, requiring rehabilitation or placement in skilled care facilities [8]. Understanding these challenges enables healthcare practitioners to optimize care and maximize functional outcomes and quality of life for this complex and growing population.

Physiologic Changes with Aging

A myriad of physiologic and anatomic changes occur during aging that influence patterns of injury and the ability of the body to recover from major trauma. Pretrauma frailty, which loosely correlates with age, has been shown to be a major predictor of posttraumatic injury outcomes [9,10]. Diminished reserve and impaired ability to recover from complications after injury result from the normal aging process. Understanding these changes aids in optimizing outcomes in elderly trauma patients, as well as providing guidance in planning of posttrauma rehabilitation and prognosis.

Neurologic function declines in aging, leading to increased rates of gait instability and subsequent falls in the elderly population. Alterations in cognition, vision, reflexes, muscular strength, and proprioception contribute to the propensity for injury. Cortical atrophy results in greater rates of significant brain injury due to increased shear of bridging parasagittal veins leading to subdural and subarachnoid hemorrhage. Increased mobility of the brain within the cranial vault results in higher rates of contusion and countercoup injury after blunt trauma.

Cardiovascular function and reserve also deteriorate over time due to both natural and disease-related factors. Normal aging results in cardiovascular decline due to myocyte loss with a compensatory increase in myocyte volume. The decrease in myocardial compliance results from fat cell infiltration into the ventricular walls and septum, causing decreased diastolic relaxation and slower filling. Decreased maximal cardiac output (due to a decrease in maximal heart rate with preserved stroke volume) and ejection fracture are seen with progressive aging. Loss of myocytes also leads to stiffening of large vessels, which, combined with progressive intimal hyperplasia, increases afterload and impairs early diastolic filling. Deterioration of the conducting system increases rates of arrhythmias in a patient population increasingly dependent on the atrial contribution to maintain end-diastolic volume. The increased use of beta-blockers blunts the body's response to trauma and stress and confounds evaluation for shock.

Calcification of costal cartilage and muscular atrophy contribute to decreased thoracic compliance over time. Forced vital capacity and forced expiratory volume in 1 second (FEV_1) decrease with aging. Oxygen diffusion decreases due to thickening of the alveolar basement membrane. Decreased airway sensitivity and mucociliary clearance leads to higher susceptibility to aspiration and subsequent pneumonia.

Aging is associated with progressive renal cortical loss with glomerulosclerosis and tubular senescence, resulting in decreased glomerular filtration rate and impaired reabsorption and secretion of fluids and electrolytes. Renal reserve decreases, increasing the likelihood of acute kidney injury after trauma due to relative hypoperfusion.

Progressive loss of muscle mass and strength increases the risk of injury in the aging population. Degeneration of myocytes and collagen, combined with cartilaginous and ligamentous stiffening of joints, predisposes patients to accident and injury. Osteoporosis increases the risk of fractures and subsequent disability [11].

Immunologic response to traumatic injury is blunted in the elderly population. Impaired sympathetic response and diminished thermoregulation increase the risk of complications after injury. Aging is associated with decreased immunologic function secondary to decreases in T-lymphocyte response and natural killer cell activity. An increased cytokine response occurs with aging, resulting in an increased incidence of systemic inflammatory response syndrome [12].

Mechanisms and Patterns of Injury

In the elderly, blunt mechanisms of injury predominate. In 2015, motor vehicle collisions (MVCs) were the most common mechanism of injury leading to hospitalization, with greater mortality and severity of injury among patients aged 65 or older compared with their younger counterparts [13–15]. As the population ages, the overall number of elderly drivers and passengers will continue to increase, further adding to the growing problem of elderly victims of motor vehicle–related injuries. Behavioral intervention and risk-reduction strategies are encouraging tools in the prevention of these injuries but are poorly studied [16].

Falls are the leading cause of injury and injury-related mortality for individuals over age 75 and second only to MVCs in those aged 65 to 74. Nearly 2.5 million older adults receive treatment yearly in emergency departments for falls, and yet fewer than half of falls are reported to medical personnel [17]. This results in over 700,000 hospital admissions per year, including over 250,000 for hip fractures. While most falls are from ground level, in the elderly population these are still associated with high incidences of morbidity and mortality [18].

Management of Specific Injuries

Neurotrauma

Traumatic brain injuries (TBIs) are a significant contributor of morbidity and mortality in the elderly. In a study by Haring et al. between 2000 and 2010, patients aged 65 to 69 accounted for 13.0 percent of all TBI-related hospitalizations, and patients older than age 85 accounted for 30.3 percent of all admissions. Overall mortality in this population was 11.4 percent over this study period [19]. Common injuries include subarachnoid, subdural, and epidural hemorrhages. This is due to the more adherent dura, cerebral atrophy, and cerebrovascular atherosclerosis seen during the aging process. Confounding these data are the patients who present with intracranial bleeds prior to a traumatic injury (fall, MVC, etc.), which may be mistriaged as TBIs. In addition to age-related physiologic and anatomic factors, a major contributor to TBI outcomes is the use of anticoagulants in this patient population [20]. Further confounding this issue is the rapid adoption of the use of direct oral anticoagulants (DOACs) in the elderly population. The inability to monitor the degree of anticoagulation and limited options for reversal of these agents make the management of TBI patients receiving these agents difficult. Prothrombin complex concentrate (PCC) use for the reversal of warfarin rapidly reverses coagulopathy and decrease the progression of intracranial hemorrhage, but reversal agents for DOACs are still under development and poorly studied [21,22]. Idarcizumab (Praxbind) was approved in 2015 by the Food and Drug Administration (FDA) for the reversal of dabigatran, and other agents such as andexanet alfa show promise in reversing the effects of factor Xa inhibitors [23].

Spinal Trauma

Spine trauma is a significant contributor to morbidity and mortality in the elderly. Cervical spinal fractures are among the top five fractures in elderly patients. Fractures in this population are associated with a significant rate of high cervical fractures with dens involvement. Fortunately, neurologic involvement is still infrequent [24]. Management of these fractures in the elderly is debatable. High rates of surgical complications and mortality with surgical treatment are weighed against the high rate of nonunion in older patients with cervical spine injuries treated nonoperatively with rigid cervical collars [25]. Lower spinal compression fractures are extremely common in the elderly population. Greater than one-fourth of postmenopausal women have vertebral compression fractures due to inadequate accumulation of bone mass in childhood and early adulthood and resorption after menopause. Nonoperative management, including analgesia, bracing, and physical therapy, is effective in the majority of cases, with surgery reserved for chronic, severe pain, instability, or neurologic compromise [26].

Thoracic Trauma

Elderly patients are especially susceptible to pulmonary complications after blunt thoracic trauma. Rib fractures are associated with poor outcomes. Elderly patients who sustain rib fractures have increased ventilator days, intensive care unit (ICU) and hospital lengths of stay, and rates of pneumonia and twice the mortality and thoracic morbidity than their younger counterparts. Each additional rib fracture increases mortality by 19 percent and risk of pneumonia by 27 percent [27]. Additional factors contributing to poorer outcomes in these elderly patients include decreased physiologic reserves and preexisting comorbidities but require further study [28]. Optimal pain control and pulmonary toileting are essential to optimize outcomes in these patients. In elderly patients, use of epidural analgesia over intravenous narcotic analgesia decreases morbidity, as well as hospital length of stays and overall hospital costs, but may be associated with increased deep venous thrombosis [29–31]. Frequent treatment with anticoagulants further complicates the placement of epidural and paravertebral catheters for analgesia.

Abdominal Trauma

Most intra-abdominal solid-organ injuries are managed nonoperatively. Specifically, the majority of hepatic and splenic injuries are managed with observation, with angioembolization and surgery reserved for those with active bleeding or hemodynamic instability. Risks of splenectomy include morbidity from laparotomy as well as the risk of postsplenectomy sepsis, although the true risk is unknown. Initial concerns regarding advanced age (defined as older than age 55) being a predictor of failure in nonoperative management of splenic injury have not borne out; therefore, advanced age should not be used as the sole determinant in the decision to pursue nonoperative management [32–35]. Improved imaging and interventional techniques have shown good results in the management of both liver and spleen injuries without surgical exploration. However, overall mortality for patients managed both operatively or nonoperatively is elevated compared with their younger counterparts [36]. Therefore, decision making regarding operative versus nonoperative management of solid-organ injury is based on hemodynamic status and transfusion requirements. Patients who are hemodynamically appropriate or respond rapidly to volume resuscitation are appropriate candidates for a trial of nonoperative management. These candidates require close hemodynamic monitoring, serial examinations, and hematocrit determinations. Patient who continue to have hemodynamic instability or have ongoing transfusion requirements should be managed surgically or with angiography and angioembolization.

Thermal Injury

For unclear reasons, elderly patient do particularly poorly after sustaining burn injuries [37]. The LD_{50} for burn size for patients older than age 65 has remained at 35 percent, whereas gains have in made in younger patients [38,39]. This relationship appears to be linear, however, without a clear inflection point and relates to preexisting conditions as opposed to age alone. Likely higher rates of preexisting pulmonary disease, immobility, and decreased pulmonary reserve contribute to this finding. Elderly patients have longer lengths of stays and higher rates of multisystem organ failure but not infections or sepsis. This may be explained by alterations in the inflammatory response (metabolic, glycemic, immune, wound healing) in the aging population and requires a multimodal approach [40].

Musculoskeletal Trauma

Elderly patients are at particular risk of morbidity and mortality secondary to musculoskeletal trauma. Increased risk of falls, relative skeletal fragility, degenerative joint disease, stress fractures, periprosthetic fractures, and pathologic fractures contribute to increased rates and poorer outcomes. In patients older than age 80, those with hip fractures suffer up to three times the annual mortality compared with those without hip fractures [41]. This difference in outcomes is likely due to preexisting medical comorbidities, lower bone mineral density, and less muscular mass.

Orthopedic injuries should be managed in the safest and most expedient manner. While early operative fixation (<24 hours from injury) has been shown to be beneficial in younger patients, failure to manage preexisting conditions leads to higher mortality in the elderly population [42,43]. Medical consultation, optimization of medications, and stabilization of medical condition prior to repair of orthopedic injuries (up to 72 hours) leads to better outcomes with no increase in 30-day or long-term mortality, infectious complications, myocardial infarction, or thromboembolism. Perioperative antibiotics should address coverage of *Staphylococcus aureus*, and methicillin-resistant *Staphylococcus aureus*, and *Staphylococcus epidermis* in institutions with high rates of colonization. Thromboembolic prophylaxis is an area of controversy, but current American College of Chest Physicians (ACCP) guidelines recommend use of low-molecular-weight heparin, fondaparinux, low-dose unfractionated heparin, a vitamin K antagonist, aspirin, or intermittent leg compression devices in the perioperative period [44]. Ultimately, risk of surgery must be weighed against optimizing the best chance of return to pretrauma functional status and quality of life.

Outcomes

The outcome of trauma patients is associated with the appropriate triage of patients to the appropriate facilities that are best able to manage the complexity and severity of their injuries. Patients younger than age 55 are at an increased risk of undertriage to appropriate trauma centers [45–47]. A recent study reviewing the data from the National Trauma Data Bank (NTDB) showed that elderly trauma patients who were triaged to centers that managed a higher proportion of elderly patients had a 34 percent decrease in mortality risk (odds ratio [OR] 0.66, 95 percent confidence interval [CI] 0.54–0.97) [48]. This difference appears to be attributable to the ability of high elderly volume centers to salvage elderly patients after occurrence of complications as opposed to higher initial survival after traumatic injury [49,50].

Resuscitation Goals

Cardiovascular aging contributes to the difficulties in compensating for stress and increased demands after shock and trauma. Diminished cardiac output with decreased maximal heart rate, in addition to common use of antihypertensive and heart rate–controlling medications, makes the diagnosis of shock and hypoperfusion challenging in this population. In a prospective, randomized trial of elderly hip fracture patients, early use of invasive monitoring with pulmonary artery catheters was shown to decrease mortality rates [51]. Increased base deficit (−6 mEq/liter or less) or lactic academia (>2.2 mg/dl) has been shown to be associated with increased mortality [52,53]. Early use of pulmonary artery catheters to guide resuscitation to target cardiac indices or oxygen consumption may be beneficial in optimizing outcomes, but recent intraoperative studies suggest that goal-directed resuscitation appears to be less effective in elderly patients [54,55].

Contribution of Frailty to Outcome

Research involving the geriatric trauma population is difficult to interpret. There is a lack of consensus on the definition and characteristics of geriatric trauma patients and a lack of randomized, prospective, controlled trials examining this age group specifically. The overall mortality rate for elderly trauma patients is approximately 15 percent [56]. This rate increases in a linear fashion with increasing age until age 84, after which rates decline [57]. Research does support that advanced age alone is not a predictor of poor outcomes, and advanced age should not be used as the sole criterion for denying or limiting care [58]. Excellent outcomes are possible because most geriatric trauma patients return home, and up to 85 percent will return to independent function [59,60].

The presence and severity of preexisting conditions are major determinants of outcomes after trauma [61,62]. A combination of factors including preexisting conditions, medications, nutritional status, functional ability, and general state of health contributes to the ability to survive and recover from traumatic injury. Up to 38 percent of geriatric trauma patients are frail, with an increased risk of fractures and discharge to an institution.

Increasing frailty is a risk factor for postoperative morbidity, mortality, and hospital length of stay [63–66]. In geriatric trauma patients, preinjury frailty assessment, using one of a number of available tools, may be a useful predictor of postinjury functional status and mortality [67]. The Trauma-Specific Frailty Index (TSFI) uses a scale based on 50 variables associated with poorer outcomes, has been validated in a trial of 200 patients, and is a fast and reliable tool for use in trauma patients [68]. Routine assessment of pretrauma status may be a useful tool in early determination of postdischarge needs and functional recovery. While posttrauma ambulation is a significant predictor of outcomes, pretrauma ambulation status is a predictor of long-term survivorship in the elderly with hip fractures [69]. Use of tools such as the Geriatric Trauma Outcome Score {age + [2.5 × Injury Severity Score (ISS)] + 22 (if transfused packed red blood cells)} may provide a more accurate estimation of mortality after trauma [70]. Use of these scores can assist practitioners in discussions with families in determining treatments and goals of care and may help to identify patients in need of early involvement of palliative care services.

While most patients do return to independent living, a significant proportion experiences diminution in quality of life across multiple domains [71]. On average, elderly patients experience the equivalent of loss of one activity of daily living (ADL) 1 year after their injury [72]. This predisposes them to further loss of function, independence, and death. A multidisciplinary approach is required in the management of these complex patients. Early geriatric consultation can improve functional recovery after trauma injury in older patients [73].

Optimal care of these patients requires not only appropriate management of their traumatic injuries but also prevention of further injury and harm. One-third of patients over age 65 suffer a fall annually, and one-third of those either returned to the emergency department or died within 1 year [74,75]. Risk factors for additional falls include prior falls, independent living, use of walking aids, depression, cognitive deficits, and use of greater than six medications. Screening and identification of these risk factors in elderly patients may be an opportunity for intervention to prevent further falls in the future. Targeted educational programs addressing these factors prevent recurrent injury and falls and may benefit long-term outcomes [76].

Special Considerations

Elderly abuse is a common and underreported cause of significant morbidity and mortality in the elderly population. It is estimated that 10 percent of older adults are victims of abuse, but fewer than 1 in 24 cases are ever reported to the authorities [77,78]. Abuse occurs in many forms, including physical, sexual, emotional, psychological, neglect, and financial exploitation. In physical abuse, the most common injuries involve blunt trauma with fists or household objects and are reported as "falls" [79]. Injuries to the upper extremities, face, and neck are uncommon following ground-level falls but are common in victims of elder abuse [80]. Healthcare providers must maintain a low threshold for suspicion of elder abuse in order to intervene early in this vulnerable population.

Palliative Care

Excellent outcomes are possible with appropriate triage, aggressive monitoring and resuscitation, and a multidisciplinary, collaborative approach to management of these patients. Goals of care must include optimization of functional recovery and quality of life, in addition to discreet morbidity and mortality rates [81,82]. Especially in this high-risk population, reasonable discussions are necessary regarding limitations of care and withdrawal of care but are often inadequate or missing. Use of tools such as the TSFI and Geriatric Trauma Outcome (GTO) scores may help to identify patients in need of early palliative care consultation and evaluation for end-of-life needs [83]. Complex issues such as the competence of patients to partake in these discussions, surrogate decision making, minimizing suffering, and family and social dynamics all require careful consideration and measured communication. Engaging all members of the healthcare team including physicians, nurses, religious ministries, social workers, rehabilitation and physical medicine services, palliative care services, and hospital ethics committees may help to facilitate communication and decision making in difficult cases.

References

1. United States Census Bureau. *United States Quickfacts*, 2015, available at www.census .gov/quickfacts/table/PST045215/00.html (accessed January 18, 2016).

2. Campbell PR. *Population Projections for States by Age, Sex, Race and Hispanic Origin: 1995 to 2025*. Washington, DC: US Bureau of the Census, Population Division, 1996.

3. Centers for Disease Control and Prevention (CDC), Web-Based Injury Statistics Query and Reporting System (WISQAR), 2015, available at http://webappa.cdc.gov/sasweb/ ncipc/nfirates2001.html (accessed January 18, 2016).

4. Taylor MD, Tracy JK, Meyer W, Pasquale M, Napolitano LM. Trauma in the elderly: intensive care unit resource use and outcome. *J Trauma* 2002; **53**(3):407–14.

5. MacKenzie EJ, Morris JA Jr, Smith GS, Fahey M. Acute hospital costs of trauma in the United States: implications for regionalized systems of care. *J Trauma* 1990; **30**(9):1096–101; discussion 101–3.

6. Perdue PW, Watts DD, Kaufmann CR, Trask AL. Differences in mortality between elderly and younger adult trauma patients: geriatric status increases risk of delayed death. *J Trauma* 1998; **45**(4):805–10.

7. Tornetta P, Mostafavi H, Riina J, et al. Morbidity and mortality in elderly trauma patients. *J Trauma* 1999; **46**:702–6.

8. van Aalst JA, Morris JAJ, Yates HK, et al. Severely injured geriatric patients return to independent living: a study of factors influencing function and independence. *J Trauma* 1991; **31**:1096–101.

9. McDonald VS, Thompson KA, Lewis PR, et al. Frailty in trauma: a systematic review of the surgical literature for clinical assessment tools. *J Trauma Acute Care Surg* 2016.

10. Dayama A, Olorunfemi O, Greenbaum S, Stone ME Jr, McNelis J. Impact of frailty on outcomes in geriatric femoral neck fracture management: an analysis of National Surgical Quality Improvement Program dataset. *Int J Surg* 2016; **28**: 185–90.

11. Cummings SR, Melton LJ. Epidemiology and outcomes of osteoporotic fractures. *Lancet* 2002; **359**(9319):1761–67.

12. Aalami OO, Fang TD, Song HM, et al. Physiological features of aging persons. *Arch Surg* 2003; **138**:1068–76.

13. Nance ML, ed. National Trauma Data Bank Report, 2015, available at www.facs.org/~/ media/files/quality%20programs/trauma/nt db/ntdb%20annual%20report%202014 .ashx (accessed January 2016).

14. Hui T, Avital I, Soukiasian H, Margulies DR, Shabot MM. Intensive care unit outcome of vehicle-related injury in elderly trauma patients. *Am Surg* 2002; **68**(12):1111–14.

15. Mosenthal AC, Livingston DH, Lavery RF, et al. The effect of age on functional outcome in mild traumatic brain injury: 6-month report of a prospective multicenter trial. *J Trauma* 2004; **56**(5): 1042–48.

16. Crandall M, Streams J, Duncan T, et al. Motor vehicle collision-related injuries in the elderly: an Eastern Association for the Surgery of Trauma evidence-based review of risk factors and prevention. *J Trauma Acute Care Surg* 2015; **79**(1):152–58.

17. Centers for Disease Control and Prevention, National Center for Injury Prevention and Control. Web-Based Injury Statistics Query and Reporting System (WISQARS), 2016, available at www.cdc.gov/injury/wisqars/index.html.

18. Joseph B, Pandit V, Khalil M, et al. Managing older adults with ground-level falls admitted to a trauma service: the effect of frailty. *J Am Geriatr Soc* 2015; **63**:745–49.

19. Haring RS, Narang K, Canner JK, et al. Traumatic brain injury in the elderly: morbidity and mortality trends and risk factors. *J Surg Res* 2015; **195**:1–9.

20. Peck KA, Calvo RY, Schechter MS, et al. The impact of preinjury anticoagulants and prescription antiplatelet agents on outcomes in older patients with traumatic brain injury. *J Trauma Acute Care Surg* 2014; **76**:431–36.

21. Edavettal M, Rogers A, Rogers F, et al. Prothrombin complex concentrate accelerates international normalized ratio reversal and diminishes the extension of intracranial hemorrhage in geriatric trauma patients. *Am Surg* 2014; **80**:372–76.

22. Moorman ML, Nash JE, Stabi KL. Emergency surgery and trauma in patients treated with the new oral anticoagulants: dabigatran, rivaroxaban, and apixaban. *J Trauma Acute Care Surg* 2014; **77**:486–94.

23. Siegal DM, Curnutte JT, Connolly SJ, et al. Andexanet alfa for the reversal of factor Xa inhibitor activity. *N Engl J Med* 2015; **373** (25):2413–24.

24. Harris MB, Reichmann WM, Bono CM et al. Mortality in elderly patients after cervical spine fractures. *J Bone Joint Surg* 2010; **92**:567–74.

25. Delcourt R, Begue T, Saintyves G et al. Management of upper cervical spine fractures in elderly patients: current trends and outcomes. *Injury Int J Care Injured* 2015; **46**(Suppl 1):S24–27.

26. Kim DH, Vaccaro AR. Osteoporotic compression fractures of the spine: current options and considerations for treatment. *Spine J* 2006; **6**(5):479–87.

27. Bulger EM, Arneson MA, Mock CN. et al. Rib fractures in the elderly. *J Trauma* 2000; **48**(6):1040–47.

28. Bergeron E, Lavoie A, Clas D, et al. Elderly trauma patients with rib fractures are at greater risk of death and pneumonia. *J Trauma* 2003; **54**:478–85.

29. Wisner DH. A stepwise logistic regression analysis of factors affecting morbidity and mortality after thoracic trauma: effect of epidural analgesia. *J Trauma* 1990; **30**:799–804.

30. Ullman DA, Fortune JB, Greenhouse BB, et al. The treatment of patients with multiple rib fractures using continuous thoracic epidural narcotic infusion. *Reg Anesth* 1989; **14**:43–47.

31. Zaw AA, Murry J, Hoang D et al. Epidural analgesia after rib fractures. *Am Surg* 2015; **81**(10):950–54,

32. Peitzman AB, Harbrecht BG, Rivera L, Heil B. Contributions of age and gender to outcome of blunt splenic injury in adults: multicenter study of the Eastern Association for the Surgery of Trauma. *J Trauma* 2001; **51**(5):887–95.

33. Falimirski ME, Provost D. Nonsurgical management of solid abdominal organ injury in patients over 55 years of age. *Am Surg* 2000; **66**(7):631–35.

34. Cocanour CS, Moore FA, Ware DN. Age should not be a consideration for nonoperative management of blunt splenic injury. *J Trauma* 2000; **48**(4):606–10; discussion 610–12.

35. Bhangu A, Nepogodiev D, Lai N, Bowley DM. Meta-analysis of predictive factors and outcomes for the failure of non-operative management of blunt splenic trauma. *Injury* 2012; **43**(9): 1337–46.

36. Harbrecht BG, Peitzman AB, Rivera L, et al. Contribution of age and gender to outcome of blunt splenic injury in adults: a multicenter study of the Eastern

Association for the Surgery of Trauma. *J Trauma* 2001; **51**:887–95.

37. Wearn C, Hardwicke J, Kitsios A, et al. Outcomes of burns in the elderly: revised estimates from the Birmingham Burn Centre. *Burns* 2015; **41**(6):1161–68.

38. Kraft R, Herndon DN, Al-Mousawi AM, et al. Burn size and survival probability in paediatric patients in modern burn care: a prospective observational cohort study. *Lancet* 2012; **379**(9820):1013–21.

39. Pereira CT, Barrow RE, Sterns AM, et al. Age dependent differences in survival after severe burns: a unicentric review of 1,674 patients and 179 autopsies over 15 years. *J Am Coll Surg* 2006; **202**(3):536–48.

40. Jeschke MG, Patsouris D, Stanojcic M, et al. Pathophysiologic response to burns in the elderly. *EBioMedicine* 2015; **2**(10):1536–48.

41. Haentjens P, Magaziner J, Colon-Emeric CS, et al. Meta-analysis: excess mortality after hip fracture among older women and men. *Ann Intern Med* 2010; **152**:380–90.

42. Grimes JP, Gregory PM, Noveck H, et al. The effects of time-to-surgery on mortality and morbidity in patient following hip fracture. *Am J Med* 2002; **112**:702–9.

43. Kenzora JE, McCarthy RE, Lowel JD, et al. Hip fracture mortality: relation to age, treatment, preoperative illness, time of surgery and complications. *Clin Orthop* 1984; **1984**:45–56.

44. Falck-Ytter Y, Francis CW, Johanson NA et al. Prevention of VTE in orthopedic surgery patients: Antithrombotic Therapy and Prevention of Thrombosis, 9th edn: American College of Chest Physicians Evidence-Based Clinical Practice Guidelines. *Chest* 2012; **141**(Suppl 2): e278S.

45. Ma MH, MacKenzie EJ, Alcorta R, Kelen GD. Compliance with prehospital triage protocols for major trauma patients. *J Trauma* 1999; **46**:168–75.

46. Phillips S, Rond PC, Kelly SM, Swartz PD. The failure of triage criteria to identify geriatric patients with trauma: results from the Florida Trauma Triage Study. *J Trauma* 1996; **40**:278–83.

47. Zimmer-Gembeck MJ, Southard PA, Hedges JR, et al. Triage in an established trauma system. *J Trauma* 1995; **39**:922–28.

48. Zafar SN, Obirieze A, Schneider ED, et al. Outcomes of older trauma care at centers treating a higher proportion of older patients. *J Trauma Acute Care Surg* 2015; **78**(4):852–59.

49. Zafar SN, Shah AA, Zogg CK, et al. Morbidity or mortality? Variations in trauma centres in the rescue of older injured patients. *Injury* 2015, available at http://dx.doi.org/10.1016/j.injury.2015.11.044.

50. Sheetz KH, Krell RW, Englesbe MJ, et al. The importance of the first complication: understanding failure to rescue after emergent surgery in the elderly. *J Am Coll Surg* 2014; **219**(3):365–70.

51. Schultz RJ, Whitfield GF, LaMura JJ, et al. The role of physiologic monitoring in patients with fractures of the hip. *J Trauma* 1985; **25**:309–16.

52. Davis JW, Kaups KL, Base deficit in the elderly: a marker of severe injury and death. *J Trauma* 1998; **45**:873–77.

53. Schulman AM, Claridge JA, Young JS. Young versus old: factors affecting mortality after blunt traumatic injury. *Am Surg* 2002; **68**:942–47.

54. Scalea TM, Simon HM, Duncan AO, et al. Geriatric blunt multiple trauma: improved survival with early invasive monitoring. *J Trauma* 1990; **30**(2):129–34; discussion 134–36.

55. Bertha E, Arfwedson C, Imnell A, Kalman S. Towards individualized perioperative, goal-directed haemodynamic algorithms for patients of advanced age: observations during a randomized, controlled trial. *Br J Anaesth* 2016; **116**(4):486–92.

56. Hashmi A, Ibrahim-Zada I, Rhee P, et al. Predictors of mortality in geriatric trauma patients: a systematic review and meta-analysis. *J Trauma Acute Care Surg* 2014; **76**(3):894–901.

57. Friese RS, Wynne J, Joseph B, et al. Age and mortality after injury: is the association linear? *Eur J Trauma Emerg Surg* 2014; **40** (5):567–72.

58. Jacobs DG, Plaisier BR, Barie PS, et al. Practice management guidelines for geriatric trauma: the EAST Practice Management Guidelines Work Group. *J Trauma* 2003; **54**:391–416.

59. Carrillo EH, Richardson JD, Malias MA, Cryer HM, Miller FB. Long term outcome of blunt trauma care in the elderly. *Surg Gynecol Obstet* 1993; **176**(6):559–64.

60. Day RJ, Vinen J, Hewitt-Falls E. Major trauma outcomes in the elderly. *Med J Aust* 1994; **160**(11):675–78.

61. Morris JA Jr, MacKenzie EJ, Edelstein SL. The effect of preexisting conditions on mortality in trauma patients. *JAMA* 19901; **263**(14):1942–46.

62. Smith DP, Enderson BL, Maull KI. Trauma in the elderly: determinants of outcome. *South Med J* 1990; **83**(2):171–77.

63. Rockwood K, Song X, MacKnight C, et al. A global clinical measure of fitness and frailty in elderly people. *Can Med Assoc J* 2005; **173**(5):489–95.

64. Fried LP, Ferrucci L, Darer J, et al. Untangling the concepts of disability, frailty, and comorbidity: implications for improved targeting and care. *J Gerontol A Biol Sci Med Sci* 2004; **59**(3):255–63.

65. Robinson TN, Wu DS, Pointer L, et al. Simple frailty score predicts postoperative complications across surgical specialties. *Am J Surg* 2001; **213**(1):37–42.

66. Makary MA, Segev DL, Pronovost PJ, et al. Frailty as a predictor of surgical outcomes in older patients. *J Am Coll Surg* 2010; **210** (6):901–8.

67. Maxwell CA[1], Mion LC, Mukherjee K, et al. Pre-injury physical frailty and cognitive impairment among geriatric trauma patients determines post-injury functional recovery and survival. *J Trauma Acute Care Surg* 2015.

68. Joseph B, Pandit V, Zangbar B, et al. Validating trauma-specific frailty index for geriatric trauma patients: a prospective analysis. *J Am Coll Surg* 2014; **219**:10–17.

69. Iosifidis M, Iliopoulos E, Panagiotou A, et al. Walking ability before and after a hip fracture in elderly predict greater long-term survivorship. *J Orthop Sci.* 2016; **21**(1):48–52.

70. Zhao FZ, Wolf SE, Nakonezny PA, et al. Estimating geriatric mortality after injury using age, injury severity, and performance of a transfusion: the geriatric trauma outcome score. *J Palliat Med* 2015; **18**: 677–81.

71. Inaba K, Goecke M, Sharkey P, Branneman F. Long term outcomes after injury in the elderly. *Trauma* 2003; **54**(3): 486–91

72. Kelley-Quon, L., Min, L., Morley, et al. Functional status after injury: a longitudinal study of geriatric trauma. *Am Surg* 2010; **76**(10):1055–58.

73. Tillou A, Kelley-Quon L, Burruss S, et al. Long-term postinjury functional recovery: outcomes of geriatric consultation. *JAMA Surg* 2014; **149**:83–89.

74. Liu SW, Obermeyer Z, Chang Y, Shankar KN. Frequency of ED revisits and death among older adults after a fall. *Am J Emerg Med* 2015; **33**: 1012–1018.

75. Tan MP, Kamaruzzaman SB, Zakaria MI, et al. Ten-year mortality in older patients attending the emergency department after a fall. *Geriatr Gerontol Int* 2015 Jan 22. doi:10.1111/ggi.12446. [Epub ahead of print]

76. Corman, E. Including fall prevention for older adults in your trauma injury prevention program – introducing farewell to falls. *J Trauma Nurs.* 2009; **16**(4): 206–7.

77. Acierno R, Hernandez MA, Amstadter AB, et al. Prevalence and correlates of emotional, physical, sexual, and financial abuse and potential neglect in the United States: the National Elder Mistreatment Study. *Am J Public Health* 2010; **100**: 292–97.

78. Pillemer K, Finkelhor D. The prevalence of elder abuse: a random sample survey. *Gerontologist* 1988; **28**:51–57.

79. Friedman LS, Avila S, Tanouye K, et al. A case-control study of severe physical abuse of older adults. *J Am Geriatr Soc* 2011; **59**:417–22.

80. Rosen T, Bloemen EM, LoFaso VM, et al. Emergency department presentations for injuries in older adults independently known to be victims of elder abuse. *J Emerg Med* 2016.

81. Peschman J, Brasel K. End-of-life care of the geriatric surgical patient. *Surg Clin North Am* 2015; **95**:191–202.

82. Stevens Cl, Torke AM. Geriatric trauma: a clinical and ethical review. *J Trauma Nurs* 2016; **23**(1):36–41.

83. Huijberts S, Buurman BM, de Rooij SE. End-of-life care during and after an acute hospitalization in older patients with cancer, end-stage organ failure, or frailty: a sub-analysis of a prospective cohort study. *Palliat Med* 2016; **30**(1):75–82.

Chapter 10

Immune Response and Infections in the Elderly

Nicole Bryan and Arif R. Sarwari

Key Points

- The study of the aging immune system is currently in its early phases, and the term *immunosenescence* has been used to identify this phenomenon.
- For individuals older than age 65, infections are a major source of morbidity and mortality.
- The innate immune system consists of neutrophils and macrophages, epithelial barriers, natural killer cells, dendritic cells, complement proteins, and the nonspecific defenses such as the production of mucus and antimicrobial peptides and mucociliary function. With aging, changes in the innate immune system result in chronic inflammation.
- The adaptive immune system consists of B and T lymphocytes, which, respectively, affect humoral and cellular immune responses. Both show age-related decreases in number and diversity.
- The impact of aging seems to be larger on the adaptive immune system than on the innate immune system.
- Elderly patients frequently demonstrate diminished protection following receipt of routine vaccinations compared with younger populations.

Introduction

With an aging global population, the geriatric patient is increasingly likely to be encountered not only in the ambulatory setting but also in the critical care units. The study of the aging immune system is currently in its early phases, but there is some consensus on its impact on infection, malignancy, and autoimmunity. The term *immunosenescence* has been used to identify this phenomenon. Of note, it is difficult to separate a true change in immune function from other fundamental host defenses associated with aging. These defenses include alterations in barriers such as the skin, decreased acidity of the stomach, impairment in mucociliary clearance in the airways, impaired cough reflexes, malnutrition, changes in the urinary stream causing obstruction, and the impact of other comorbidities such diabetes. Of these, malnutrition has the potential to have a significant impact on immunosenescence and is not uncommon in the geriatric population.

To better understand the aging immune system, it can be subdivided into the traditional categories of an innate (neutrophils, macrophages, etc.) and adaptive system (B and

T lymphocytes, immunoglobulins, etc.). While both are affected by aging, the impact seems to be larger on the adaptive system. However, there is some impact of aging on both neutrophil and macrophage oxidative burst and phagocytic activity.

The innate immune system, in addition to neutrophils and macrophages, consists of our epithelial barriers, natural killer cells, dendritic cells, complement proteins, and the nonspecific defenses such as the production of mucus and antimicrobial peptides and mucociliary function. With aging, changes in the innate immune system result in chronic inflammation. The adaptive immune system may be simplistically thought of as consisting of B and T lymphocytes, which, respectively, affect humoral and cellular immune responses. Both show age-related decreases in number and diversity.

Immunosenescence

The aging process is accompanied by a decline in numerous physiologic activities, and the immune system is no exception. The gradual deterioration in physiologic functions is referred to as *senescence*, which is derived from the Latin term *senescere*, meaning "to grow old." The term *immunosenescence* refers to the alterations in immune system function that occur because of the normal biologic aging process, independent of any underlying diseases. This process affects all facets of the immune system, including both the innate and adaptive responses, with significant clinical implications in the development of infection, responsiveness to vaccination, and malignancy [1].

For individuals older than age 65, infections are a major source of morbidity and mortality. Interestingly, not all components of the immune system are adversely affected. Specifically, the ability to mount an effective response against previously encountered infectious organisms appears to remain intact, whereas activation of the immune system when faced with a novel pathogen diminishes over time. Clinically, these changes may manifest as deviations from the typical presentation of severe infection, including lack of fever in up to 30 percent of patients [2] as well as few localizing signs, and instead present with nonspecific symptoms including altered mental status, generalized weakness, and falls [3]. These findings likely represent a diminished capacity to mount an inflammatory response in response to an infection.

The decreased responsiveness of the aging immune system to novel infectious agents also carries implications for vaccination in this population. Elderly patients frequently demonstrate diminished protection following receipt of routine vaccinations compared with younger populations. As a result, several different strategies have been developed to maximize vaccine effectiveness. These include administering higher doses [4], use of routine boosters [5], optimization of vaccine adjuvants [6], and altering the route of administration [7]. These strategies will be discussed in detail later in this chapter.

In addition to increased susceptibility to infection, immunosenescence has also been associated with an increase in the incidence of cancer that is also observed with aging, particularly between the ages 65 and 85 years. This observed increase is multifactorial in nature and includes environmental factors (increased exposure to carcinogens over time) as well as biologic factors, which favor a selective advantage to tumorigenic cells. In addition, the immune system plays a key role in protection against the development of malignancy through the process of immunosurveillance, by which the immune system identifies cancerous or precancerous cells and eliminates them before they cause disease. However, alterations in the immune response that occur with aging, particularly the adaptive immune system, can result in tumor cells avoiding detection and the resulting immune activation [8].

Aging and Hematopoietic Stem Cell Production

Hematopoietic stem cells (HSCs) serve as the key progenitor cell from which all cellular constituents of the immune system are derived. While they make up only 0.01 percent of the cellular bone marrow population, they are the key to maintaining all mature components of the immune system, including both the innate and adaptive arms. It is their ability for long-term self-renewal as well as differentiation into multiple cell lineages that makes them essential for maintaining an immune system comprised of relatively short-lived mature effector cells. Studies have demonstrated that the process of aging affect both the number and the function of HSCs. Flow cytometry studies performed in different mice strains reveal that the HSC population may be either increased or decreased during the aging process, with unknown genetic factors likely playing a key role. However, with regard to function, multiple animal studies have demonstrated a marked decrease in the capacity of HSCs from aged animals to repopulate a fully functional immune system compared with younger animals following HSC or bone marrow transplantation. Additionally, the aging process also affect whether a given HSC will develop along a myeloid or a lymphoid differentiation pathway. Specifically, the myeloid pathway is favored over the lymphoid pathway, resulting in an overall decrease in the number of B and T lymphocytes relative to the myeloid cells. One potential explanation for these findings is a decrease in the expression of the interleukin 7 receptor (IL-7R) in older HSCs because IL-7 is key in initiating and maintaining lymphoid differentiation [9].

Changes in Specific Components of the Immune System

Innate Immunity

The innate immune system, which is also referred to as the *ancestral part*, consists of multiple cellular and noncellular defense mechanisms. These include neutrophils, monocytes/macrophages, natural killer (NK) cells, complement components, and mucosal barriers and cytokines. Thus the impact of aging on the innate immune system is characterized by complex changes of multiple individual components. Interestingly, while some innate functions do diminish with age, others exhibit enhanced activity. These asymmetric changes ultimately result in an overall increase in the inflammatory state and have led many to describe the age-related changes as immune dysregulation rather than pure senescence [10]. Neutrophils are the predominant immune cells present in the circulation, and they provide a defense against bacterial and fungal infections. In general, they have a very short lifespan compared with hematopoietic cells, with a half-life of only 8 to 12 hours. Their lifespan may be extended by inflammatory cytokines such as granulocyte-macrophage colony-stimulating factor and interferon, as well as by bacterial products such as lipopolysaccharide (LPS), which maximizes their killing potential. They are summoned to infection sites by chemokines, where they use a host of mechanisms to destroy invading pathogens. These include ingestion of microorganisms through phagocytosis and subsequent killing via generation of reactive oxygen species (ROS) as well as proteolytic enzymes [11].

The aging process significantly affect multiple facets of neutrophil function. First, the chemotactic response becomes aberrant, likely impairing the ability of neutrophils to hone to a specific site of infection [12]. However, in vivo this manifests as a decreased ability to resolve inflammation. One possible explanation for these findings is that there is diminished chemotactic response once the neutrophil reaches the infected tissue, which results in increased inflammation in surrounding tissues due to the lack of directional movement [11]. In addition, neutrophils exhibit diminished phagocytic capacity with aging [10,13], as well as impaired respiratory burst, which may manifest as increased or decreased superoxide production depending on the stimulus [10]. Finally, the ability of proinflammatory stimuli (LPS, granulocyte colony-stimulating factors, IL-6) to extend the lifespan of neutrophils also deteriorates with the aging process, which further impairs the ability of neutrophils to clear invading microbial pathogens [14].

Monocytes/macrophages constitute another key component of the innate immune system. Monocytes arise from myeloid progenitor cells and are present throughout the circulation. They subsequently differentiate into tissue-associated macrophages, which are present in multiple organ systems throughout the body, including brain, liver, lungs, skin, and bones. Their functional role varies depending on the specific organ where they reside. However, in general, they phagocytose and kill microorganisms and eliminate cellular debris. In addition, they also secrete myriad of cytokines, which may serve to direct and enhance the innate immune response and interact with the adaptive immune system by serving as key antigen-presenting cells [10].

The effect of aging on the number and function of monocytes and macrophages is varied. While there appears to be no impact on the number of circulating blood monocytes with advanced age, there does appear to be a decrease in the number of macrophages in the bone marrow isolated from older individuals [15,16]. With regard to the phagocytic function of macrophages, current data are conflicting, with some studies demonstrating a decreased phagocytic capacity with aging and others showing opposite results. These discrepancies may be secondary to differences in the activation state of the cells, their tissue source, or other experimental conditions [10].

Another key macrophage function that is disrupted by the aging process is antigen presentation. Activation of the adaptive arm of the immune system relies on a complex system of antigen recognition by either T or B lymphocytes. T-cell receptors rely on an interaction with the major histocompatibility complex class II (MHC class II) to recognize degraded products presented by macrophages and other antigen-presenting cells. Once T cells are activated, they further regulate cellular and humoral immune responses, including those which form the basis for immunologic memory. In addition, MHC class II complexes are also the key in generating the T-cell repertoire in the thymus. With advanced age, there is a significant decrease in MHC class II expression in macrophages, which is most likely secondary to decreased gene transcription following activation [17]. Given the vital role MHC class II molecules play in activation of T lymphocytes, their decreased expression contributes to the dysfunction of the adaptive immune system with aging.

Natural killer (NK) cells are a population of cytotoxic lymphocytes that are responsible for MHC- independent killing of virally infected cells as well as tumor cells. They are divided into two separate populations based on their surface marker CD56. CD56^{bright} cells comprise approximately 10 percent of the circulating NK cells and function primarily in the secretion of inflammatory cytokines, particularly interferon-gamma (IFN-γ). CD56^{dim} cells, in contrast, constitute up to 90 percent of circulating lymphocytes and exhibit a predominantly cytotoxic function with minimal cytokine production. Interestingly, the total number of NK cells increases with aging, which is unlike what is seen with other lymphocyte populations. However, both subpopulations do not increase at the same rate; rather, there is a larger increase in the CD56^{dim} population resulting in a change in the overall ratio between CD56^{dim} and CD56^{bright} cells. This increase in the number of NK cells appears to be a compensatory mechanism for declining function because decreased killing capacity has been observed when examined on a per-cell basis [18]. In addition, cytokine production, including IFN-γ, is also diminished by the aging process. This impaired cytokine production is likely not overcome by increasing cell numbers and potentially contributes to higher infection risk and mortality in elderly individuals [11,19,20].

Adaptive Immunity

The adaptive immune system consists of B and T lymphocytes. These cells are responsible for antigen neutralization via antibody production as well as cell-mediated immunity directed against intracellular pathogens such as viruses and neoplastic cells, respectively. In addition, they also interact closely with the innate immune system to further hone the inflammatory response to pathogenic invasion. Both cell types become fully mature and activated via antigen recognition of cell surface receptors. In the case of B cells, these receptors consist of membrane-bound immunoglobulins, which are subsequently secreted once the cells fully mature into plasma cells. T cells, in contrast, recognize complementary antigen-MHC complexes that exist on the surfaces of antigen-presenting cells and further require costimulation with CD3 and other costimulatory molecules in order to become fully activated effector cells. The aging process has a significant impact on the total number and cellular subtypes, as well as receptor diversity, for both T and B lymphocytes. The overall impact of these changes is a decreased ability to recognize and mount an effective immune response. Interestingly, memory lymphocytes appear to be more resilient to the aging process, and long-term immunity is mostly preserved [21].

Aging of T Lymphocytes. Naive T cells originate in the bone marrow and subsequently migrate to the thymus, where they undergo further selection prior to maturation in secondary lymphoid tissues. The thymus is most active early in life and subsequently undergoes a functional decline in a process termed *involution* [22]. The size of the thymus peaks in the first year of life and then steadily decreases. As part of this process, the active portion of the thymus is slowly replaced by fatty tissue, which is nearly complete by 40 to 50 years of age [23]. By age 70, only 10 percent of the thymus is involved in active replication [21].

Because of thymic involution, there is a marked decrease in the number of naive T lymphocytes and by extension T-cell receptor (TCR) diversity. One study estimated that between the ages of 25 and 60 years, there are 20 million different TCR β-chains compared with only 200,000 after age 70 [24]. In addition, markedly low levels of recent thymic emigrants were identified in centenarians when compared with young (ages 20–45 years) or middle-aged volunteers, suggesting a marked depletion in the naive T-cell population with advanced age [25]. This diminished naive T-cell population and TCR diversity significantly limits the ability of elderly patients to respond to new infections, placing them at higher risk for morbidity and mortality. In addition, it also contributes to diminished vaccine responsiveness in this population.

In addition to a decrease in the naive T-cell population and, by extension, TCR diversity, the aging process also induces changes in the number and composition of the circulating T-lymphocyte population. Studies have consistently demonstrated that there is an overall decline in the total T-cell population in elderly individuals, as measured by a decline in $CD3^+$ cells. Furthermore, longitudinal studies have shown that an inversion of the CD4: CD8 ratio may occur over time, which is associated with increased mortality within 1 to 2 years [26].

Also, there is an emergence of a discrete subpopulation of T cells, which are $CD28^-$ cells, that predominantly affects $CD8^+$ cells. CD28 is a very potent costimulatory molecule localized on the surface membrane of T lymphocytes. Activation of this receptor in the setting of TCR recognition of a MHC-antigen complex triggers the release of IL-2, which is key for T-cell proliferation. Furthermore, it also facilitates maturation into effector T cells, which no longer require costimulation. The cause of the emergence of this $CD28^-$ population remains unknown. However, it is hypothesized that this population derives from $CD28^+$ lymphocytes, which undergo repetitive antigenic stimulation, resulting in loss of the CD28 receptor and entry into a quiescent state of replication [27,28]. Interestingly, this phenomenon has been observed in other settings as well, including HIV infection, autoimmune disorders, and following treatment with radiochemotherapies [28].

Another key phenomenon observed in aging T-cell populations is decreased production of IL-2. As mentioned earlier, IL-2 is a key cytokine that drives the expansion of T-lymphocyte populations as well as their differentiation. It is particularly key to mediating the CD4 response because it is the only cytokine capable of driving cell cycle progression. Furthermore, IL-1 is also responsible for maintaining survival in fully differentiated effector cells because they rapidly undergo apoptosis in its absence. With aging, the ability of $CD4^+$ T lymphocytes to produce IL-2 following stimulation of the TCR is significantly reduced. This ultimately results in a diminished T-helper population in terms of both numbers and functional capacity. Furthermore, because T-helper cells are the key to a robust antibody response via stimulation of B lymphocytes, there is also a defect in the humoral response [29,30].

Aging of B Lymphocytes. B lymphocytes originate and mature in the bone marrow, with further affinity maturation occurring in the germinal centers of B-cell follicles before they begin circulating in the bloodstream. They are responsible for generating humoral immunity in the form of secreted immunoglobulins, and as noted earlier, they rely heavily on interactions with T cells to fully differentiate and become activated as plasma cells. Immature B lymphocytes express immunoglobulin on their cell surface. Following antigenic exposure, they begin to produce secreted immunoglobulins, which initially consists of IgM, but later switch to one of the more mature phenotypes, including IgG, IgA, or IgE, in a process referred to as *class switching*. Additionally, immunoglobulins can also undergo a process of somatic hypermutation to further improve their specificity for a given antigen to more effectively neutralize it. The ability to recognize antigens and generate a robust antibody response is the primary functional role of these cells.

The aging process has a significant impact on both the number of B lymphocytes and the functional capacity to generate and secrete a diverse array of immunoglobulin. Studies of bone marrow specimens have revealed a decrease in the number of B-cell precursors present, thereby limiting the number of cells available to mature and secrete immunoglobulin [31]. Interestingly, B lymphocytes also exhibit a decrease in the number of newly generated memory cells and an increase in the number of circulating naive cells. Furthermore, B cells isolated from elderly individuals exhibit a decreased ability to undergo class switching from IgM to secondary isotypes, such as IgG [32].

In addition to a decrease in class switching and conversion to memory cells, there is a decline in the diversity of the B-lymphocyte population, as discussed with T-lymphocytes. This decrease in the B-cell repertoire may be secondary to diminished production of precursors in the bone marrow and is associated with a poor overall health status in elderly individuals [33].

Memory Cells. The ability to provide long-lasting immunity to a specific pathogen is one of the key features of the adaptive immune response. This phenomenon was observed as early as 430 BC in Athens, where it was noted that "the same man was never attacked twice" with regard to a plague. It has since been demonstrated throughout the centuries with multiple pathogens, including measles, polio, and yellow fever. Further observation also determined that ongoing antigenic challenge is not necessary in order to maintain protection [34]. This aspect of immunity was observed more recently during the 2009 H1N1 influenza pandemic, during which persistent antibody responses to the virus were identified in older individuals. As discussed earlier, the ability to generate an effective memory B or T lymphocyte from a naive cell diminishes with age. However, functional memory cells, which were generated from antigenic exposure earlier in life, can provide ongoing lifelong protection [35]. This observation likely explains the discrepancy between the immune response to novel pathogens compared with that of previously encountered organisms in individuals of advanced age.

Vaccine Implications in the Elderly

One of the most potent tools in our repertoire for prevention of infections is immunizations. However, the age-related changes in the immune system that render elderly individuals susceptible to novel pathogens also affect their responsiveness to vaccines. As a result, different strategies are employed in an effort to maximize the protection provided by a given vaccine, and the CDC has issued guidelines specifically for individuals over age 65. One strategy is the use of different adjuvants. Specifically, the use of protein conjugates appears to elicit a more robust response than polysaccharide conjugates. This strategy has been employed in pneumococcal vaccination and provides the basis for the current CDC recommendation for the use of the 14-valent protein-conjugated vaccine (PCV14) in individuals age 65 and older prior to receipt of the 23-valent polysaccharide vaccine (PPV23) [6]. Another strategy that has been employed is the use of higher-dose vaccines. Influenza studies have demonstrated enhanced production of protective antibody after receiving a higher-dose vaccine compared with the standard dose [36]. These findings led to FDA approval of higher-dose influenza vaccines for older adults. Other strategies under investigation include use of novel adjuvants [37], refining vaccine schedules [5], and changing the routes of administration [7].

References

1. Ginaldi L, Loreto MF, Corsi MP, Modesti M, De Martinis M. Immunosenescence and infectious diseases. *Microbes Infect* 2001; 3(10): 851–57.

2. Norman DC. Fever in the elderly. *Clin Infect Dis* 2000; 31(1):148–51.

3. Gavazzi G, Krause KH. Ageing and infection. *Lancet Infect Dis* 2002; 2(11):659–66.

4. Falsey AR, Treanor JJ, Tornieporth N, et al. Randomized, double-blind controlled phase

3 trial comparing the immunogenicity of high-dose and standard-dose influenza vaccine in adults 65 years of age and older. *J Infect Dis* 2009; **200**(2):172–80.

5. Kaml M, Weiskirchner I, Keller M, et al. Booster vaccination in the elderly: their success depends on the vaccine type applied earlier in life as well as on pre-vaccination antibody titers. *Vaccine* 2006; **24**(47–48): 6808–11.

6. de Roux A, Schmöle-Thoma B, Siber GR, et al. Comparison of pneumococcal conjugate polysaccharide and free polysaccharide vaccines in elderly adults: conjugate vaccine elicits improved antibacterial immune responses and immunological memory. *Clin Infect Dis* 2008; **46**(7):1015–23.

7. Holland D, Booy R, De Looze F, et al. Intradermal influenza vaccine administered using a new microinjection system produces superior immunogenicity in elderly adults: a randomized controlled trial. *J Infect Dis* 2008; **198**(5):650–58.

8. Malaguarnera L, Cristaldi E, Malaguarnera M. The role of immunity in elderly cancer. *Crit Rev Oncol Hematol* 2010; **74**(1):40–60.

9. Geiger H, Rudolph KL. Aging in the lympho-hematopoietic stem cell compartment. *Trends Immunol* 2009; **30** (7):360–65.

10. Gomez CR, Nomellini V, Faunce DE, Kovacs EJ. Innate immunity and aging. *Exp Gerontol* 2008; **43**(8):718–28.

11. Panda A, Arjona A, Sapey E, et al. Human innate immunosenescence: causes and consequences for immunity in old age. *Trends Immunol* 2009; **30**(7):325–33.

12. Wenisch C, Patruta S, Daxböck F, Krause R, Hörl W. Effect of age on human neutrophil function. *J Leukoc Biol* 2000; **67** (1):40–45.

13. Butcher SK, Chahal H, Nayak L, et al. Senescence in innate immune responses: reduced neutrophil phagocytic capacity and CD16 expression in elderly humans. *J Leukoc Biol* 2001; **70**(6):881–86.

14. Fortin CF, Larbi A, Dupuis G, Lesur O, Fülöp T Jr. GM-CSF activates the Jak/STAT pathway to rescue polymorphonuclear neutrophils from spontaneous apoptosis in young but not elderly individuals. *Biogerontology* 2007; **8** (2):173–87.

15. Ogawa T, Kitagawa M, Hirokawa K. Age-related changes of human bone marrow: a histometric estimation of proliferative cells, apoptotic cells, T cells, B cells and macrophages. *Mech Ageing Dev* 2000; **117**(1–3):57–68.

16. Takahashi I, Ohmoto E, Aoyama S, et al. Monocyte chemiluminescence and macrophage precursors in the aged. *Acta Med Okayama* 1985; **39**(6):447–51.

17. Herrero C, Sebastián C, Marqués L, et al. Immunosenescence of macrophages: reduced MHC class II gene expression. *Exp Gerontol* 2002; **37**(2–3):389–94.

18. Borrego F, Alonso MC, Galiani MD, et al. NK phenotypic markers and IL-2 response in NK cells from elderly people. *Exp Gerontol* 1999; **34**(2):253–65.

19. Ogata K, An E, Shioi Y, Nakamura K, et al. Association between natural killer cell activity and infection in immunologically normal elderly people. *Clin Exp Immunol* 2001; **124**(3):392–97.

20. Krishnaraj R, Bhooma T. Cytokine sensitivity of human NK cells during immunosenescence: 2. IL2-induced interferon gamma secretion. *Immunol Lett* 1996; **50**(1–2):59–63.

21. Agarwal S, Busse PJ. Innate and adaptive immunosenescence. *Ann Allergy Asthma Immunol* 2010; **104**(3):183–90; quiz 190–92, 210.

22. Mackall CL, Fleisher TA, Brown MR, et al. Age, thymopoiesis, and CD4$^+$ T-lymphocyte regeneration after intensive chemotherapy. *N Engl J Med* 1995; **332**(3): 143–49.

23. Flores KG, Li J, Sempowski GD, Haynes BF, Hale LP. Analysis of the human thymic perivascular space during aging. *J Clin Invest* 1999; **104**(8):1031–39.

24. Naylor K, Li G, Vallejo AN, et al. The influence of age on T cell generation and TCR diversity. *J Immunol* 2005; **174**(11):7446–52.

25. Nasi M, Troiano L, Lugli E, et al. Thymic output and functionality of the IL-7/IL-7 receptor system in centenarians: implications for the neolymphogenesis at the limit of human life. *Aging Cell* 2006; **5**(2):167–75.

26. Ferguson FG, Wikby A, Maxson P, et al. Immune parameters in a longitudinal study of a very old population of Swedish people: a comparison between survivors and nonsurvivors. *J Gerontol A Biol Sci Med Sci* 1995; **50**(6):B378–82.

27. Fagnoni FF, Vescovini R, Mazzola M, et al. Expansion of cytotoxic CD8⁺ CD28⁻ T cells in healthy ageing people, including centenarians. *Immunology* 1996; **88**(4):501–7.

28. Sansoni P, Vescovini R, Fagnoni F, et al. The immune system in extreme longevity. *Exp Gerontol* 2008; **43**(2):61–65.

29. Haynes L, Eaton SM, Swain SL. The defects in effector generation associated with aging can be reversed by addition of IL-2 but not other related gamma(c)-receptor binding cytokines. *Vaccine* 2000; **18**(16):1649–53.

30. Haynes L, Maue AC. Effects of aging on T cell function. *Curr Opin Immunol* 2009; **21**(4):414–17.

31. McKenna RW, Washington LT, Aquino DB, et al. Immunophenotypic analysis of hematogones (B-lymphocyte precursors) in 662 consecutive bone marrow specimens by 4-color flow cytometry. *Blood* 2001; **98**(8):2498–507.

32. Frasca D, Landin AM, Lechner SC, et al. Aging down-regulates the transcription factor E2A, activation-induced cytidine deaminase, and Ig class switch in human B cells. *J Immunol* 2008; **180**(8):5283–90.

33. Gibson KL, Wu YC, Barnett Y, et al. B-cell diversity decreases in old age and is correlated with poor health status. *Aging Cell* 2009; **8**(1):18–25.

34. Ahmed R, Gray D. Immunological memory and protective immunity: understanding their relation. *Science* 1996; **272**(5258):54–60.

35. Haynes L, Eaton SM, Burns EM, et al. CD4 T cell memory derived from young naive cells functions well into old age, but memory generated from aged naive cells functions poorly. *Proc Natl Acad Sci USA* 2003; **100**(25):15053–58.

36. Busse WW, Peters SP, Fenton MJ, et al. Vaccination of patients with mild and severe asthma with a 2009 pandemic H1N1 influenza virus vaccine. *J Allergy Clin Immunol* 2011; **127**(1):130–7, e1–3.

37. Couch RB, Bayas JM, Caso C, et al. Superior antigen-specific CD4⁺ T-cell response with AS03-adjuvantation of a trivalent influenza vaccine in a randomised trial of adults aged 65 and older. *BMC Infect Dis* 2014; **14**:425.

Transfusion Therapy and Common Hematologic Problems in the Critically Ill Elderly

Aryeh Shander, Faraz Syed and Mazyar Javidroozi

Key Points

- Physiologic changes with aging are generally expected to increase the risk of anemia while limiting the physiologic adaptations to anemia.
- Anemia is common in elderly patients and is often multifactorial.
- Anemia is an independent risk factor for worse outcomes and should never be left untreated.
- While transfusion is commonly considered to be the default treatment of anemic elderly patients, it is important to consider management strategies other than transfusion.
- Allogeneic blood transfusions have been linked to several unfavorable outcomes and must be used only when clearly indicated.
- Several control trials have demonstrated that restrictive transfusion strategies are associated with reduced use of blood while achieving similar or better outcomes than liberal transfusion strategies.
- Some evidence suggests that certain patient populations (e.g., those with cardiovascular morbidities) might face some risk when managed with restrictive transfusion strategies, but more studies are needed.
- Despite the general assumption that elderly patients might benefit from more liberal transfusion strategies, this notion is not supported by the available evidence.
- Other strategies including preventive measures – discussed under the concept of patient blood management – should be considered in all critically ill elderly patients who are anemic or at risk of becoming anemic.

Introduction

Advanced age is associated with significant changes within the hematologic and cardiovascular systems (along with other organs), including how these systems interact with one another. When it comes to the clinical manifestations of these changes and their impact on patient outcomes, the lines often become blurred, and the clinical impact of many of the cellular and subcellular changes that are associated with senescence remains debatable.

Aging is associated with marked changes in bone marrow cellularity. These changes are hallmarked by a gradual reduction in the hematopoietic cell populations and associated cytokine levels, while the fat cell counts increase. From a cellular perspective, all populations in the hematopoietic lineage from stem cells to more differentiated cells are affected [1]. As a result, the frequency of hematologic disorders – namely anemia – increases with aging, while the capacity of bone marrow to respond to hematological stress – namely increased production of red blood cells (RBCs) in response to bleeding – declines [2]. Age-related changes affecting coagulation systems are observed in platelets as well as coagulation factors, with a general shift toward *hypercoagulability* in the aged patients, which contributes to an increased incidence of thrombotic events in this population [3]. It is important to remember that these and many other changes of aging are gradual in nature and that there is no magic age beyond which all the changes appear abruptly. Similarly, there are many elderly patients who may not experience decline in hemoglobin levels or in other functions of the hematologic system [4].

As with many other cancers, the prevalence of hematopoietic malignancies increases with advanced age. This phenomenon is attributed to several factors, including an accumulation of mutations in stem cells over time [5]. It has been shown that hematopoiesis becomes increasingly "clonal" as we age, meaning that fewer populations of hematopoietic stem cells become dominant and give rise to the bulk of blood cells produced in the bone marrow. Clonal hematopoiesis is more common in elderly patients, and it may lead to leukemia in some [1].

Aging affects the immune system and is associated with impairments in function affecting both innate and adaptive immunity [6] (see Chapter 10). The clinical consequences of these changes (collectively referred to as *immunosenescence*) [7] may emerge as increased infections and infective complications. Sepsis is therefore more common in the elderly, and it is increasingly associated with worse outcomes, including a higher risk of mortality [8]. Aging is generally recognized as a proinflammatory state, and the term *inflamm-aging* is used to describe the low-grade inflammation that is often present in the aged body [9]. The consequences of this ongoing inflammation are a matter of debate, and some have linked it with the increased frequency of other chronic diseases that are seen more frequently in the elderly, from diabetes and cardiovascular problems to neurodegenerative diseases and malignancies [7].

Aging is also associated with a gradual decline in the physiologic functional capacity of the cardiovascular and respiratory systems (and their reserve capacity). Perfusion is tightly controlled throughout the body to ensure a reliable supply of oxygen to the cells to meet demands. Several aspects of the regulatory mechanisms that are in place to maintain this balance are compromised during aging – as a direct result of the aging process itself or the result of the presence of concurrent ailments that are more common in the elderly (e.g., hypertension, atherosclerosis) [10]. Furthermore, the declining reserve capacity of the cardiovascular and respiratory systems in aging is expected to limit the adaptability of body to changing conditions that limit supply or increase demand, increasing the risk of becoming decompensated in situations that are normally tolerated in younger patients [11].

Widespread changes in other organs also may affect the hematologic system. For example, age-related changes in the gastrointestinal system include disruption of the mucosal defense barrier, which can lead to an increased risk of inflammation and infection. This mucosal disruption and the ensuing inflammatory processes may interfere with absorption of nutrients, causing malnutrition and potentially leading to nutritional anemia [12].

Discussion of the pathophysiologic characteristics and changes associated with aging often leads us to the concept of *frailty*. While there is no standard definition for frailty, it generally can be described clinically as a state of increased vulnerability to acute stressors that is a result of a progressive decline in the functional status and reserve capacities of various physiologic systems in the body [13]. From a practical point of view, the presence of at least three of the five criteria suggested by Fried et al. is highly suggestive of frailty in an elderly patient: low energy, low grip strength, low physical activity, slowed walking speed, and unintended weight loss [14].

Key Concepts

Anemia in the Elderly

The interaction between aging and the hematologic system is multidimensional and can have far-reaching implications. Advanced age (and frailty) can increase the risk of developing anemia or worsening of this condition, while reduced reserve capacity of other systems (and the expected impaired physiologic adaptations to anemia) [15] might lead to increased susceptibility to hypoxia and may reduce the tolerance to anemia. Additionally, reduced hematopoietic capacity in the elderly may delay the recovery from acute blood loss, for example, following trauma or surgery [2].

Anemia in the elderly is often multifactorial, and etiologies include inflammation, renal insufficiency, blood loss, nutritional deficiencies (iron, folate, vitamin B_{12}), declined hematopoietic capacity, increased cell death (erythrocyte apoptosis or eryptosis), and iatrogenic causes such as drug-induced anemia [16–19] In a substantial number of elderly patients, the cause(s) of anemia might not be readily identified, giving rise to the term *unexplained anaemia of the elderly* (UAE) or *anemia of unknown etiology* (AUE) in this population. In a study from the 3rd National Health and Nutrition Examination Survey (NHNES), the primary cause of anemia in older patients was attributed to iron deficiency in one-third of patients and chronic renal disease or chronic inflammation in another one-third of patients, whereas the remaining one-third of anemic patients were classified as having AUE [20]. With increasing knowledge of the causes of anemia, it might be a matter of time until the underlying causes are identified in some of the AUE patients [18]. However, in some other patients, AUE appears to be a distinct entity characterized by a normocytic anemia developing in the absence of nutrition deficiency, inflammation, or renal dysfunction [21]. In a large study comparing elderly patients with AUE with matched cohorts of nonanemic and anemic individuals with determined causes, interleukin 6 (IL-6) and hepcidin were not different, suggesting that inflammation or iron restriction was not a primary cause [22]. Reduced testosterone levels and a blunted erythropoietin response (characterized by raised levels of erythropoietin but not raised as much as expected for the level of anemia present) were seen more frequently in patients with AUE [22].

Anemia is more frequent in elderly populations [19]. Table 11.1 provides a summary of the reported prevalence of anemia among various aged populations [20,23–32]. As can be seen, there is often a trend toward increase prevalence of anemia in older populations.

Anemia in the elderly is an independent risk factor for unfavorable outcomes. It has been linked to a decline in quality of life [33], cognitive function [29,32,34], activities of daily living [35], mobility [36,37], and strength [37,38]. Anemia also leads to an increased risk of physical impairments [30,31], falls [39,40], depression [41], hospitalization and nursing home placement [42,43], frailty [30], and mortality [31,32,35,42–44]. Table 11.1 summarized the negative outcomes of anemia reported in a number of studies.

Table 11.1 Prevalence of Anemia in the Elderly and Its Reported Consequences

Study	Population	Definition of anemia	Prevalence of anemia	Outcomes of anemia
Contreras et al. (2015) [31]	328 people older than 85 years of age living in a community	WHO criteria	24 percent	Anemia was associated with more dependence and higher comorbidity and mortality.
Deal et al. (2009) [25]	A representative sample of 436 community-dwelling women aged 70 to 80 years in the United States	Hb < 12 g/dl	8.8 percent	Anemia was associated with poorer baseline performance and faster rates of decline on cognitive tests.
Guralnik et al. (2004) [20]	US population aged 65 or older from the 3rd National Health and Nutrition Examination Survey (1988–94)	WHO criteria	11.0 percent of men and 10.2 percent of women ≥ 65 years of age; >20 percent in those ≥85 years of age	–
Hong et al. (2013) [29]	2,552 elderly subjects (mean age 76.1 years) participating in the Health, Aging, and Body Composition study	WHO criteria	15.4 percent	Anemia at baseline was independently associated with increased risk of dementia.
Jorgensen et al. (2010) [23]	5,286 residents of Tromsø, Norway, 55–77 years of aged	WHO criteria	3.4 percent	Lower Hb was associated with higher risk of fracture. Anemic men (but not women) had a 2.15 higher risk of nonvertebral fractures than men with high Hb levels.
Juarez-Cedillo et al. (2014) [30]	1,933 older community-dwelling adults enrolled in the Study on Aging and Dementia in Mexico	WHO criteria	8.3 percent	Anemia and low Hb were independently associated with increased risk of frailty.
Nakashima et al. (2012) [27]		WHO criteria	29 percent	–

Rosnick et al. (2010) [28]	Random sample of 124 adults younger than 60 years of age in long-term care facilities in Maringa, Brazil	WHO criteria	54 percent	Anemia was associated with worse physical performance; patients with anemia associated with chronic kidney disease had lower self-efficacy and outcome expectations for functional activities than those without anemia.
Samper-Ternent et al. (2011) [26]	451 residents from 12 nursing homes with an average age of 83.7 ± 8.2 years	WHO criteria	10.3 percent	–
Zakai et al. (2013) [32]	5,605 adults older than 60 years of age from the Mexican National Health and Nutrition Survey	WHO criteria	9 percent developed anemia during the 3-year follow-up	Hb decline and anemia were associated with worsening of cognitive function and mortality.

Note: World Health Organization (WHO) criteria for the definition of anemia is based on a hemoglobin concentration of less than 13 g/dl in adult men and less than 12 g/dl in adult nonpregnant women [24] (Hb = hemoglobin).

Some evidence suggests that the impact of anemia and hemoglobin levels on outcome in the elderly patients is more complicated [21]. In a study of nonhospitalized elderly disabled women, there was a sharp increase in the risk of 5-year mortality with declining levels of hemoglobin. Interestingly, high hemoglobin levels were also found to be associated with increased risk of long-term mortality (although the magnitude of the risk was far smaller compared than that associated with lower levels of hemoglobin) [45]. Another finding in this study was that lowest mortality rates were associated with a hemoglobin level of 14 to 14.5 g/dl, and there was a linear increase in the risk of death as hemoglobin levels decreased from that range. The suggestion that hemoglobin decline rather than presence or absence of anemia might be a more accurate predictor of unfavorable outcomes in the elderly is supported by other studies [32]. The effect of critical illness as a significant risk factor for the development of anemia [46] and anemia as a significant contributor to the worsening of outcome further complicate the issue [17,47]. A similar association between anemia and worse outcome can be seen in critically ill elderly patients [48].

Blood Transfusion Strategies and Outcomes

Blood transfusion has been traditionally considered to be the standard treatment for anemia across populations including the elderly. Transfusion provides a seemingly simple and readily available treatment to quickly raise the hemoglobin level and restore blood oxygen-carrying capacity and hemodynamic status of the patient to avoid tissue hypoxia and ischemia. In reality, a unit of allogeneic red blood cells (RBCs) is a complex and heterogeneous mixture of various cells and bioactive factors, antigens, vesicles, metabolites, and mediators that could be constantly changing [49]. Transfusion of allogeneic blood should be viewed as a live-tissue transplantation in essence and treated with the same level of caution and scrutiny [50].

Historically, infectious risks and complications have been the leading concerns related to allogeneic blood transfusions. Following implementation of various screening, testing, and processing (e.g., pathogen inactivation) strategies, the risk of transmission of infections through donated blood has been reduced to extremely low levels – typically less than 0.1 per million units of blood components for hepatitis C and B and human immunodeficiency virus – in the developed nations [51]. Nonetheless, new infectious agents remain a potential risk given the unavoidable delay between the first emergence of an infection and the time measures to screen for it or methods to inactivate the pathogen are implemented [52]. Despite the wide publicity and significant cost to the healthcare systems [53], the health burden of transfusion-transmitted infections is dwarfed compared with the noninfectious risk of blood transfusion.

Not surprisingly, many of the complications of blood transfusion are rooted in the immunogenicity of allogeneic blood and its interactions with the immune system of the recipient. Examples include alloimmunization [54], immunomodulation [55], febrile reactions [56], transfusion-related acute lung injury (TRALI) [57], and graft-versus-host disease (GVHD) [58].

Ex vivo storage and processing of donated blood units and the changes that occur during storage (storage lesion) are other mechanisms that have been suggested for the negative effects of blood transfusion [59,60]. Nonetheless, clinical trials to date have not been able to demonstrate a clear superiority for the transfusion of fresh blood units versus aged blood units (but still within the accepted shelf life of the component) in terms of improved clinical outcomes [61,62].

The number of studies linking allogeneic blood transfusions with unfavorable clinical outcomes including multiorgan dysfunction, cardiac complications, thromboembolic events, respiratory distress and failure, prolonged ventilator dependency, stroke, renal injury, sepsis and infection, mortality, and prolonged hospital stay in various patient population has been growing continuously [63,64]. This has given rise to efforts to restrict the use of blood transfusion and limit it only to patients in whom it is clearly indicated.

In their landmark study (Transfusion Requirements in Critical Care [TRICC] trial), Hebert et al. randomized anemic critically ill patients to a restrictive transfusion strategy (transfusing when hemoglobin fell below 7 g/dl to maintain hemoglobin between 7 and 9 g/dl) versus a liberal transfusion strategy (transfusing when hemoglobin fell below 10 g/dl to maintain it between 10 and 12 g/dl) [65]. They reported that the restrictive transfusion strategy was associated with reduced mortality compared with a liberal transfusion strategy among patients who were less acutely ill and those who were younger than 55 years of age, while there was a nonsignificant trend toward increased mortality risk among patients with acute cardiac ischemia and infarction [65]. Given that the survival benefits of restricting transfusions was clearly seen in younger patients, one must ask whether there is a potential for harm from restrictive transfusion strategies to elderly critically ill patients.

The results of the TRICC trial have been largely corroborated by trials conducted since then. A meta-analysis of data from over 3,700 participants in 17 clinical trials concluded that a restrictive transfusion strategy can achieve a 37 percent reduction in the risk of being transfused and a 0.75 unit smaller amount of blood being transfused on average per patient. Analysis of the pooled data indicated that using a restrictive transfusion strategy was associated with a significant reduction in the risk of infection [66]. In another meta-analysis of published data from over 6,200 participants in 19 clinical trials, restrictive transfusion strategy was found to be associated with a 30 percent reduction in transfusion rate and 1.19 absolute reduction in the number of units transfused, in addition to reducing the risk of in-hospital mortality rates (relative risk [RR] 0.77, 95 percent confidence interval [CI] 0.62–0.95) [67].

Holst et al. evaluated data from 31 trials in patients undergoing cardiovascular surgery and concluded that adhering to a restrictive transfusion strategy (hemoglobin threshold of 7 to 9 g/dl or hematocrit level of 24–25 percent depending on the study) compared with a less restrictive transfusion strategy (hemoglobin threshold of 8 to 10 g/dl or hematocrit of 30–32 percent) was associated with a significant reduction in transfusion use, while there was no statistically significant impact on the risk of myocardial infarction, stroke, renal failure, or mortality [68].

Among 1,000 patients with septic shock and a hemoglobin level of 9 g/dl or less in the intensive care unit (ICU) who were randomized to receive 1 unit of RBCs when hemoglobin was below 7 g/dl (lower threshold) or 9 g/dl (higher threshold), 90-day mortality, ischemic events, and the need for life support were similar [69]. In post hoc analyses of subgroups of patients with chronic lung disease, hematologic malignancy, metastatic cancers, or post-operative patients, no survival benefit was observed for transfusion at higher versus lower hemoglobin thresholds [70]. Long-term follow-up of these patients did not reveal any significant differences in mortality and health-related quality of life between the study arms [71].

Another group looked at the impact of transfusion strategies on risk of mortality in adult patients undergoing surgeries and critically-ill adult patients and concluded that a liberal transfusion strategy may improve survival in patients undergoing surgery but not in the critically ill [72]. It should be noted that the reported survival benefit of transfusion in this meta-analysis was heavily influenced by two studies that have faced methodologic criticism [73,74].

Ripolles et al. analyzed the data from six trials with a total of 2,156 patients, focusing on critically ill patients and those admitted with acute coronary syndrome, and they observed a trend toward less mortality among the critically ill patients randomized to restrictive transfusion strategies (RR 0.86, 95% CI 0.73–1.01) [75]. Recently, Carson et al. reviewed the data from over 12,500 participants in 31 clinical trials comparing restrictive transfusion triggers (usually hemoglobin 7–8 g/dl) with liberal transfusion triggers (hemoglobin 9–10 g/dl) [76]. Use of restrictive transfusion triggers was associated with 43 percent reduction in transfusion rates, whereas there was no negative impact on 30-day mortality or morbidity [76]. The authors concluded that while more studies are needed in particular patient populations such as those with acute coronary syndrome, acute neurologic disorders, stroke, cancers (including hematologic malignancies), and bone marrow failure, the available evidence supports the notion that allogeneic blood transfusions are generally not needed in patients with hemoglobin levels greater than 7–8 g/dl [76]. The authors did not specifically address elderly patients in their analysis. However, it is expected that with the higher prevalence of the comorbidities in the elderly, more research is needed in this specific population.

The impact of the presence of cardiovascular comorbidities on the outcomes of transfusion strategies was specifically addressed by a meta-analysis of 11 trials on over 3,000 patients undergoing noncardiac surgery [77]. Overall pooled risk of 30-day mortality was not statistically significantly different between the restrictive and liberal transfusion strategies, whereas restrictive transfusion strategy (based on a hemoglobin threshold of 8 g/dl or less) was associated with an increased risk of acute coronary syndrome (pooled risk ratio 1.78; 95% CI 1.18–2.70) [77]. In their subgroup analysis of data from trials on patients with acute myocardial infarction, Ripolles et al. reported a nonsignificant trend toward increased risk of mortality in patients assigned to restrictive transfusion strategies (RR 3.85, 95% CI 0.82–18.0) [75].

In a study on 2,003 patients with a hemoglobin concentration of less than 9 g/dl following cardiac surgery who were randomized to a liberal transfusion strategy (based on a postoperative hemoglobin threshold of less than 9 g/dl) or restrictive transfusion strategy (based on a hemoglobin threshold of less than 7.5 g/dl), the restrictive transfusion strategy was associated with significant reductions in resource use and costs without negatively affecting the primary composite outcome of any serious infection or ischemic events within the 3-month period following surgery [78]. However, all-cause mortality rates were higher in the restrictive transfusion arm (4.2 percent versus 2.6 percent in liberal transfusion group; hazards ratio [HR] 1.64, 95% CI 1.00–2.67). This observation led the investigators to refrain from recommending restrictive transfusion strategies without any reservations for patients following cardiac surgery, and they called for additional studies and meta-analyses of the data from existing studies in this population [78].

Hovaguimian et al. have recently published a meta-analysis of data from trials comparing liberal and restrictive transfusion strategies in which they pooled and analyzed data from trials within four predefined context-specific subgroups: patients undergoing cardiovascular surgery (3,323 patients from eight trials), elderly patients undergoing orthopedic surgery (3,777 patients from nine trials), medical or surgical acute care patients (emergency or critical care unit; 4,129 patents from 10 trials), and patients with acute brain trauma on intracranial bleeding (244 patients from two trials) [79]. The authors concluded that based on their analysis, there was a possibility that restrictive transfusion strategies in patients undergoing cardiovascular surgery were associated with an increased risk of complications related to inadequate oxygen supply (RR 1.09, 95% CI 0.97–1.22) and early mortality (RR 1.39, 95% CI 0.95–2.04). However, no such association was reported in critically ill patients or those with acute cerebral bleeding [79].

While controlled, randomized trials (and the meta-analyses that pool the results from several trials) are generally considered to provide the highest grade of evidence on the safety and efficacy of medical treatments, including transfusions, it is important to recognize the limitation of these studies. There is often the possibility of issues related to outcome-specific risk adjustment in trials (and meta-analyses that draw on them). Reported associations between restrictive transfusion strategies and increased risk of ischemic cardiac events often lack adequate assessment and analysis for the potential role of baseline risk factors for their outcomes. Additionally, clinical trials of transfusion strategies often focus on transfusions performed in a prespecified time period during the course of care and might overlook any transfusions given outside that window. As such, a patient who was assigned to the restrictive transfusion arm of a study focusing on the postoperative period might still have receive liberal transfusions before or during the surgery, confounding the observed association between the outcomes and transfusion strategies. The same issues can persist and even propagate when data from large trials suffering from these issues is pooled in meta-analyses [80].

Based on the available evidence, a transfusion hemoglobin threshold of 7 to 8 g/dl appears to be safe and reasonable for most critically ill patients and in the absence of other indications of transfusion (e.g., symptoms of hypoxia). However, extra caution might be warranted in the presence of certain comorbidities such as ischemic cardiac disease and brain injury, and more studies are needed in these patient populations [81]. This approach is rather based on an abundance of caution and not necessarily supported by available evidence. Hence alternative treatment options (primarily and prevention and treatment of anemia) should be considered whenever possible (see below) [82].

Blood Transfusion in the Elderly

A recurring theme in retrospective transfusion studies is the observation that transfused patients are generally significantly older that their nontransfused peers. When it comes to transfusion decisions, factors most commonly considered by clinicians include the hemoglobin level, comorbidities, and age [83]. Nonetheless, the underlying evidence to support the idea that advanced age, in absence of other comorbidities, is an independent factor that makes the patient more in need of transfusion (or more liberal transfusion strategies) is generally lacking. While elderly patients are among the largest patient populations across various hospital wards and outpatient clinics, the number of studies specifically addressing transfusion in this population is very limited.

Wu et al. conducted a retrospective review of data from approximately 79,000 patients hospitalized with acute myocardial infarction aged 65 years or older [84]. As expected, they observed that lower hemoglobin levels at the time of admission were associated with increased risk of mortality within 30 days. The impact of transfusion on mortality depended on the hemoglobin level: transfusion was associated with a reduced risk of mortality within

30 days in patients who had lower hemoglobin levels at admission (odds ratio [OR] 0.22, 95% CI 0.11–0.45 in patients with hematocrit levels of 5 to 24 percent and OR 0.69, 95% CI 0.53–0.89 in those with admission hematocrit levels of 30.1 to 33 percent) [84]. However, the conclusion that elderly patients with acute coronary artery disease may benefit from transfusion at hematocrit levels as high as 30 percent (or 33 percent on admission) was inconclusive and challenged by others [85].

In a smaller cohort study on 919 elderly patients undergoing surgery for hip fracture, one-third of the patients were transfused during hospital stay [86]. Although transfusion did not affect survival up to 6 months following admission, the risk of infection (of chest, urinary tract, or wound) was significantly higher in transfused patients (hazard ratio [HR] 1.91, 95% CI 1.41–2.59), and transfused patients had significantly longer duration of stay in hospital compared with patients who were not transfused [86]. The association between restrictive transfusion strategies and reduced risk of infection in hospitalized patients has been confirmed in a meta-analysis of 21 randomized, controlled trials (risk ratio [RR] 0.82, 95% CI 0.72–0.95) [87].

Gregersen et al. studied the association between transfusion strategies and various outcomes in 157 patients 65 years of age or older who underwent surgery for hip fracture [88]. They randomized patients to transfusion strategies based on a hemoglobin threshold of less than 9.7 g/dl (restrictive) or less than 11.3 g/dl (liberal) during the 30-day period following surgery. No significant differences were detected between the study groups with regard to overall quality of life (QoL) a month or a year later. However, the authors reported improved recovery of activities of daily living (ADLs) in patients randomized to their liberal transfusion strategy [88]. In a related study including 284 elderly patients following hip fracture surgery, despite the similarity of measures of ADLs, patients randomized to restrictive transfusion strategy had increased mortality at 30 days (HR 2.4, 95 percent CI 1.1–5.2) and 90 days (only among nursing home residents; HR 2.0, 95% CI 1.1–5.2) [89]. Subsequent analysis of the same group of patients indicated that there was no significant difference in the infection rates among patients randomized to liberal versus restrictive transfusion strategies (66 versus 72 percent, respectively; RR 1.08, 95% CI 0.93–1.27) [90]. While these related studies suggest that liberal transfusion strategies might offer some advantages over restrictive transfusion strategies in elderly patients, it must be emphasized that the restrictive transfusion strategy used in these studies was based on a hemoglobin threshold of 9.7 g/dl, which is in the ballpark of liberal hemoglobin thresholds in most other studies. In other words, what is being compared in these studies might be more appropriately labeled "liberal" and "more liberal" transfusion strategies, which resulted in almost 9 of every 10 patients being transfused regardless of study arm allocation [88–90].

In a clinical trial to study the impact of liberal blood transfusion on recovery in elderly patients undergoing surgery for hip fracture, Carson et al. randomized over 2,000 patients 50 years of age or older (mean age 81 years of age) to either a restrictive transfusion strategy (hemoglobin threshold < 8 g/dl or when symptoms of anemia were present) or a liberal transfusion strategy (hemoglobin threshold 10 g/dl) [91]. Almost all patients in the liberal arm were transfused (median of 2 units of RBCs), whereas 41 percent of patients in the restrictive arm received transfusions. The primary outcome of death or inability to walk unassisted across a room on 60-day follow-up occurred in 35.2 and 34.7 percent of the patients in the liberal and restrictive strategy arms, respectively (OR 1.01; 95% CI 0.84–1.22). There was no significant difference in the occurrence of other complications between the study arms [91].

In the meta-analysis by Hovaguimian et al. [79], elderly orthopedic surgery was one of the four context-specific subgroups. Of note, over half the patients whose data were pooled were from the trial by Carson et al. discussed earlier [91]. Based on their pooled data analysis, they concluded that restrictive transfusion strategies were associated with an increased risk of events reflective of inadequate oxygen supply (RR 1.41, 95% CI 1.03–1.92). However, there was no increase in the risk of early mortality (RR 1.09, 95% CI 0.80–1.49). In contrast, elderly patients assigned to restrictive transfusion strategies were less likely to suffer infectious complications (RR 0.75, 95% CI 0.53–1.04) [79].

With limited evidence available on the impact of transfusion strategies on outcomes of elderly patients (and even more limited evidence from critically ill elderly patients), it is difficult to make transfusion recommendations specific to this population. While advanced age remains a traditional factor to consider when making transfusion decisions [83], the actual clinical implication of age with regard to transfusion requirements is not clearly defined yet, and it remains to be established whether older age can independently justify more liberal transfusion strategies. Until then, a hemoglobin threshold of 7 to 8 g/dl for transfusion of blood can be considered for these patients in the absence of other indications of transfusion [21,81]. The presence of comorbidities – which tend to more be prevalent at older age – is a distinct consideration that might justify transfusion at higher hemoglobin thresholds, while more studies are needed to better define the optimal transfusion strategies in these patients. In the meanwhile, currently available transfusion guidelines, including those specifically addressing transfusion in critically ill patients, can be applied in the critically ill elderly patients [92–101] (Table 11.2).

Thinking beyond Transfusions

The ongoing heated debates over various transfusion strategies and their impact on outcomes should not divert our attention from the key notion that a blood transfusion is more often than not just a reactive and desperate measure to temporarily and hastily control and ameliorate a low hemoglobin level and avoid tissue hypoxia. However, barring the acute catastrophes such as massive blood loss, it is easy to overlook the underlying processes that often take place over time and gradually push a patient to a state where a blood transfusion becomes the only viable option. As such, a blood transfusion in many cases can be viewed as a "management failure" that deserves a complete failure mode and effects analysis (FMEA) [102].

Recognition of modifiable risk factors of transfusion is the key. Anemia is among the leading risk factors for blood transfusion across populations, and thus anemia must be addressed [103, 104] As discussed previously, the prevalence of anemia increases with age. There are ample publications on strategies to detect, diagnose, and determine the type, cause(s), and proper management of anemia [17,47,105–107]. Figure 11.1 provides an algorithm to diagnose and treat anemia that is generalizable to the elderly and elderly critically ill as well [17].

There has been a shift away from focus on the use of blood components and transfusions toward an emphasis on patient outcomes and measures to improve them. This notion is central to the concept of *patient blood management* (PBM). PBM is defined as the timely application of evidence-based medical and surgical concepts designed to maintain hemoglobin concentration, optimize hemostasis, and minimize blood loss in an effort to improve patient outcomes [82, 108, 109]. Various modalities under a comprehensive PBM strategy

Table 11.2 Summary of Blood Transfusion Guidelines

Guidelines	American Society of Anesthesiology (2006) [96]	Society of Thoracic Surgeons (2007) [92]	Italian Society of Transfusion Medicine and Immunohematology (2011) [93–95]	American Association of Blood Banks (2016) [97]	National Clinical Guideline Center (UK) (2015) [98]	American College of Physicians (2013) [99]	British Committee for Standards in Hematology (2013) [100]	American College of Critical Care Medicine (2009) [101]
Patient population	General surgery	Cardiovascular surgery	General surgery	Hemodynamically stable adult hospitalized patients including critically ill	General patient populations	Adult patients with heart disease	Critically ill patients	Adult trauma and critically ill patients.
Blood transfusion is usually indicated	Hemoglobin < 6 g/dl	Hemoglobin < 6 g/dl Hemoglobin < 7 g/dl in postoperative period Possibly higher hemoglobin levels when risk of end-organ ischemia exists	Hemoglobin < 6 g/dl Hemoglobin 6–8 g/dl in presence of risk factors Hemoglobin 6–10 g/dl if symptoms of hypoxia are present	Hemoglobin ≤ 7 g/dl in general including critically ill Hemoglobin ≤ 8 g/dl in patients undergoing orthopedic surgery, cardiac surgery, and those with preexisting cardiovascular disease	Hemoglobin ≤ 7 g/dl in absence of major bleeding, acute coronary syndrome, or transfusion-dependent chronic anemia Hemoglobin ≤ 8 g/dl for patients with acute coronary syndrome	Hemoglobin < 7–8 g/dl in hospitalized patients with coronary heart disease	Hemoglobin ≤ 7 g/dl Target hemoglobin 9–10 g/dl in early-onset severe sepsis with evidence of hypoxia Target hemoglobin > 7 g/dl in late-onset severe sepsis Target hemoglobin 9 g/dl in traumatic brain injury and/or cerebral ischemia Target hemoglobin > 8–10 g/dl in subarachnoid hemorrhage	Patients with evidence of hemorrhagic shock. Patients with evidence of acute hemorrhage and hemodynamic instability or inadequate oxygen delivery (DO_2). Hemoglobin < 7 g/dl in critically ill patients requiring mechanical ventilation. Hemoglobin < 7 g/dl in resuscitated critically ill trauma patients

							Target hemoglobin 8–9 g/dl in acute coronary syndrome Target hemoglobin > 7 g/dl in stable angina	Hemoglobin < 7 g/dl in critically ill patients with stable cardiac disease. Hemoglobin ≤ 8 g/dl on hospital admission in patients with acute coronary syndrome.
Blood transfusion rarely indicated	Hemoglobin > 10 g/dl	Hemoglobin > 10 g/dl	Hemoglobin > 10 g/dl	Hemoglobin > 10 g/dl	–	Hemoglobin > 10 g/dl	Hemoglobin > 9 g/dl	Hemoglobin > 10 g/dl
Areas of uncertainty	Hemoglobin 6–10 g/dl	–	–	Patients with acute coronary syndrome, severe thrombocytopenia (patients treated for hematologic or oncologic reasons who are at risk of bleeding), chronic transfusion-dependent anemia (not recommended due to insufficient evidence)	–	–	–	Patients with sepsis, patients at risk of acute lung injury and acute respiratory distress syndrome, patients with neurologic injury and diseases.
Other factors to consider	Ischemia, extent/rate of bleeding, volume status, risk factors for hypoxia complications	Age, severity of illness, cardiac function, ischemia, extent/rate of blood loss, mixed	Rate of blood loss, risk factors, symptoms of hypoxia/ischemia	Symptoms of hypoxia (chest pain, orthostatic hypotension, unresponsive	–	–	More caution with hemoglobin trigger of 7 g/dl if patient is elderly with significant cardiorespiratory	While transfusion at a hemoglobin threshold of < 7 g/dl is as effective as a hemoglobin threshold of < 10

Table 11.2 (cont.)

Guidelines	American Society of Anesthesiology (2006) [96]	Society of Thoracic Surgeons (2007) [92]	Italian Society of Transfusion Medicine and Immunohematology (2011) [93–95]	American Association of Blood Banks (2016) [97]	National Clinical Guideline Center (UK) (2015) [98]	American College of Physicians (2013) [99]	British Committee for Standards in Hematology (2013) [100]	American College of Critical Care Medicine (2009) [101]
		venous oxygen saturation (SVO_2)		tachycardia, heart failure)			comorbidities (target hemoglobin 7–9 g/dl)	g/dl in patients with hemodynamically stable anemia except those with acute myocardial infarction or unstable myocardial ischemia, use of hemoglobin levels as trigger for transfusion should be avoided; decision for RBC transfusion should be based on an individual patient's intravascular volume status, evidence of shock, duration and extent of anemia, and cardiopulmonary physiologic parameters.

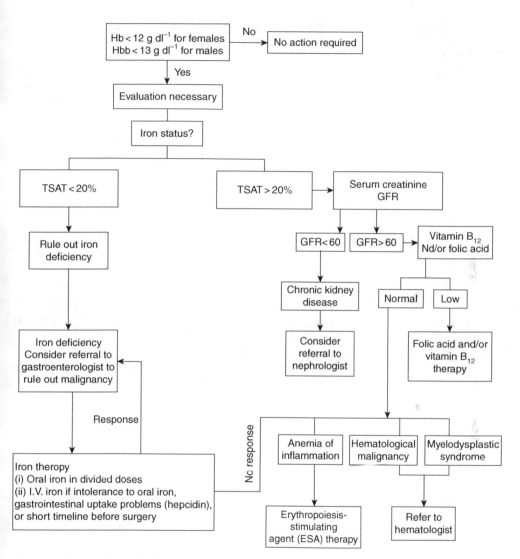

Figure 11.1 General algorithm for detection, diagnosis, and treatment of anemia. (*Source:* Modified from Shander et al. [17].)

can be considered in all elderly patients, including those who are critically ill. Examples include various treatments for anemia tailored to the patient's specific etiologies and minimization of blood loss due to iatrogenic causes and diagnostic phlebotomy [110]. These and other similar PBM approaches are particularly important in the critically ill patient given the high incidence of hospital-acquired anemia and its negative consequences – including increased risk of transfusion – in this vulnerable patient population [111–113].

Availability and Application of Clinical Guidelines for Very Old Patients

No specific guidelines for timing and use of transfusion or BPM are currently available for patients over 80 years of age. While substantial variations in practice exist and some clinicians may advocate a more liberal transfusion strategy in very old patients out of an abundance of caution, this is not based on objective evidence. Further research is needed in this very specific and growing patient population to better define the risks of anemia and transfusion and indications for allogeneic blood as well as other PBM modalities.

References

1. Shlush LI, Zandi S, Itzkovitz S, Schuh AC. Aging, clonal hematopoiesis and preleukemia: not just bad luck? *Int J Hematol* 2015; **102**:513–22.

2. Tuljapurkar SR, McGuire TR, Brusnahan SK, et al. Changes in human bone marrow fat content associated with changes in hematopoietic stem cell numbers and cytokine levels with aging. *J Anat* 2011; **219**:574–81.

3. Franchini M. Hemostasis and aging. *Crit Rev Oncol Hematol* 2006; **60**:144–51.

4. Patel KV. Epidemiology of anaemia in older adults. *Semin Hematol* 2008; **45**: 210–17.

5. Moehrle BM, Geiger H. Aging of hematopoietic stem cells: DNA damage and mutations? *Exp Hematol* 2016; **44**:895–901.

6. Pinti M, Appay V, Campisi J, et al. Aging of the immune system: focus on inflammation and vaccination. *Eur J Immunol* 2016; **46**: 2286–301.

7. Fulop T, Dupuis G, Witkowski JM, Larbi A. The role of immunosenescence in the development of age-related diseases. *Rev Invest Clin* 2016; **68**:84–91.

8. Starr ME, Saito H. Sepsis in old age: review of human and animal studies. *Aging Dis* 2014; **5**:126–36.

9. Franceschi C, Garagnani P, Vitale G, Capri M, Salvioli S. Inflammaging and "garb-aging." *Trends Endocrinol Metab* 2017; **28**:199–212.

10. Nagata K, Yamazaki T, Takano D, et al. Cerebral circulation in aging. *Ageing Res Rev* 2016; **30**:49–60.

11. Sprung J, Gajic O, Warner DO. Review article: age related alterations in respiratory function – anesthetic considerations. *Can J Anaesth* 2006; **53**:1244–57.

12. Soenen S, Rayner CK, Jones KL, Horowitz M. The ageing gastrointestinal tract. *Curr Opin Clin Nutr Metab Care* 2016; **19**:12–18.

13. Xue QL. The frailty syndrome: definition and natural history. *Clin Geriatr Med* 2011; **27**:1–15.

14. Fried LP, Tangen CM, Walston J, et al. Frailty in older adults: evidence for a phenotype. *J Gerontol A Biol Sci Med Sci* 2001; **56**:M146–56.

15. Madjdpour C, Spahn DR, Weiskopf RB. Anemia and perioperative red blood cell transfusion: a matter of tolerance. *Crit Care Med* 2006; **34**:S102–8.

16. Shander A, Javidroozi M, Ashton ME. Drug-induced anemia and other red cell disorders: a guide in the age of polypharmacy. *Curr Clin Pharmacol* 2011; **6**:295–303.

17. Shander A, Goodnough LT, Javidroozi M, et al. Iron deficiency anemia: bridging the knowledge and practice gap. *Transfus Med Rev* 2014; **28**:156–66.

18. Makipour S, Kanapuru B, Ershler WB. Unexplained anemia in the elderly. *Semin Hematol* 2008; **45**:250–54.

19. Rohrig G. Anemia in the frail, elderly patient. *Clin Interv Aging* 2016; **11**:319–26.

20. Guralnik JM, Eisenstaedt RS, Ferrucci L, Klein HG, Woodman RC. Prevalence of anemia in persons 65 years and older in the United States: evidence for a high rate of unexplained anaemia. *Blood* 2004; **104**: 2263–68.

21. Goodnough LT, Schrier SL. Evaluation and management of anemia in the elderly. *Am J Hematol* 2014; **89**:88–96.

22. Waalen J, von Löhneysen LK, Lee P, Xu X, Friedman JS. Erythropoietin, GDF15, IL6, hepcidin and testosterone levels in a large cohort of elderly individuals with anaemia of known and unknown cause. *Eur J Haematol* 2011; **87**:107–16.

23. Jorgensen L, Skjelbakken T, Lochen ML, et al. Anaemia and the risk of non-vertebral fractures: the Tromso Study. *Osteoporos Int* 2010; **21**:1761–68.

24. Blanc B, Finch CA, Hallberg L. Nutritional aneamias: report of a WHO Scientific Group. *WHO Tech Rep Ser* 1968; **405**: 1–40.

25. Deal JA, Carlson MC, Xue QL, Fried LP, Chaves PH. Anemia and 9-year domain-specific cognitive decline in community-dwelling older women: the Women's Health and Aging Study II. *J Am Geriatr Soc* 2009; **57**:1604–11.

26. Samper-Ternent R, Michaels-Obregon A, Wong R. Coexistence of obesity and anaemia in older Mexican adults. *Ageing Int* 2011; **37**:104–17.

27. Nakashima AT, de Moraes AC, Auler F, Peralta RM. Anemia prevalence and its determinants in Brazilian institutionalized elderly. *Nutrition* 2012; **28**:640–43.

28. Resnick B, Sabol V, Galik E, Gruber-Baldini AL. The impact of anemia on nursing home residents. *Clin Nurs Res* 2010; **19**:113–30.

29. Hong CH, Falvey C, Harris TB, et al. Anemia and risk of dementia in older adults: findings from the Health ABC Study. *Neurology* 2013; **81**:528–33.

30. Juarez-Cedillo T, Basurto-Acevedo L, Vega-Garcia S, et al. Prevalence of anemia and its impact on the state of frailty in elderly people living in the community: SADEM Study. *Ann Hematol* 2014; **93**: 2057–62.

31. Contreras MM, Formiga F, Ferrer A, et al. [Profile and prognosis of patients over 85 years old with anaemia living in the community: Octabaix STUDY.] *Rev Esp Geriatr Gerontol* 2015; **50**:211–15.

32. Zakai NA, French B, Arnold AM, et al. Hemoglobin decline, function, and mortality in the elderly: the Cardiovascular Health Study. *Am J Hematol* 2013; **88**:5–9.

33. Thein M, Ershler WB, Artz AS, et al. Diminished quality of life and physical function in community-dwelling elderly with anemia. *Medicine (Baltimore)* 2009; **88**:107–14.

34. Lucca U, Tettamanti M, Mosconi P, et al. Association of mild anemia with cognitive, functional, mood and quality of life outcomes in the elderly: the "Health and Anemia" study. *PLoS One* 2008; **3**:e1920.

35. Denny SD, Kuchibhatla MN, Cohen HJ. Impact of anemia on mortality, cognition, and function in community-dwelling elderly. *Am J Med* 2006; **119**:327–34.

36. Chaves PH, Ashar B, Guralnik JM, Fried LP. Looking at the relationship between hemoglobin concentration and prevalent mobility difficulty in older women: should the criteria currently used to define anemia in older people be reevaluated? *J Am Geriatr Soc* 2002; **50**: 1257–64.

37. Penninx BW, Guralnik JM, Onder G, et al. Anemia and decline in physical performance among older persons. *Am J Med* 2003; **115**:104–10.

38. Penninx BW, Pahor M, Cesari M, et al. Anemia is associated with disability and decreased physical performance and muscle strength in the elderly. *J Am Geriatr Soc* 2004; **52**:719–24.

39. Dharmarajan TS, Avula S, Norkus EP. Anemia increases risk for falls in hospitalized older adults: an evaluation of falls in 362 hospitalized, ambulatory, long-term care, and community patients. *J Am Med Dir Assoc* 2006; **7**:287–93.

40. Penninx BW, Pluijm SM, Lips P, et al. Late-life anemia is associated with increased risk of recurrent falls. *J Am Geriatr Soc* 2005; **53**: 2106–11.

41. Son SJ, Lee KS, Na DL, et al. Anemia associated with depressive symptoms in mild cognitive impairment with severe white matter hyperintensities. *J Geriatr Psychiatry Neurol* 2011; **24**:161–67.

42. Penninx BW, Pahor M, Woodman RC, Guralnik JM. Anemia in old age is associated with increased mortality and hospitalization. *J Gerontol A Biol Sci Med Sci* 2006; **61**:474–79.

43. Salive ME, Cornoni-Huntley J, Guralnik JM, et al. Anemia and hemoglobin levels in older persons: relationship with age, gender, and health status. *J Am Geriatr Soc* 1992; **40**:489–96.

44. Zakai NA, Katz R, Hirsch C, et al. A prospective study of anemia status, hemoglobin concentration, and mortality in an elderly cohort: the Cardiovascular Health Study. *Arch Intern Med* 2005; **165**: 2214–20.

45. Chaves PH, Xue QL, Guralnik JM, et al. What constitutes normal hemoglobin concentration in community-dwelling disabled older women? *J Am Geriatr Soc* 2004; **52**:1811–16.

46. Astin R, Puthucheary Z. Anemia secondary to critical illness: an unexplained phenomenon. *Extrem Physiol Med* 2014; **3**:4.

47. Shander A. Anemia in the critically ill. *Crit Care Clin* 2004; **20**:159–78.

48. Mukhopadhyay A, Tai BC, See KC, et al. Risk factors for hospital and long-term mortality of critically ill elderly patients admitted to an intensive care unit. *Biomed Res Int* 2014; **2014**:960575.

49. Perros AJ, Christensen AM, Flower RL, Dean MM. Soluble mediators in platelet concentrates modulate dendritic cell inflammatory responses in an experimental model of transfusion. *J Interferon Cytokine Res* 2015; **35**:821–30.

50. Mincheff MS, Meryman HT. Blood transfusion, blood storage and immunomodulation. *Immunol Invest* 1995; **24**:303–9.

51. Funk MB, Heiden M, Volkers P, Lohmann A, Keller-Stanislawski B. Evaluation of risk minimization measures for blood components: based on reporting rates of transfusion-transmitted reactions (1997–2013). *Transfus Med Hemother* 2015; **42**:240–46.

52. Shander A, Lobel GP, Javidroozi M. Transfusion practices and infectious risks. *Expert Rev Hematol* 2016; **9**:597–605.

53. Jackson BR, Busch MP, Stramer SL, AuBuchon JP. The cost-effectiveness of NAT for HIV, HCV, and HBV in whole-blood donations. *Transfusion* 2003; **43**:721–29.

54. Brown CJ, Navarrete CV. Clinical relevance of the HLA system in blood transfusion. *Vox Sang* 2011; **101**:93–105.

55. Refaai MA, Blumberg N. Transfusion immunomodulation from a clinical perspective: an update. *Expert Rev Hematol* 2013; **6**:653–63.

56. Hirayama F. Current understanding of allergic transfusion reactions: incidence, pathogenesis, laboratory tests, prevention and treatment. *Br J Haematol* 2013; **160**: 434–44.

57. Kenz HE, Van der Linden P. Transfusion-related acute lung injury. *Eur J Anaesthesiol* 2014; **31**:345–50.

58. Fast LD. Developments in the prevention of transfusion-associated graft-versus-host disease. *Br J Haematol* 2012; **158**:563–68.

59. Orlov D, Karkouti K. The pathophysiology and consequences of red blood cell storage. *Anaesthesia* 2015; **70**(Suppl 1):29–12.

60. Qu L, Triulzi DJ. Clinical effects of red blood cell storage. *Cancer Control* 2015; **22**:26–37.

61. Lacroix J, Hebert PC, Fergusson DA, et al. Age of transfused blood in critically ill adults. *N Engl J Med* 2015; **372**:1410–18.

62. Steiner ME, Ness PM, Assmann SF, et al. Effects of red-cell storage duration on patients undergoing cardiac surgery. *N Engl J Med* 2015; **372**:1419–29.

63. Shander A, Javidroozi M, Ozawa S, Hare GM. What is really dangerous: anaemia or transfusion? *Br J Anaesth* 2011; **107**(Suppl 1):i41–59.

64. Chatterjee S, Wetterslev J, Sharma A, Lichstein E, Mukherjee D. Association of blood transfusion with increased mortality in myocardial infarction: a meta-analysis and diversity-adjusted study sequential

analysis. *JAMA Intern Med* 2013; **173**: 132–39.

65. Hebert PC, Wells G, Blajchman MA, et al. A multicenter, randomized, controlled clinical trial of transfusion requirements in critical care. Transfusion Requirements in Critical Care Investigators, Canadian Critical Care Trials Group. *N Engl J Med* 1999; **340**:409–17.

66. Carless PA, Henry DA, Carson JL, et al. Transfusion thresholds and other strategies for guiding allogeneic red blood cell transfusion. *Cochrane Database Syst Rev.* 2010; **4**:CD002042.

67. Carson JL, Carless PA, Hebert PC. Transfusion thresholds and other strategies for guiding allogeneic red blood cell transfusion. *Cochrane Database Syst Rev.* 2012; **4**:CD002042.

68. Holst LB, Petersen MW, Haase N, Perner A, Wetterslev J. Restrictive versus liberal transfusion strategy for red blood cell transfusion: systematic review of randomised trials with meta-analysis and trial sequential analysis. *BMJ* 2015; **350**: h1354.

69. Holst LB, Haase N, Wetterslev J, et al. Lower versus higher hemoglobin threshold for transfusion in septic shock. *N Engl J Med* 2014; **371**:1381–91.

70. Rygard SL, Holst LB, Wetterslev J, Johansson PI, Perner A. Higher vs lower haemoglobin threshold for transfusion in septic shock: subgroup analyses of the TRISS trial. *Acta Anaesthesiol Scand.* 2017; **61**:166–75.

71. Rygard SL, Holst LB, Wetterslev J, et al. Long-term outcomes in patients with septic shock transfused at a lower versus a higher haemoglobin threshold: the TRISS randomised, multicentre clinical trial. *Intensive Care Med* 2016; **42**:1685–94.

72. Fominskiy E, Putzu A, Monaco F, et al. Liberal transfusion strategy improves survival in perioperative but not in critically ill patients: a meta-analysis of randomised trials. *Br J Anaesth* 2015; **115**:511–19.

73. Hajjar LA, Vincent JL, Galas FR, et al. Transfusion requirements after cardiac

surgery: the TRACS randomized controlled trial. *JAMA* 2010; **304**:1559–67.

74. Murphy GJ, Pike K, Rogers CA, et al. Liberal or restrictive transfusion after cardiac surgery. *N Engl J Med* 2015; **372**:997–1008.

75. Ripolles MJ, Casans FR, Espinosa A, et al. Restrictive versus liberal transfusion strategy for red blood cell transfusion in critically ill patients and in patients with acute coronary syndrome: a systematic review, meta-analysis and trial sequential analysis. *Minerva Anestesiol* 2016; **82**: 582–98.

76. Carson JL, Stanworth SJ, Roubinian N, et al. Transfusion thresholds and other strategies for guiding allogeneic red blood cell transfusion. *Cochrane Database Syst Rev.* 2016; **10**:CD002042.

77. Docherty AB, O'Donnell R, Brunskill S, et al. Effect of restrictive versus liberal transfusion strategies on outcomes in patients with cardiovascular disease in a non-cardiac surgery setting: systematic review and meta-analysis. *BMJ* 2016; **352**: i1351.

78. Reeves BC, Pike K, Rogers CA, et al. A multicentre randomised controlled trial of transfusion indication threshold reduction on transfusion rates, morbidity and health-care resource use following cardiac surgery (TITRe2). *Health Technol Assess* 2016; **20**:1–260.

79. Hovaguimian F, Myles PS. Restrictive versus liberal transfusion strategy in the perioperative and acute care settings: a context-specific systematic review and meta-analysis of randomized controlled trials. *Anesthesiology* 2016; **125**:46–61.

80. Trentino K, Farmer S, Gross I, Shander A, Isbister J. Observational studies: should we simply ignore them in assessing transfusion outcomes? *BMC Anesthesiol* 2016; **16**:96.

81. Holst LB. Benefits and harms of red blood cell transfusions in patients with septic shock in the intensive care unit. *Dan Med J* 2016; **63**:B5209.

82. Shander A, Isbister J, Gombotz H. Patient blood management: the global view. *Transfusion.* 2016; 56(Suppl 1):S94–102.

83. Shander A, Fink A, Javidroozi M, et al. Appropriateness of allogeneic red blood cell transfusion: the International Consensus Conference on Transfusion Outcomes. *Transfus Med Rev* 2011; **25**: 232–46.

84. Wu WC, Rathore SS, Wang Y, Radford MJ, Krumholz HM. Blood transfusion in elderly patients with acute myocardial infarction. *N Engl J Med* 2001; **345**: 1230–36.

85. Perlman S, Moskowitz D, Bennett H. Transfusion in elderly patients with myocardial infarction. *N Engl J Med* 2002; **346**:779–82.

86. Shokoohi A, Stanworth S, Mistry D, et al. The risks of red cell transfusion for hip fracture surgery in the elderly. *Vox Sang* 2012; **103**:223–30.

87. Rohde JM, Dimcheff DE, Blumberg N, et al. Health care-associated infection after red blood cell transfusion: a systematic review and meta-analysis. *JAMA* 2014; **311**: 1317–26.

88. Gregersen M, Borris LC, Damsgaard EM. Blood transfusion and overall quality of life after hip fracture in frail elderly patients: the transfusion requirements in frail elderly randomized controlled trial. *J Am Med Dir Assoc* 2015; **16**:762–66.

89. Gregersen M, Borris LC, Damsgaard EM. Postoperative blood transfusion strategy in frail, anemic elderly patients with hip fracture: the TRIFE randomized controlled trial. *Acta Orthop* 2015; **86**: 363–72.

90. Gregersen M, Damsgaard EM, Borris LC. Blood transfusion and risk of infection in frail elderly after hip fracture surgery: the TRIFE randomized controlled trial. *Eur J Orthop Surg Traumatol* 2015; **25**: 1031–38.

91. Carson JL, Terrin ML, Noveck H, et al. Liberal or restrictive transfusion in high-risk patients after hip surgery. *N Engl J Med* 2011; **365**:2453–62.

92. Ferraris VA, Ferraris SP, Saha SP, et al. Perioperative blood transfusion and blood conservation in cardiac surgery: the Society of Thoracic Surgeons and the Society of Cardiovascular Anesthesiologists Clinical Practice Guideline. *Ann Thorac Surg* 2007; **83**:S27–86.

93. Liumbruno GM, Bennardello F, Lattanzio A, Piccoli P, Rossetti G. Recommendations for the transfusion management of patients in the peri-operative period: I. The pre-operative period. *Blood Transfus* 2011; **9**:19–40.

94. Liumbruno GM, Bennardello F, Lattanzio A, Piccoli P, Rossetti G. Recommendations for the transfusion management of patients in the peri-operative period: II. The intra-operative period. *Blood Transfus* 2011; **9**:189–217.

95. Liumbruno GM, Bennardello F, Lattanzio A, Piccoli P, Rossetti G. Recommendations for the transfusion management of patients in the peri-operative period: III. The post-operative period. *Blood Transfus.* 2011; **9**:320–35.

96. Practice guidelines for perioperative blood transfusion and adjuvant therapies: an updated report by the American Society of Anesthesiologists Task Force on Perioperative Blood Transfusion and Adjuvant Therapies. *Anesthesiology* 2006; 105:198–208.

97. Carson JL, Guyatt G, Heddle NM, et al. Clinical practice guidelines from the AABB: red blood cell transfusion thresholds and storage. *JAMA* 2016; **316**: 2025–35.

98. National Clinical Guideline Center (UK). *Blood Transfusion*, 2015, available at www .ncbi.nlm.nih.gov/pubmed/26632625.

99. Qaseem A, Humphrey LL, Fitterman N, Starkey M, Shekelle P. Treatment of anemia in patients with heart disease: a clinical practice guideline from the American College of Physicians. *Ann Intern Med* 2013; **159**:770–79.

100. Retter A, Wyncoll D, Pearse R, et al. Guidelines on the management of anaemia and red cell transfusion in adult critically ill patients. *Br J Haematol* 2013; **160**:445–64.

101. Napolitano LM, Kurek S, Luchette FA, et al. Clinical practice guideline: red blood cell transfusion in adult trauma and critical care. *Crit Care Med* 2009; **37**:3124–57.

102. Lu Y, Teng F, Zhou J, Wen A, Bi Y. Failure mode and effect analysis in blood transfusion: a proactive tool to reduce risks. *Transfusion* 2013; **53**:3080–87.

103. Gombotz H, Rehak PH, Shander A, Hofmann A. Blood use in elective surgery: the Austrian benchmark study. *Transfusion* 2007; **47**:1468–80.

104. Gombotz H, Rehak PH, Shander A, Hofmann A. The second Austrian benchmark study for blood use in elective surgery: results and practice change. *Transfusion* 2014; **54**:2646–57.

105. Goodnough LT, Shander A, Spivak JL, et al. Detection, evaluation, and management of anemia in the elective surgical patient. *Anesth Analg* 2005; **101**:1858–61.

106. Goodnough LT, Maniatis A, Earnshaw P, et al. Detection, evaluation, and management of preoperative anaemia in the elective orthopaedic surgical patient:

NATA guidelines. *Br J Anaesth* 2011; **106**:13–22.

107. Shander A. Preoperative anaemia and its management. *Transfus Apher Sci* 2014; **50**:13–15.

108. Shander A, Hofmann A, Isbister J, Van AH. Patient blood management: the new frontier. *Best Pract Res Clin Anaesthesiol* 2013; **27**:5–10.

109. Shander A, Nemeth J, Cruz JE, Javidroozi M. Patient blood management: a role for pharmacists. *Am J Health Syst Pharm* 2017; **74**:e83–89.

110. Fischer DP, Zacharowski KD, Meybohm P. Savoring every drop: vampire or mosquito? *Crit Care* 2014; **18**:306.

111. Koch CG, Li L, Sun Z, et al. Hospital-acquired anemia: prevalence, outcomes, and healthcare implications. *J Hosp Med* 2013; **8**:506–12.

112. Koch CG, Li L, Sun Z, et al. From bad to worse: anaemia on admission and hospital-acquired anaemia. *J Patient Saf* 2014.

113. Kurniali PC, Curry S, Brennan KW, et al. A retrospective study investigating the incidence and predisposing factors of hospital-acquired anaemia. *Anaemia* 2014; **2014**:634582.

Stress Response to Surgery in the Elderly

Nazish K. Hashmi and Mihai V. Podgoreanu

Key Points

- Major surgery is a global healthcare burden and is further compounded by unprecedented population aging, a major risk factor for perioperative organ injury and poor long-term outcomes.
- Surgical trauma triggers a robust stress response, the characteristics of which are generally altered with aging, becoming the primary mechanism driving further injury and perioperative organ dysfunction in older adults.
- A new field of geroscience has identified seven pillars of aging that distinguish the key processes to understanding and treating biologic aging, principal among which is *adaptation to stress*.
- With aging, the allostatic response becomes impaired, and there may be an exaggerated or inadequate peak response, as well as a sluggish return to baseline.
- Aging increases vulnerability to surgical stress, ischemia-reperfusion injury, and critical illness that is related to decreases in *physical resilience* characterized by immunosenescence, loss of mitochondrial function and nutrient sensing, and impaired recovery following surgical stressors.
- Increasing evidence suggests that prehabilitation, healthy diet, nutrition, and exercise for seniors in anticipation of surgical stressors are effective interventions to promote physical resilience.
- Provocative tests or biomarkers to predict increased vulnerability or, conversely, physical resilience are poorly developed, and our understanding of which patient subgroups may experience substantial benefit from interventions remains limited. Furthermore, pharmacologic resilience enhancers or boosters are currently not available.
- The influence of age as a modifier of subsequent insults and "second hits" (e.g., postoperative infection) and its impact on outcome trajectories are extremely complex. The intestinal microbiota decreases in abundance and function following surgical trauma, and a virulent and resistant pathobiome emerges, rendering the stressed host more vulnerable to infection.
- Postoperative pain trajectories differ by age and are amenable to interventions aimed at elderly patients.

Major Surgery in an Aging Population: A Global Healthcare Burden

The life expectancy for the US population in 2014 had increased to 78.8 years as death rates declined for children and young adults [1]. The number of adults aged 65 or older was estimated to be 46.2 million, which is 28 percent (or 10 million) more than in 2004 [2]. This number is expected to grow from 13 percent of the total population to over 20 percent in 2030, with adults older than age 85 expected to triple in the next four decades to 19 million [3]. Major surgery is a global healthcare burden, with around 244 million procedures performed annually, up to 4 percent of patients suffering perioperative deaths, up to 15 percent having serious postoperative morbidity, and 5 to 15 percent being readmitted within 30 days [4,5].

The implication of an aging population in the perioperative setting is obvious: the elderly comprises more than 40 percent of all surgical patients in the United States [6]. With the growing popularity of transcatheter aortic valve replacement (TAVR) and other minimally invasive procedures for malignancies, we can only expect to see a further increase in the number of elderly surgical patients. Among the very elderly, there is a threefold increased risk of death, including anesthesia-related deaths [7]; more than 40 percent will experience significant postoperative complications requiring extended intensive care unit (ICU) stays [8,9], with over 50 percent of patients older than age 65 [10] and 22 percent older than age 85 [11] receiving ICU care; and there will be an exponential increase in the use of state-of-the-art life support technologies. In octogenarians, planned surgical admissions to the ICU are associated with 12 and 25 percent ICU and hospital mortality, respectively. However, unplanned surgical admissions to the ICU are associated with a higher 1-year mortality of 67 percent [12]. Even more important, many elderly ICU survivors continue to display excess mortality and a high incidence of post-ICU syndrome following hospital discharge [11,13,14] such that only *one-quarter* of patients aged 80 and older return to their baseline level of physical function at 1 year [15].

General Characteristics of the Surgical Stress Response

The systemic host response to major surgery can be conceptualized as an acute "controlled trauma." It is an evolutionarily conserved, complex series of neuroendocrine, metabolic, coagulation, inflammatory, and immune system events that maximize an organism's ability to heal. This stereotyped multilevel stress response is modified by two categories of influences: *host (endogenous) factors*, such as age, gender, prior health status, and the genome, and *procedural (exogenous) factors*, including type, duration, and invasiveness of surgery, anesthetic management, fluid administration, and need for extracorporeal circulation and perioperative analgesia. The interactions between endogenous and exogenous factors ultimately contribute to variability in postoperative outcomes and recovery trajectories [16–21] (Figure 12.1). As it will be discussed in greater detail in this chapter, aging is a particular concern because many older surgical patients present with multiple comorbidities, are frail, and have decreased reserves and resilience to cope with surgical stress [22–24].

Classically described by Sir David Cuthbertson, the immune, inflammatory, and metabolic responses to traumatic injury characteristically display three distinct phases – *ebb, flow*, and *recuperation* – which were subsequently extrapolated to surgery and the

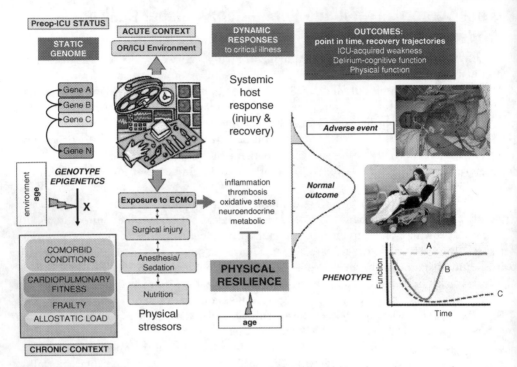

Figure 12.1 Variability in patient responses to perioperative stressors is driven by endogenous and exogenous factors. (*Source:* Modified from Podgoreanu et al. [11].)

perioperative setting [19,25,26]. During the ebb phase, an intense vasoconstrictive response shunts blood and substrate toward vital organs, geared toward the organism's survival by reducing posttraumatic energy depletion. This leads to the flow phase, a hypermetabolic state accompanied by increases in physiologic parameters such as cardiac output, minute ventilation, and oxygen consumption, aimed at providing substrate and energy for reparative mechanisms. As recovery occurs, the recuperation phase of the stress response aims to downregulate previously revved-up physiologic processes and return the organism to its preinjury state [17].

It is now appreciated that early drivers of the surgical stress response are sterile local tissue injury, inflammation, afferent nerve cell stimuli, neuroendocrine responses, and endothelial dysfunction, leading to a succession of rapidly cascading events from a local to a systemic phenomenon [27] (Figure 12.2). Damage signals generated from local tissue injury are detected by pattern-recognition receptors on resident and nonresident immune cells, resulting in activation of effector systems, including key proinflammatory cytokines, complex interactions with complement, and acute coagulopathy and hyperfibrinolysis. The primary goal of the acute immune response is wound healing and prevention of pathogen invasion through a restorative process that involves coagulation, inflammation, proliferation, and remodeling. Each phase of repair is complexly orchestrated by immune cells, cytokines, chemokines, changes in gene transcription, and posttranslational modifications.

At the same time, local tissue trauma with peripheral nerve injury, activation of nociceptors, and pain during major surgery induce afferent mediators and

BRIEF OVERVIEW OF THE SURGICAL STRESS RESPONSE

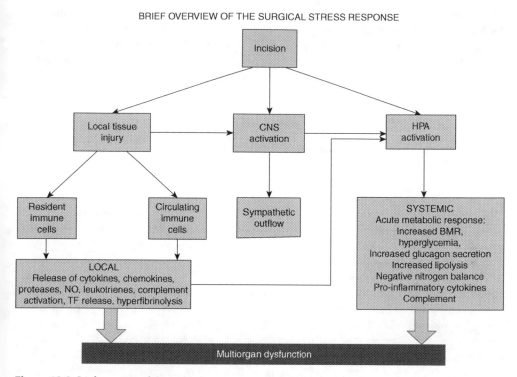

Figure 12.2 Brief overview of the surgical stress response showing the complex interplay between the central nervous system (CNS) and the mediators released at the time of local tissue injury, resulting in an inflammatory response (HPA = hypothalamic-pituitary axis).

neurotransmitters to the spinal cord and central nervous system (CNS), activating the hypothalamic-pituitary-adrenal (HPA) axis and the nucleus tractus solitarius and ultimately exacerbating the stressed clinical phenotype in surgical patients through release of stress hormones, altered circadian entrainment, and neuroinflammation. The magnitude of the systemic response is proportional to the degree of surgical insult, with cardiac surgery being an extreme example where the consequences of surgical trauma are compounded by ischemia-reperfusion and physiologic responses to cardiopulmonary bypass [27]. While normally self-limiting and resolving, the stress response to surgical injury can in some instances "overshoot" and exceed the body's internal tolerances, becoming the primary mechanism driving further perioperative organ injury such as cognitive and cardiac dysfunction, endothelial activation, vascular instability, systemic inflammation, coagulopathy, and possibly immunosuppression with increased risk of infection [26–28].

In surgical patients, acute sterile stressors are often followed by secondary insults that may be either sterile or pathogen induced (such as postoperative infection). Consequently, the so-called two-hit model of inflammatory insult has become the commonly accepted paradigm for stressful injury. The components of host response from the initial surgical insult are more clearly defined than those resulting from secondary events. What has become clear is that the cognate signals from either sterile surgical injury or pathogen-induced sources converge on the same recognition/response pathways. Interestingly, while host responses to the initial sterile hit of surgery are modified primarily by the magnitude of the insult and patient-specific (*endogenous*) factors, including age, *exogenous factors* such as postoperative management and pathogen virulence more prominently influence the overall responsiveness to secondary insults [29].

Aging Modifies the Host Response to Surgical Injury

Inflammation and Immune System

There is increasing evidence that specific cellular and molecular changes are direct contributors to all manifestations of aging, including altered responses to surgical stress. A dizzying composite of *phenotypes of aging* include changes in mitochondrial, nuclear, and ribosomal DNA; genomic and chromatin instability; increasing levels of oxidative stress (particularly mitochondrial damage); increasing systemic inflammation, paradoxically concomitant with declining immunocompetence; increasing glycation of proteins, which potentiates inflammation; increasing cellular senescence and loss of telomeres; dysregulation of apoptosis (programmed cell death is over- or underrecruited); impaired protein turnover and reduced removal of damaged and glycated proteins (impaired autophagy); endocrine dyscrasia; and altered stem cell repair and rejuvenation [30].

The relationship between age-related immune competence and confounding illness is more complex than commonly appreciated [31,32]. Epidemiologic data suggest that aging centrally involves changes in both innate and adaptive immunity (in the direction of declining adaptive immunity and compensatory upregulation of innate immunity), combined with increasing systemic inflammation. This proinflammatory heightened innate immune responsiveness in older subjects [33], often in the absence of an inflammatory threat – dubbed *inflamm-aging* – is characteristically more systemic, chronic, and often asymptomatic [30]. The aging population exhibits increased cytokine markers of low-grade inflammation (e.g., interleukin 6 [IL-6]), and this is associated with increased risk for the development of both infection [34] and other stressful events [35]. Elderly subjects challenged with lipopolysaccharides (LPS) also exhibit a more prolonged febrile response and hypotension [33,36,37] and have prolonged and enhanced cytokine responses during pneumococcal pneumonia [38]. Recently, *inflammasome* activation has also been mechanistically implicated in inflamm-aging [39]. As a component of the innate immune system, inflammasomes are intracellular structures triggered by the presence of pathogens or cellular stress and are responsible for the maturation of inflammatory cytokines IL-1β and IL-18. Specifically, in individuals 85 years of age and older, elevated and persistent expression of particular inflammasome gene modules correlates with the occurrence of hypertension, arterial stiffness, chronic increases in levels of inflammatory cytokines, metabolic dysfunction, oxidative stress, and all-cause mortality [39]. Although some theories of aging suggest that innate immune response capacity is sustained, at least in part, by the accumulated influences of noxious challenges, such as oxidative stress [40], there may be other interacting factors that promote proinflammatory competence during aging. For instance, the diminution of autonomic variability, in particular of vagal activity, that accompanies advancing age [41] may promote enhanced tumor necrosis factor α (TNF-α) activity during initial stress. By contrast, physical conditioning enhances parasympathetic system signaling and provides a survival advantage to physically fit elderly patients during acute inflammatory stress by attenuating cytokine excesses [29]. Furthermore, age-related imbalances in the composition of gut microbes (the gut microbiome) appear to drive increased intestinal permeability, age-associated inflammation, and decreased macrophage function [42]. With increasing evidence supporting the central role of the microbiome and dysbiosis in outcomes and recovery following surgical stress, sepsis, and critical illness [43], the implications of aging in increasing translocation of microbial pathogens from the intestine to the systemic circulation following shock, ischemia-reperfusion, and hemorrhage cannot be overemphasized [44]. In this regard, the main goal of early enteral nutrition in the postoperative course and critical illness is to promote nonnutritional benefits such as gut integrity and modulation of immunity (*immunonutrition*) and only later on to address maintenance of lean muscle mass and avoidance of malnutrition. Given our better understanding of the gut microbiome and its implications for surgical stress response and outcomes, the role of perioperative probiotics and other acute nutritional interventions (such as fecal transplantation) to help preserve of restore beneficial intestinal microbial communities is an active area of investigation [44,45]. Meta-analyses found an approximately 40 percent reduction in operative site infections and postoperative sepsis with systematic probiotic use, as well as a consistent reduction in the incidence of multiple-organ-dysfunction syndrome after trauma, but convincing evidence for their therapeutic efficacy is lacking [46].

The process of *immunosenescence*, or age-related defects in the human immune system, appears to affect principally the adaptive immune response [32,33]. There is a gradual loss of T-cell repertoire from naive CD8 T cells and a reduced response to neoantigens in elderly subjects. Concomitantly, there is a gradual shift from a type 1 cytokine response (IL-2, interferon-gamma [IFN-γ], and TNF-α) toward a type 2 response (IL-4, IL-6, IL-10, and IL-15) that further impairs cell-mediated immunity [29]. The net result is reduced pathogen recognition, chemotaxis, and phagocytosis with an inadequate T-cell antibody response and cytotoxicity.

Two recent studies shed some new light on the role of immune responsiveness in predicting recovery after surgery. By cataloging the detailed phenotypic and functional immune responses to surgical trauma in individual immune cell types using mass cytometry, Gaudilliere et al. identified a uniform surgical immune signature as well as novel predictors of specific aspects of surgical recovery such as functional impairment and pain [47]. Specifically, cell signaling responses, but not cell counts, were linked to recovery. Furthermore, the correlated signaling responses occurred most notably in CD14[+] monocytes and dendritic cells, with signaling induced by toll-like receptor 4 (TLR4) activation demonstrating a very strong predictive ability for individual postoperative recovery trajectories. In a follow-up study from the same group, the authors demonstrated that the preoperative "immune phenotype" of individual patients, assessed in vitro as the strength of LPS-induced signaling in CD14[+] monocytes in samples collected before surgery, also predicts the speed of postoperative recovery in some domains [48].

Coagulation System

An increasingly *procoagulant and prothrombotic milieu* arises with aging. Surgical tissue injury results in the release of tissue factor (TF), which, in turn, results in activation of the coagulation cascade via the extrinsic pathway. This leads to clot formation via thrombin generation and fibrin deposition. Uncontrolled activation of tissue factor can result in perioperative coagulopathy [49] There is an age-related increase in plasma concentrations of many coagulation factors. An element of this heightened procoagulant status may reflect the ongoing inflammatory processes mentioned earlier, given some markers, notably factor VIII and fibrinogen. The hemostasis factor affected most by age is the increase in von Willebrand factor. Furthermore, thrombin generation and platelet activation both increase with aging [50]. Increased platelet activation results in upregulation of specific binding to leukocytes that promote a proinflammatory state and inhibit resolution of inflammation. Thus in older people there is an increase in platelet P-selectin expression, proinflammatory leukocyte phenotypes, and platelet-leukocyte interactions [51] that have significant influences in mediating organ injury following surgical stress. This increase in leukocytes bound to platelets has been attributed to a decrease in the biologic activity of nitric oxide and cyclic guanosine monophosphate (cGMP) in platelets [52]. Plasminogen activator inhibitor 1 (PAI-1) is a principal inhibitor of fibrinolysis and is induced in thrombotic, fibrotic, and cardiovascular diseases, which, in turn, primarily afflict the older population. PAI-1 expression is elevated in aged individuals and is significantly upregulated in a variety of pathologies associated with the process of aging, including myocardial and cerebral infarction, atherosclerosis, cardiac and lung fibrosis, metabolic syndromes, cancer, and inflammatory responses. Thus PAI-1 may play a critical role in the development of aging-associated pathologic changes. Intriguingly, PAI-1 is also recognized as a marker and mediator of senescence and a key member of a group of proteins collectively known as the *senescence-messaging secretome* [53].

Hyperfibrinolysis also can occur as a result of surgical stress and is seen in trauma and cardiac and major spine surgery. Hyperfibrinolysis can result in the need for massive transfusion and may lead to prolonged ICU and hospital lengths of stay and even death [54]. In contrast, postoperative immobility and the systemic inflammation accompanying surgical stress response can lead to an increased risk of postoperative thromboembolism in older adults in the setting of acquired thrombophilia associated with aging [55].

Neuroendocrine-Metabolic Systems

The *endocrine response* to surgery includes secretion of growth hormone, adrenocorticotropic hormone (ACTH), prolactin, and vasopressin from the pituitary; increased cortisol, catecholamines, and aldosterone from the adrenals; and increased glucagon release and decreased insulin release from the pancreas. There is also a decrease in testosterone, estrogen, and triiodothyronine following surgery. The complex interplay between these hormones induces a catabolic state characterized by insulin resistance, hyperglycemia, lipolysis, and skeletal muscle wasting resulting in a negative nitrogen balance. The magnitude of these catabolic changes is likely not very different in the elderly compared with young adults, but elderly patients have reduced muscle mass at the outset and are more prone to protein catabolism [56]. Skeletal muscle wasting can result in frailty and delayed return to baseline functional status [57], need for discharge to intermediate care institutions such as nursing facilities, and worst of all, death.

Though, effect of age on responses to the initial surgical insult are somewhat described in the literature, our understanding of the influence of age as a modifier of subsequent insults and second hits (e.g., postoperative infection) and its impact on outcome trajectories remains extremely limited. Most models of infection pathogenesis, including postoperative infection, do not incorporate host stress. It is now well established that following acute insults to the host such as surgery, trauma, myocardial infarction, or burn surgery, the intestinal microbiota decreases in abundance and function, and a virulent and resistant pathobiome emerges, rendering the stressed host more vulnerable to infection [58]. This is particularly complex because the intervention or treatment-related effects appear to interact with endogenous determinants such as age in the context of prolonged postoperative stress and systemic inflammatory response. Age-related diminutions of immune and endocrine functions [59] and autonomic signal attenuation all may contribute to adverse outcomes among elderly patients. There is currently limited insight across the age spectrum as to how prominently these endogenous factors contribute to loss of adaptability during prolonged stress [29].

Geroscience Concepts Applied to Surgical Stress Response

With the underlying rationale that aging itself is the predominant risk factor for most diseases and conditions that limit health life expectancy or "healthspan," a new field of *geroscience* is seeking to understand the integrated aging-related changes in biologic systems and develop novel multidisease preventative and therapeutic approaches. Kennedy et al. have recently described seven highly intertwined processes driving aging (hence termed the *pillars of aging*) – including adaptation to stress, epigenetics, inflammation, macromolecular damage, metabolism, proteostasis, and stem cells and regeneration [60]. Importantly, understanding the interplay among these seven pillars is critical and should inform our approaches to study perioperative stress responses and how they may underlie surgical resilience across organ systems. Several key concepts pertaining to aging as a modifier of surgical stress response will be outlined next – these include allostasis and allostatic load, hormesis, frailty, and resilience.

Allostasis, Allostatic Load, and Surgical Stress Response

Allostasis, a concept introduced by Sterling and Eyer in 1988, describes the effect of stressors on an organism. It refers to the organism's ability to respond to stressors or external stimuli with continuous change in an effort to maintain dynamic equilibrium. The goal of allostasis is preservation of somatic stability. When stress is perceived by the organism, it results in the activation of the hypothalamic-pituitary-adrenal (HPA) axis with a resulting increase in serum cortisol, norepinephrine, and epinephrine. When the stressor dissipates, this response is turned off, and the serum cortisol and other stress hormones return to baseline in an efficient manner. As the organism ages, the allostatic response becomes impaired, and there may be an exaggerated or inadequate peak response, as well as a sluggish return to baseline [61,62]. Repeated and prolonged exposure of the organism to these mediators can have deleterious effects, resulting in a buildup of wear and tear, a term described as *allostatic load*. The allostatic load therefore is the price the organism pays for adaptation to physiologic stressors [63]. The original primary mediators of allostatic load are catecholamines, cortisol, and dihydroepiandrosterone sulfate (DHEA-S). Other hormones and proteins were later included to assess allostatic load, such as insulin-like growth factor 1 (IGF-1), IL-6, serotonin, and C-reactive protein (CRP) [64,65]. These primary mediators result in physiologic changes and outcomes, including elevated systolic and diastolic blood pressure, blood glucose, lipid levels, and measures of body habitus, including waist-hip ratio. These are termed *secondary mediators of stress*. The eventual outcome of allostatic load is an increased propensity to develop chronic diseases, including atherosclerosis and diabetes mellitus.

Four types of allostatic load have been described as being important to the well-being of the individual. First, in the case of frequent exposures to stress such as repeated episodes of uncontrolled hypertension, the susceptible elderly individual can experience adverse outcomes such as a myocardial infarction or hemorrhagic stroke. Second, when exposed to similar stressors, there is failure of adaptation of the stress response resulting in prolonged exposure to stress mediators. The third type of allostatic load revolves around the inability of the individual to terminate the allostatic response once the stressful stimulus has subsided. An example of this type of allostatic load is the decreased bone mineral density in chronically depressed women, who continue to have an elevated serum cortisol level, which, in turn, inhibits new bone formation. In the fourth type of allostatic load, there is an inadequate allostatic response that then leads to hyperactivity of inflammatory cytokines, which are typically suppressed by glucocorticoids. This typically manifests as an increased susceptibility to autoimmune and inflammatory diseases [61].

As an organism ages, changes occur in many organ systems that are linked to the development of chronic degenerative diseases. One important process is aging of the immune system, manifested as an overall increase in proinflammatory cytokines such as IL-6, TNF-α, CRP, and IL-1β, with an accompanying reduction in anti-inflammatory cytokines such as IL-10. This "inflammaging" has been implicated in the pathogenesis of diabetes, dementia, and cardiovascular diseases and is associated with a higher mortality [66]. It is interesting to note that the cytokine profile of centenarians remains similar to that of young adults, supporting the idea that "inflammaging" is associated with decreased longevity [67].

Telomere length is another marker of allostatic load. Telomeres are tandemly repeating short DNA strands at the ends of eukaryotic chromosomes. Telomeres and their associated proteins are responsible for protection of the genomic DNA. At the end of each cell division, telomeres shorten in length, leaving the cell more vulnerable to genomic instability. The enzyme telomerase can add DNA repeating sequences at the end of the chromosome to compensate for attrition [68]. Shorter telomere length is associated with risk factors for cardiovascular disease and may be a predictor of mortality in patients with chronic kidney disease, Alzheimer's disease, and stroke. Shortened telomere length is seen in people exposed to chronic stress such as caregivers [69]. In postmenopausal women caring for patients with dementia who were exposed to an acute stressor, a higher cortisol level associated with the acute stressor was associated with shorter telomeres. The long-term consequence of repeated high-stress exposure is likely accelerated cellular senescence [70].

Hormesis as a Potential Modifier of Surgical Stress Response in the Elderly

Hormesis, a term used most extensively in the fields of toxicology and radiation biology, refers to a generalized, evolutionarily conserved biphasic pattern of adaptive cellular responses to stressors whereby a beneficial effect (e.g., stress tolerance, improved "healthspan," or longevity) results from exposure to *low doses* of agents or intensities of environmental factors that are otherwise toxic or lethal when given at higher concentrations or intensities. First described in 1946, hormetic responses were largely ignored in biomedical research until the discovery that transient heat stress invoked the appearance of a protected phenotype in cells, tissues, or organisms such that they were able to withstand the harmful effects induced by otherwise lethal stressors. Interest in this area was boosted to new heights with the discovery that antecedent exposure to short bouts of sublethal ischemia followed by reperfusion conferred cardioprotection in hearts subsequently exposed to lethal ischemia-reperfusion (I/R), a phenomenon termed *ischemic preconditioning* (IPC). Subsequent to that came the discoveries that the heart and other organs could be protected by subjecting distant organs or tissues (e.g., the small intestine, kidneys, and limbs) to IPC – which is referred to as *remote, interorgan*, or *distant site ischemic preconditioning* (RIPC) – or by using gradual and hemodynamically controlled reperfusion (multiple short bouts of I/R) to salvage previously ischemic but viable myocardium (a phenomenon designated *ischemic postconditioning*) [71]. More recently, the neuroprotective effects of cold-shock response have been reported. A protein released during hypothermia has been found to affect the progression of neurodegenerative disease in mice by sparing neurons from death and preserving synaptic plasticity [72]. These early findings support the concept that adaptive intrinsic pleiotropic cell survival programs can be activated by a variety of mildly noxious stimuli or pharmacologic agents to confer protection against the deleterious effects of I/R, which have tremendous translational relevance for surgical stress response and perioperative organ protection. In addition to heat and cold-shock response, examples of such conserved prosurvival and longevity hormetic inducible pathways include mitochondrial responses to increased oxidative stress, the unfolded protein response to endoplasmic reticulum stress, immunomodulation of signaling via TLR4, and metabolic control in response to diet restriction, caloric restriction, exercise, DNA repair/genetic stability in response to heat and radiation [73], and hibernation [74]. A prosurvival pathway shared by intermittent fasting, caloric restriction, exercise, and hibernation involves activation of a family of protein deacetylases called *sirtuins* (chief among which is sirtuin-3), which results in both antioxidant and metabolic reprogramming hormetic effects [74,75]. Consequently, candidate hormetic mimetics are key regulators of such prosurvival pathways and include stimulated DNA repair, endogenous antioxidants, restoration of protein structure and function, energy endurance, immunoregulation, and systemic and metabolic responses to ischemia. Several examples include hormetic heat mimetics (molecular chaperones such as HSP70, ethanol, and quercetin) and diet-restriction mimetics (metformin, resveratrol, and PPAR-delta agonists). Several points of intervention exist for limiting postischemic tissue injury that may be targeted by the adaptive endogenous programs invoked by conditioning stimuli. The mechanistic rationale for developing pharmacologic conditioning strategies that mimic the remarkably powerful effects of ischemic conditioning is sound. Lifestyle interventions, including exercise, caloric restriction or intermittent fasting, dietary manipulations, and consumption of alcoholic beverages and/or phytochemicals, may induce hormetic responses – and are relevant to perioperative management. One such area of controversy surrounds preoperative nutritional recommendations, particularly in elderly surgical patients. The current trend in preoperative nutrition away from preoperative fasting and toward carbohydrate loading embedded in enhanced recovery after surgery (ERAS) nutritional guidelines has to be counterbalanced against evidence that short-term dietary restriction and fasting (or pharmacological diet-restriction mimetics) preconditions against surgical stress via both upstream nutrient-sensing mechanisms and effector mechanisms implicating increased prosurvival insulin signaling and elevated endogenous hydrogen sulfite production [76].

Despite promising preclinical studies, the efficacy of many hormetic interventions has proven ineffective in the presence of aging and cardiovascular risk factors and/or is adversely affected by coincident use of cardiovascular drugs, anesthetics (especially propofol), and opioids. Obstacles to its practical application in patients remain, as evidenced by the recent failures of remote ischemic preconditioning (RIPC) randomized, controlled trials to reduce mortality and morbidity in cardiac surgery [77]. Thus, uncovering the mechanisms responsible for such impaired responses to preconditioning stimuli and differentiating hormesis from toxic stress will be imperative to successful clinical application of hormetic interventions in relevant surgical patient populations, including the elderly.

Frailty as a Modifiable Predictor of Postoperative Outcomes in Older Adults

Frailty is defined as a multidimensional syndrome characterized by progressive reduction in physical reserve, energy, cognitive reserve, and an overall lack of physiologic reserve across several organ systems that results in a state of vulnerability by impairing an individual's ability to cope with stressors. It is prevalent among the elderly and a known risk factor for falls, institutionalization, and morbidity [78]. Clinical frailty in older adults is associated with worse perioperative outcomes across many surgical subspecialties. The frail elderly patient is more likely to experience serious complications [79–81], prolonged hospital stay [82], higher 30-day readmission rate following elective cardiac and noncardiac surgery [79], loss of independent activity with increased discharge to an institutional facility [83], and reduced 1-year survival [84]. Makary et al. measured frailty prospectively in patients older than age 65 presenting for elective surgery [82] and found frail patients to have more than 2.5-fold higher risk of complications compared with nonfrail patients. They were also more likely to have increased length of stay and had a higher likelihood of discharge to an assisted-living facility [82,85]. Moreover, preexisting cognitive impairment is emerging as a predictor of poor outcomes following surgical stress in seniors. In subjects older than age 65, the prevalence of dementia is estimated at 5 to 10 percent, and that of mild cognitive impairment, a frequently undetected problem, is as high as 35 to 50 percent. Importantly, preexisting cognitive impairment is a predictor and modifier of common cognitive complications of surgery – namely postoperative delirium (20–80 percent incidence) and postoperative cognitive dysfunction (12–15 percent incidence) [86]. The morbidity and higher economic burden of frailty call for a simplified preoperative assessment and adequate optimization of all elderly patients undergoing surgery (see Chapter 15). Indeed, a comprehensive geriatric assessment may be a stronger predictor of postoperative outcomes in this patient population than the time-honored American Society of Anesthesiology score [87].

To optimize the quality of care for elderly surgical patients, the American College of Surgery and the American Geriatric Society developed best practice guidelines for perioperative management of geriatric patients in 2012 [88]. These guidelines focus on problems specific to the elderly surgical patient, including frailty, cognitive dysfunction, and polypharmacy. They also include recommendations for assessment of nutritional status, social support, and decision-making capacity. The group compiled the recommendations in the form of a checklist (Table 12.1) that would enable a thorough and optimal preoperative workup and identify high-risk patients for further assessment. Surgery departments at various institutions have adopted and modified these guidelines to fit their patient populations. Wozniak et al. implemented these guidelines at the Sinai Center for Geriatric Surgery and modified them by including a hearing screen, oral screen, performance status, Charlson

Table 12.1 Checklist for the Optimal Preoperative Assessment of Geriatric Surgical Patients

In addition to conducting a complete history and physical examination of the patient, the following assessments are strongly recommended:

1. Assess the patient's *cognitive ability* and *capacity* to understand the anticipated surgery.
2. Screen the patient for *depression*.
3. Identify the patient's risk factors for developing *postoperative delirium*.
4. Screen for *alcohol* and other *substance abuse/dependence*.
5. Identify the patient's risk factors for postoperative *pulmonary complications* and implement appropriate strategies for prevention.
6. Perform a preoperative *cardiac evaluation* according to the American College of Cardiology/American Heart Association algorithm for patients undergoing noncardiac surgery.
7. Document *functional status* and *history of falls*.
8. Determine baseline *frailty score*.
9. Assess patient's *nutritional status* and consider preoperative interventions if the patient is at severe nutritional risk.
10. Take an accurate and detailed *medication history* and consider appropriate perioperative adjustments; monitor for *polypharmacy*.
11. Determine the patient's *treatment goals* and *expectations* in the context of the possible treatment outcomes.
12. Determine patient's *family* and *social support system*.
13. Order appropriate preoperative *diagnostic tests* focused on elderly patients.

(*Source:* Chow et al. [88].)

Comorbidity Index, pressure ulcer risk, and caregiver burden interview [89]. It was performed by an experienced nurse practitioner and added 20 minutes to their standard preoperative assessment. Other surgical specialties, including urology, have also acknowledged the surgical risk of an elderly adult and emphasized the importance of achieving good functional outcomes [90], which are incredibly important to elderly surgical patients. While no specific practice guidelines aimed at geriatric surgical patients have been issued by the American Society of Anesthesiology, there is a growing body of literature addressing some of the current controversies in this arena, including choice of anesthesia and prevention of postoperative delirium [91].

Physical Resilience in Older Adults

Understanding how advanced age modifies surgical stress is important because improved surgical outcomes in the elderly depend on instituting appropriate perioperative measures to reduce the stress response, with the ultimate goal of early return to the preoperative physical state. However, postoperative patient trajectories, and in particular the ability to maintain or recover appropriate function following major surgery, remain poorly described, lacking both a precise phenotypic framework and mechanistic understanding. What little we do know about recovery from surgery as a primary outcome relies on cross-sectional incidence data with infrequent assessments, which limits characterization of speed of recovery and underlying mechanisms. An emerging concept separates responses to physical stressors (such as surgical trauma) into two key steps – deviation from the original (*baseline*) state and return to the original state (*recovery*). Consequently, stress resistance can be characterized by two different components, respectively: (1) ability to resist deviation from homeostasis (*robustness*), as measured by the magnitude of deviation from the original preoperative state following surgical stress and time to a peak value, and (2) ability to fully recover after such deviation (*resilience*), as measured by time to recovery and completeness of functional recovery [92]. Preliminary evidence suggests that a number of biomarkers of surgical resilience (such as neuropeptide Y, testosterone, and dehydroepiandrosterone) correlate with better recovery trajectories after surgery and can be used as prognostic indicators [93] in conjunction with "prehabilitation" strategies to lessen the risks of adverse perioperative outcomes. In this regard, knowledge of the dose-response relationships to the magnitude of surgical stressors is particularly important because of the potential of threshold effects, further complicated by combinations of either concurrent or sequential stressors [94].

Modifying the Surgical Stress Response and Improving Outcomes

The goal of anesthesia is to blunt the surgical stress response by reducing the production and release of *stress mediators*. Although small studies found better immunologic and neurohumoral-metabolic responses to surgical stress in patients receiving total intravenous anesthesia (e.g., remifentanil and propofol) versus volatile anesthesia (e.g., sevoflurane) [95], very limited and sometimes controversial evidence exists with respect to optimal anesthetic choice for elderly frail patients, mostly from orthopedic hip surgery. Neuman et al. reported a 29 percent lower adjusted risk of mortality and a 24 percent decrease in pulmonary complications in patients receiving regional anesthesia for hip surgery [96], whereas others found a higher incidence of perioperative complications following hip surgery in patients who had spinal anesthesia [97]. A 2004 Cochrane review did not reveal important differences in outcomes between the two techniques, and the 2014 Guidelines on the Management of Hip Fractures in the Elderly by the American Association of Orthopedic Surgeons propose no difference in outcomes for general or neuraxial anesthesia [98]. Absent strong evidence favoring one anesthetic choice over another, anesthesiologists must use their best judgment and knowledge of the patient's comorbid diseases to decide which type of anesthetic to administer. The REGAIN trial (Regional vs General Anesthesia for Promoting Independence after Hip Surgery; ClinicalTrials.gov identifier: NCT02507505) is currently prospectively enrolling patients at multiple sites and will help improve the quality of evidence in this area.

Providing adequate analgesia is a critical component of reducing surgical stress in the elderly. It is important to realize that uncontrolled pain is common in older adults, especially those with underlying cognitive dysfunction [99,100]. Uncontrolled pain can lead to adverse outcomes, including delirium, cardiopulmonary complications, lengthier rehabilitation, need for readmission, and development of chronic pain syndromes [101]. In contrast, the elderly patients are at higher risk of having adverse events from analgesics as a result of altered pharmacokinetics, increased CNS sensitivity to drugs, and frailty, limiting their ability to compensate for medication overdose [102]. Multimodal analgesia, with increased use of nonopioid analgesics such as gabapentin, pregabalin, acetaminophen, ketorolac, and local anesthetics (infiltrated, neuraxial, or regional), can reduce pain in the immediate postoperative period and facilitate early rehabilitation and discharge [103]. Neuraxial techniques are also beneficial in the elderly for analgesia after major abdominal, vascular, and even orthopedic procedures. The geriatric surgical patient stands to gain a lot of benefit from this technique for postoperative analgesia, especially with regard to early ambulation, early return of bowel function, less sedation, and lowered cardiovascular morbidity [104].

The American Geriatric Society released a best practice report for management of postoperative delirium in the elderly. The report recommends prompt diagnosis and pharmacologic treatment of delirium [105], underscoring the importance of adequate analgesia and avoidance of certain benzodiazepines, H1 antagonists, and meperidine. There is also some evidence suggesting that titration of anesthesia to avoid burst suppression on the processed electroencephalogram may reduce the incidence of postoperative delirium [106]. This benefit of a "lighter plane of anesthesia" must be balanced against the risk of possible intraoperative awareness, movement, and sympathetic activation during surgery, all of which could be harmful in the elderly.

Conclusion

In conclusion, there is a fundamental gap in understanding how aging increases vulnerability to surgical stress, ischemia-reperfusion injury, and postoperative critical illness. A number of observations draw a link among aging, loss of mitochondrial function, nutrient sensing, "inflammasome" activation, and impaired recovery following surgical stressors – under a paradigm of age-related decreased *physical resilience* [92]. Understanding why some older adults recover function rapidly after surgical stress and critical illness and others decline, continues to pose both scientific and clinical questions. What are the driving mechanisms, and are these specific to organ systems or is there an underlying resilience trait? What is the role of pain, environment, and psychosocial factors in modulating surgical resilience? Answers to such scientific questions would inform key clinical questions. If we can predict surgical resilience, can we modify or avoid the stressor or change how we deliver care? Are there pleiotropic interventions that can boost surgical resilience in older adults? Importantly, as perioperative physicians and intensivists we should expand our focus from successful ICU and hospital discharge to a more comprehensive assessment and understanding of functional capacity as a therapeutic endpoint [107]. Tools to assess disability following surgical stress and critical illness exist [108], and preliminary studies looking at the impact of disability on ICU survivors suggest that this is indeed a prevalent and essential patient-centered outcome to improve [109].

References

1. Arias E, Kochanek K, Xu J, Murphy S. Mortality in the United States, 2014. *NCHS Data Brief* 2015; **229**:1–8.

2. Administration of Aging. Profile of Older Americans: 2015. Administration for Community Living, US Department of Health and Human Services, 2015, available at www.acl.gov/aging-and-disability-in-america/data.../profile-older-americans.

3. Vincent GK VV. *The Next Four Decades: The Older Population in the United States: 2010 to 2050*. US Department of Commerce, Economics and Statistics Administration, US Census Bureau, 2010.

4. Weiser TG, Regenbogen SE, Thompson KD, et al. An estimation of the global volume of surgery: a modelling strategy based on available data. *Lancet* 2008; **372**(9633):139–44.

5. Pearse RM, Moreno RP, Bauer P, et al. Mortality after surgery in Europe: a 7 day cohort study. *Lancet* 2012; **380**(9847): 1059–65.

6. Hall M, DeFrances C, Williams S, Golosinskiy A, Schwartzman A. National

Hospital Discharge Survey: 2007 summary. *Natl Health Stat Report* 2010; **29**:1–20, 4.

7. Li G, Warner M, Lang BH, Huang L, Sun LS. Epidemiology of anesthesia-related mortality in the United States, 1999–2005. *Anesthesiology* 2009; **110**(4):759–65.

8. Speziale G, Nasso G, Barattoni MC, et al. Operative and middle-term results of cardiac surgery in nonagenarians: a bridge toward routine practice. *Circulation* 2010; **121**(2):208–13.

9. Speziale G, Nasso G, Barattoni MC, et al. Short-term and long-term results of cardiac surgery in elderly and very elderly patients. *J Thorac Cardiovasc Surg* 2011; **141**(3):725–31, e1.

10. Angus DC, Linde-Zwirble WT, Lidicker J, et al. Epidemiology of severe sepsis in the United States: analysis of incidence, outcome, and associated costs of care. *Crit Care Med* 2001; **29**(7):1303–10.

11. Sjoding MW, Prescott HC, Wunsch H, Iwashyna TJ, Cooke CR. Longitudinal changes in ICU admissions among elderly patients in the United States. *Crit Care Med* 2016; **44**(7):1353–60.

12. Nguyen YL, Angus DC, Boumendil A, Guidet B. The challenge of admitting the very elderly to intensive care. *Ann Intensive Care* 2011; **1**(1):29.

13. Rydingsward JE, Horkan CM, Mogensen KM, et al. Functional status in ICU survivors and out of hospital outcomes: a cohort study. *Crit Care Med* 2016; **44**(5):869–79.

14. Wunsch H, Guerra C, Barnato AE, et al. Three-year outcomes for Medicare beneficiaries who survive intensive care. *JAMA* 2010; **303**(9):849–56.

15. Heyland DK, Stelfox HT, Garland A, et al. Predicting performance status 1 year after critical illness in patients 80 years or older: development of a multivariable clinical prediction model. *Crit Care Med* 2016; **44**(9):1718–26.

16. Podgoreanu MV, Schwinn DA. New paradigms in cardiovascular medicine: emerging technologies and practices: perioperative genomics. *J Am Coll Cardiol* 2005; **46**(11):1965–77.

17. Giannoudis P, Dinopoulos H, Chalidis B, Hall G. Surgical stress response. *Injury* 2006; **37**(Suppl 5):S3–9.

18. Finnerty C, Mabvuure N, Ali A, Kozar R, Herndon D. The surgically induced stress response. *JPEN J Parenter Enteral Nutr* 2013; **37**(Suppl 5):21S–29S.

19. Wilmore DW. From Cuthbertson to fast-track surgery: 70 years of progress in reducing stress in surgical patients. *Ann Surg* 2002; **236**(5):643–48.

20. Abdelmalak BB, Bonilla AM, Yang D, et al. The hyperglycemic response to major noncardiac surgery and the added effect of steroid administration in patients with and without diabetes. *Anesth Analg* 2013; **116**(5):1116–22.

21. Li L, Messina JL. Acute insulin resistance following injury. *Trends Endocrinol Metab* 2009; **20**(9):429–35.

22. Desborough JP. The stress response to trauma and surgery. *Br J Anaesth* 2000; **85**(1):109–17.

23. Jin F, Chung F. Minimizing perioperative adverse events in the elderly. *Br J Anaesth* 2001; **87**(4):608–24.

24. Cecconi M, Corredor C, Arulkumaran N, et al. Clinical review: goal-directed therapy-what is the evidence in surgical patients? The effect on different risk groups. *Crit Care* 2013; **17**(2):209.

25. Cerra F, Siegel J, Border J, Peters D, McMenamy R. Correlations between metabolic and cardiopulmonary measurements in patients after trauma, general surgery, and sepsis. *J Trauma* 1979; **19**(8):621–29.

26. Kohl B, Deutschman C. The inflammatory response to surgery and trauma. *Curr Opin Crit Care* 2006; **12**(4):325–32.

27. Dobson GP. Addressing the global burden of trauma in major surgery. *Front Surg* 2015; **2**:43.

28. Bartels K, Karhausen J, Clambey ET, Grenz A, Eltzschig HK. Perioperative

organ injury. *Anesthesiology* 2013; **119**(6): 1474–89.

29. Lowry SF. The stressed host response to infection: the disruptive signals and rhythms of systemic inflammation. *Surg Clin North Am* 2009; **89**(2):311–26, vii.

30. Watt D. The biology of aging: implications for diseases of aging and health care in the twenty-first century. In A Nair, M Sabbagh, eds., *Geriatric Neurology*. New York, NY: Wiley Online Library, 2014: 1–37.

31. Dhainaut JF, Claessens YE, Janes J, Nelson DR. Underlying disorders and their impact on the host response to infection. *Clin Infect Dis* 2005; **41**(Suppl 7):S481–89.

32. Gruver AL, Hudson LL, Sempowski GD. Immunosenescence of ageing. *J Pathol* 2007; **211**(2):144–56.

33. Opal SM, Girard TD, Ely EW. The immunopathogenesis of sepsis in elderly patients. *Clin Infect Dis* 2005; **41** (Suppl 7):S504–12.

34. Yende S, Tuomanen EI, Wunderink R, et al. Preinfection systemic inflammatory markers and risk of hospitalization due to pneumonia. *Am J Respir Crit Care Med* 2005; **172**(11):1440–46.

35. Cesari M, Penninx BW, Newman AB, et al. Inflammatory markers and onset of cardiovascular events: results from the Health ABC Study. *Circulation* 2003; **108** (19):2317–22.

36. Krabbe KS, Bruunsgaard H, Hansen CM, et al. Ageing is associated with a prolonged fever response in human endotoxemia. *Clin Diagn Lab Immunol* 2001; **8**(2): 333–38.

37. Krabbe KS, Bruunsgaard H, Qvist J, et al. Hypotension during endotoxemia in aged humans. *Eur J Anaesthesiol* 2001; **18**(9): 572–75.

38. Bruunsgaard H, Skinhoj P, Qvist J, Pedersen BK. Elderly humans show prolonged in vivo inflammatory activity during pneumococcal infections. *J Infect Dis* 1999; **180**(2):551–54.

39. Furman D, Chang J, Lartigue L, et al. Expression of specific inflammasome gene modules stratifies older individuals into

two extreme clinical and immunological states. *Nat Med* 2017; **23**(2):174–84.

40. Butcher SK, Lord JM. Stress responses and innate immunity: aging as a contributory factor. *Aging Cell* 2004; **3**(4):151–60.

41. Bonnemeier H, Richardt G, Potratz J, et al. Circadian profile of cardiac autonomic nervous modulation in healthy subjects: differing effects of aging and gender on heart rate variability. *J Cardiovasc Electrophysiol* 2003; **14**(8):791–99.

42. Thevaranjan N, Puchta A, Schulz C, et al. Age-associated microbial dysbiosis promotes intestinal permeability, systemic inflammation, and macrophage dysfunction. *Cell Host Microbe* 2017; **21**(4): 455–66, e4.

43. McDonald D, Ackermann G, Khailova L, et al. Extreme dysbiosis of the microbiome in critical illness. *mSphere* 2016; **1**(4).

44. Codner PA, Herron TJ. The shifting microbiome in surgical stress. *Curr Surg Rep* 2017; **5**(4):9.

45. Stavrou G, Kotzampassi K. Gut microbiome, surgical complications and probiotics. *Ann Gastroenterol* 2017; **30** (1):45–53.

46. Morrow LE, Wischmeyer P. Blurred lines: dysbiosis and probiotics in the ICU. *Chest* 2017; **151**(2):492–99.

47. Gaudilliere B, Fragiadakis GK, Bruggner RV, et al. Clinical recovery from surgery correlates with single-cell immune signatures. *Sci Transl Med* 2014; **6**(255):255ra131.

48. Fragiadakis GK, Gaudilliere B, Ganio EA, et al. Patient-specific immune states before surgery are strong correlates of surgical recovery. *Anesthesiology* 2015; **123**(6): 1241–55.

49. Rao LV, Pendurthi UR. Tissue factor-factor VIIa signaling. *Arterioscler Thromb Vasc Biol* 2005; **25**(1):47–56.

50. Favaloro EJ, Franchini M, Lippi G. Aging hemostasis: changes to laboratory markers of hemostasis as we age: a narrative review. *Semin Thromb Hemost* 2014; **40**(6):621–33.

51. Seidler S, Zimmermann HW, Bartneck M, Trautwein C, Tacke F. Age-dependent

alterations of monocyte subsets and monocyte-related chemokine pathways in healthy adults. *BMC Immunol* 2010; **11**:30.

52. Goubareva I, Gkaliagkousi E, Shah A, et al. Age decreases nitric oxide synthesis and responsiveness in human platelets and increases formation of monocyte-platelet aggregates. *Cardiovasc Res* 2007; **75** (4):793–802.

53. Yamamoto K, Takeshita K, Saito H. Plasminogen activator inhibitor-1 in aging. *Semin Thromb Hemost* 2014; **40**(6):652–59.

54. Dobson GP, Letson HL, Sharma R, Sheppard FR, Cap AP. Mechanisms of early trauma-induced coagulopathy: the clot thickens or not? *J Trauma Acute Care Surg* 2015; **79**(2):301–9.

55. Schlaudecker J, Becker R. Inflammatory response and thrombosis in older individuals. *Semin Thromb Hemost* 2014; **40**(6):669–74.

56. Morais JA, Chevalier S, Gougeon R. Protein turnover and requirements in the healthy and frail elderly. *J Nutr Health Aging* 2006; **10**(4):272–83.

57. Schricker T, Lattermann R. Perioperative catabolism. *Can J Anaesth* 2015; **62**(2): 182–93.

58. Alverdy JC, Luo JN. The influence of host stress on the mechanism of infection: lost microbiomes, emergent pathobiomes, and the role of interkingdom signaling. *Front Microbiol* 2017; **8**:322.

59. Chahal HS, Drake WM. The endocrine system and ageing. *J Pathol* 2007; **211**(2): 173–80.

60. Kennedy BK, Berger SL, Brunet A, et al. Geroscience: linking aging to chronic disease. *Cell* 2014; **159**(4):709–13.

61. McEwen BS. Protective and damaging effects of stress mediators. *N Engl J Med* 1998; **338**(3):171–79.

62. McEwen BS, Seeman T. Protective and damaging effects of mediators of stress: elaborating and testing the concepts of allostasis and allostatic load. *Ann NY Acad Sci* 1999; **896**:30–47.

63. McEwen BS, Stellar E. Stress and the individual: mechanisms leading to

disease. *Arch Intern Med* 1993; **153**(18): 2093–101.

64. Seplaki CL, Goldman N, Glei D, Weinstein M. A comparative analysis of measurement approaches for physiological dysregulation in an older population. *Exp Gerontol* 2005; **40**(5):438–49.

65. Dowd JB, Simanek AM, Aiello AE. Socio-economic status, cortisol and allostatic load: a review of the literature. *Int J Epidemiol* 2009; **38**(5):1297–309.

66. Bartlett DB, Firth CM, Phillips AC, et al. The age-related increase in low-grade systemic inflammation (inflammaging) is not driven by cytomegalovirus infection. *Aging Cell* 2012; **11**(5):912–15.

67. Franceschi C, Monti D, Sansoni P, Cossarizza A. The immunology of exceptional individuals: the lesson of centenarians. *Immunol Today* 1995; **16** (1):12–16.

68. Blackburn EH, Epel ES, Lin J. Human telomere biology: a contributory and interactive factor in aging, disease risks, and protection. *Science* 2015; **350**(6265): 1193–98.

69. Epel ES, Blackburn EH, Lin J, et al. Accelerated telomere shortening in response to life stress. *Proc Natl Acad Sci USA* 2004; **101**(49):17312–15.

70. Tomiyama AJ, O'Donovan A, Lin J, et al. Does cellular aging relate to patterns of allostasis? An examination of basal and stress reactive HPA axis activity and telomere length. *Physiol Behav* 2012; **106**(1):40–45.

71. Hausenloy DJ, Yellon DM. Ischaemic conditioning and reperfusion injury. *Nat Rev Cardiol* 2016; **13**(4):193–209.

72. Peretti D, Bastide A, Radford H, et al. RBM3 mediates structural plasticity and protective effects of cooling in neurodegeneration. *Nature* 2015; **518** (7538):236–39.

73. Kolb H, Eizirik DL. Resistance to type 2 diabetes mellitus: a matter of hormesis? *Nat Rev Endocrinol* 2011; **8**(3):183–92.

74. Quinones QJ, Zhang Z, Ma Q, et al. Proteomic profiling reveals adaptive responses to surgical myocardial

ischemia-reperfusion in hibernating arctic ground squirrels compared to rats. *Anesthesiology* 2016; **124**(6):1296–310.

75. Kincaid B, Bossy-Wetzel E. Forever young: SIRT3 a shield against mitochondrial meltdown, aging, and neurodegeneration. *Front Aging Neurosci* 2013; **5**:48.

76. Longchamp A, Harputlugil E, Corpataux JM, Ozaki CK, Mitchell JR. Is overnight fasting before surgery too much or not enough? How basic aging research can guide preoperative nutritional recommendations to improve surgical outcomes: a mini-review. *Gerontology* 2017; **63**(3):228–37.

77. Hausenloy DJ, Candilio L, Evans R, et al. Remote ischemic preconditioning and outcomes of cardiac surgery. *N Engl J Med* 2015; **373**(15):1408–17.

78. Xue QL. The frailty syndrome: definition and natural history. *Clin Geriatr Med* 2011; **27**(1):1–15.

79. Robinson TN, Wu DS, Pointer L, et al. Simple frailty score predicts postoperative complications across surgical specialties. *Am J Surg* 2013; **206**(4):544–50.

80. Dasgupta M, Rolfson DB, Stolee P, Borrie MJ, Speechley M. Frailty is associated with postoperative complications in older adults with medical problems. *Arch Gerontol Geriatr* 2009; **48**(1):78–83.

81. Kristjansson SR, Nesbakken A, Jordhoy MS, et al. Comprehensive geriatric assessment can predict complications in elderly patients after elective surgery for colorectal cancer: a prospective observational cohort study. *Crit Rev Oncol Hematol* 2010; **76**(3):208–17.

82. Makary MA, Segev DL, Pronovost PJ, et al. Frailty as a predictor of surgical outcomes in older patients. *J Am Coll Surg* 2010; **210**(6):901–8.

83. Robinson TN, Wallace JI, Wu DS, et al. Accumulated frailty characteristics predict postoperative discharge institutionalization in the geriatric patient. *J Am Coll Surg* 2011; **213**(1):37–42; discussion 44.

84. Bagshaw SM, Stelfox HT, McDermid RC, et al. Association between frailty and short- and long-term outcomes among critically ill patients: a multicentre prospective cohort study. *CMAJ* 2014; **186**(2):e95–102.

85. Lee DH, Buth KJ, Martin BJ, Yip AM, Hirsch GM. Frail patients are at increased risk for mortality and prolonged institutional care after cardiac surgery. *Circulation* 2010; **121**(8):973–78.

86. Culley DJ, Flaherty D, Reddy S, et al. Preoperative cognitive stratification of older elective surgical patients: a cross-sectional study. *Anesth Analg* 2016; **123**(1):186–92.

87. Zenilman ME. More powerful than the American Society of Anesthesiology score. *JAMA Surg* 2014; **149**(7):640–41.

88. Chow WB, Rosenthal RA, Merkow RP, American College of Surgeons National Surgical Quality Improvement Program, et al. Optimal preoperative assessment of the geriatric surgical patient: a best practices guideline from the American College of Surgeons National Surgical Quality Improvement Program and the American Geriatrics Society. *J Am Coll Surg* 2012; **215**(4):453–66.

89. Wozniak SE, Coleman J, Katlic MR. Optimal preoperative evaluation and perioperative care of the geriatric patient: a surgeon's perspective. *Anesthesiol Clin* 2015; **33**(3):481–89.

90. Townsend NT, Robinson TN. Surgical risk and comorbidity in older urologic patients. *Clin Geriatr Med* 2015; **31**(4):591–601.

91. Murthy S, Hepner DL, Cooper Z, Bader AM, Neuman MD. Controversies in anaesthesia for noncardiac surgery in older adults. *Br J Anaesth* 2015; **115**(Suppl 2):ii, 15–25.

92. Whitson HE, Duan-Porter W, Schmader KE, et al. Physical resilience in older adults: systematic review and development of an emerging construct. *J Gerontol A Biol Sci Med Sci* 2016; **71**(4): 489–95.

93. Graham D, Becerril-Martinez G. Surgical resilience: a review of resilience biomarkers

and surgical recovery. *Surgeon* 2014; **12** (6):334–44.

94. Hadley EC, Kuchel GA, Newman AB, et al. Report: NIA Workshop on measures of physiologic resiliencies in human aging. *J Gerontol A Biol Sci Med Sci* 2017; **72**(7):980–90.

95. Ihn CH, Joo JD, Choi JW, et al. Comparison of stress hormone response, interleukin-6 and anaesthetic characteristics of two anaesthetic techniques: volatile induction and maintenance of anaesthesia using sevoflurane versus total intravenous anaesthesia using propofol and remifentanil. *J Int Med Res* 2009; **37**(6): 1760–71.

96. Neuman MD, Silber JH, Elkassabany NM, Ludwig JM, Fleisher LA. Comparative effectiveness of regional versus general anesthesia for hip fracture surgery in adults. *Anesthesiology* 2012; **117**(1):72–92.

97. Whiting PS, Molina CS, Greenberg SE, et al. Regional anaesthesia for hip fracture surgery is associated with significantly more peri-operative complications compared with general anaesthesia. *Int Orthop* 2015; **39**(7):1321–27.

98. Brox WT, Roberts KC, Taksali S, et al. The American Academy of Orthopaedic Surgeons Evidence-Based Guideline on Management of Hip Fractures in the Elderly. *J Bone Joint Surg Am* 2015; **97** (14):1196–99.

99. Schofield PA. The assessment and management of peri-operative pain in older adults. *Anaesthesia* 2014; **69**(Suppl 1):54–60.

100. American Geriatrics Society. The management of chronic pain in older persons: AGS Panel on Chronic Pain in Older Persons. *J Am Geriatr Soc* 1998; **46** (5):635–51.

101. Falzone E, Hoffmann C, Keita H. Postoperative analgesia in elderly patients. *Drugs Aging* 2013; **30**(2):81–90.

102. McKeown JL. Pain management issues for the geriatric surgical patient. *Anesthesiol Clin* 2015; **33**(3):563–76.

103. Fabi DW. Multimodal analgesia in the hip fracture patient. *J Orthop Trauma* 2016; **30**(Suppl 1):S6–11.

104. Moraca RJ, Sheldon DG, Thirlby RC. The role of epidural anesthesia and analgesia in surgical practice. *Ann Surg* 2003; **238**(5):663–73.

105. American Geriatrics Society Expert Panel on Postoperative Delirium in Older Adults. Postoperative delirium in older adults: best practice statement from the American Geriatrics Society. *J Am Coll Surg* 2015; **220**(2):136–48, e1.

106. Radtke FM, Franck M, Lendner J, et al. Monitoring depth of anaesthesia in a randomized trial decreases the rate of postoperative delirium but not postoperative cognitive dysfunction. *Br J Anaesth* 2013; **110**(Suppl 1):i98–105.

107. Forman DE, Arena R, Boxer R, et al. Prioritizing functional capacity as a principal end point for therapies oriented to older adults with cardiovascular disease: a scientific statement for healthcare professionals from the American Heart Association. *Circulation* 2017; **135**(16):e894–918.

108. Shulman MA, Myles PS, Chan MT, et al. Measurement of disability-free survival after surgery. *Anesthesiology* 2015; **122**(3): 524–36.

109. Hodgson CL, Udy AA, Bailey M, et al. The impact of disability in survivors of critical illness. *Intensive Care Med* 2017; **43**(7):992–1001.

Chapter 13

Perioperative Care of Geriatric Patients at Risk of Developing Critical Illness

Andrea Tsai and Ruben J. Azocar

Key Points

- Admissions of geriatric patients to intensive care units (ICUs) are becoming increasingly common and are responsible for increasing healthcare costs.
- Older adults present to the ICU in two different ways: acutely and electively. Outcomes after elective ICU admission seem to be better: 1-year mortality for unscheduled surgery was 67 percent, and the 1-year mortality for emergent medical admissions was 80 percent.
- The Perioperative Surgical Home (PSH) model, aiming for a better coordination in care for the older adult, could improve outcomes and decrease costs by minimizing complications.
- The purpose of preoperative evaluation in elderly patients is to document a baseline functional status, stratify risk so that modifiable risk factors can be addressed, optimize patients prior to surgery where possible, and recognize postoperative changes objectively.
- Intraoperative management for older adults should take into account the preoperative concerns: lower doses of hypnotic, sedative, and analgesic agents due to the increased sensitivity of the elderly brain; decreased rate of redistribution leading to higher comparative blood levels of drug; and decreased metabolism of drug by the liver or kidney, leading to a longer drug half-life.
- Preoperative frailty has been strongly correlated with postoperative outcomes in the elderly patients, and a strong argument can be made for obtaining frailty scores preoperatively to predict perioperative outcomes and guide care in the ICU (especially withholding or withdrawing life support).

Introduction

The rapid growth of the population older than 65 years of age and its impact on healthcare is a well-recognized fact. Critical care services are not immune to this phenomenon; in fact, admissions of geriatric patients to intensive care units (ICUs) are increasingly common. When examining ICU admissions between1992–96 and 2002–6, a Dutch institution reported a 33 percent increase in admissions of patients older than age 75 [1]. Similarly, data from 57 ICUs in Australia and New Zealand showed a 6 percent increase per year in ICU admissions between 2000 and 2005 of patients older than 80 years of age [2]. This segment of the population represented 14 percent of all ICU admissions in this cohort. In the United States, approximately 42 to 52 percent of ICU admissions are older adult patients, with 60 percent of all ICU days attributed to this group [3]. Additionally, 11 percent of Medicare recipients spend an average of 8 days in the ICU during the final 6 months of their lives, and about 40 percent of Medicare recipients who die are admitted to the ICU during their terminal illness [4]. These ICU stays represent approximately 25 percent of total Medicare expenditures [4]. Teno et al. published data showing increases in ICU use among Medicare beneficiaries in the last 30 days of life, from 24.3 percent in 2000, to 26.3 percent in 2005, and 29.2 percent in 2009, despite a decrease in the mortality rate in acute care hospitals [5]. Considering that hospital stays that involve ICU services are two and a half times costlier than those without ($61,800 versus $25,200) [6], it is easy to infer the financial impact of the increasing number of elderly adults requiring critical care services. An additional challenge is the relative decrease in ICU beds available per capita, from 193.2 ICU beds per 100,000 elderly persons to 189.4 beds per 100,000 elderly persons, as the segment of those over 65 years continues to grow [7].

Older adults present to the ICU in two different ways: acutely and electively. An acute presentation encompasses most medical admissions as well as acute unplanned surgical admissions, e.g., trauma and surgical catastrophes. Elective, or planned, ICU admissions are generally related to surgical interventions. Outcomes in this latter group seem to be better than in the former. One study reported that postsurgical admissions had an ICU mortality of 12 percent and a hospital mortality of 25 percent, with 72 percent of those who survived being discharged home [2]. Similarly, another study found that 57 percent of elderly patients who underwent elective surgery were still living at 1 year after surgery [8]. In contrast, older patients who required emergency surgery had an 89 percent mortality rate, and those admitted for acute medical issues had a 90 percent mortality rate [8]. These findings are consistent with another study that reported that the 1-year mortality for unscheduled surgery was 67 percent and the 1-year mortality for emergent medical admissions was 80 percent [9].

Although survival after elective surgery is better than survival after emergent surgery or ICU admission for geriatric patients, unfortunately, the perioperative outcomes of this patient population are still significantly worse than those of younger adults. In a prospective observational study of 1,064 patients undergoing noncardiac surgery, those older than 65 years had a 1-year mortality rate of 10.3 percent – almost double that of younger adults (5.5 percent) [10]. These findings are no different from those of an epidemiologic study looking at surgical mortality in the United States, in which mortality increases dramatically for those older than 65 years of age [11]. A 2002–5 review of the Veterans Affairs National Surgical Quality Improvement Program (NSQIP) database examining 7,696 surgeries showed an overall 28 percent morbidity rate and 2.3 percent mortality rate, but in those older than 80 years of age the morbidity rate was 51 percent and the mortality rate was 7 percent [12].

Complications are clearly associated with mortality; very likely, an elderly patient may survive surgery but succumb to postoperative complications. Perioperative complications in older adults and their relationship with mortality have been well identified. Central nervous system (CNS) and cardiac, pulmonary, and renal systems seem to be the common systems in which complications have the greatest impact on outcomes [13–15]. A study completed at NSQIP of patients who had noncardiac surgery between 1991 and 1999 showed that in those age 80 years or older, 20 percent had one or more postoperative complications [15]. Patients who suffered complications had a higher 30-day mortality than those who did not (26 versus 4 percent, $P < 0.001$) [15].

Wunsch et al. analyzed data to determine the 3-year outcomes of 35,308 ICU Medicare beneficiaries who survived intensive care. Patients who survived the ICU had a higher 3-year mortality (39.5 percent, $n = 13,950$) than hospital controls (34.5 percent, $n = 12,173$, adjusted hazard ratio [AHR] 1.07, 95 percent confidence interval [CI] 1.04–1.10, $p < 0.001$) and general controls (14.9 percent, $n = 5,266$, AHR 2.39, 95% CI 2.31–2.48, $p < 0.001$) [16]. Interestingly, survivors who did not receive mechanical ventilation had minimal increased risk compared with hospital controls (3-year mortality 38.3 percent, $n = 12,716$ versus 34.6 percent, $n = 11,470$, respectively, AHR 1.04, 95% CI 1.02–1.07), but those who underwent mechanical ventilation had substantially increased mortality (57.6 percent, $n = 1,234$ ICU survivors versus 32.8 percent, $n = 703$ hospital controls, AHR 1.56, 95% CI 1.40–1.73), with risk concentrated in the 6 months after the quarter of hospital discharge (6-month mortality 30.1 percent, $n = 645$ for those receiving mechanical ventilation versus 9.6 percent, $n = 206$ for hospital controls, AHR 2.26, 95% CI 1.90–2.69) [16].

Examining long-term outcomes, however, should not be limited to mortality. Quality of life (QoL) is also enormously important for patients and their families. Dependency in activities of daily living (ADLs) has been associated with perioperative complications in the elderly [14]. Complications involving the CNS and cardiac, pulmonary, and renal systems have great impact on outcomes and result in unplanned admissions to the ICU [13–15]. It is also important to note that patients who survive the ICU and are discharged to a skilled care facility have higher 6-month mortality (24.1 percent for ICU survivors and hospital controls discharged to a skilled care facility versus 7.5 percent for ICU survivors and hospital controls discharged home, AHR, 2.62, 95% CI 2.50–2.74, $p < 0.001$ for ICU survivors and hospital controls combined) [16].

This growing elderly population that consumes a large segment of healthcare resources and is prone to suboptimal outcomes fits the paradigm of the American Society of Anesthesiologists' (ASA) Perioperative Surgical Home (PSH) model. This initiative is framed under the Institute for Healthcare Improvement (IHI) Triple Aim, whose goals are to enhance the patient's experience of care (quality and satisfaction) while reducing the per capita cost of healthcare [17,18]. The PSH is therefore a patient-centric, team-based model of care that emphasizes value, patient satisfaction, and reduced costs [19,20].

The key element in the conceptual frame of the PSH model is to minimize variability in perioperative care [21]. Lessons from organization management demonstrate that variability in practice increases the likelihood for errors and complications. It is suggested that variability can be reduced by ensuring continuity of care and treating the entire perioperative episode of care as one continuum rather than discrete preoperative, intraoperative, postoperative, and postdischarge episodes [21]. It appears that aiming for a better coordination in care for older adults could improve outcomes and decrease costs by minimizing complications that might lead to critical illness in this growing patient population [22].

Preoperative Assessment

In 2012, the American College of Surgeons (ACS) NSQIP and American Geriatrics Society (AGS) published best practice guidelines focusing on the optimal preoperative assessment of geriatric surgical patients [23]. These guidelines detail a comprehensive and evidence-based preoperative assessment with the goal of optimizing patients prior to surgery. Medical optimization is certainly a possibility for geriatric patients who present for elective surgeries with planned postoperative ICU admission. In contrast, the ability to optimize a geriatric patient after trauma or an unexpected surgical complication are more limited, but some degree of preoperative assessment may still be possible and is helpful for prognosis and guiding intra- and postoperative therapy. The ACS NSQIP/AGS best practice guidelines will be reviewed next, updated for more recent developments.

For the preoperative neuropsychiatric evaluation of geriatric patients, the guidelines recommend identifying risk factors for the development of delirium, assessing cognitive ability and capacity, and screening for depression as well as alcohol and other drug abuse or dependence [23]. The purpose of this evaluation is to document a baseline functional status, stratify risk so that modifiable risk factors can be addressed, optimize patients prior to surgery where possible, and ensure that postoperative changes are recognized objectively and treated.

Delirium is the most common complication in geriatric surgical patients, affecting up to 50 percent of older postoperative patients [24,25]. The guidelines recommend that risk factors for delirium be identified, and for patients at risk for postoperative delirium, the use of benzodiazepines and antihistamines should be avoided [23,26]. Risk factors for delirium are summarized in Table 13.1, with the following six risk factors highlighted by ACS NSQIP/AGS and Society of Critical Care Medicine (SCCM) guidelines: preexisting dementia, coma, history of hypertension, history of alcoholism, a high severity of illness at admission, and benzodiazepine use [23,26].

To assess cognitive ability and screen for cognitive impairment, in addition to reviewing medical records and, when possible, interviewing those familiar with the patient (e.g., family), the Mini-Cog and clock-drawing tests have emerged as rapid, effective, and recommended screening tools [23,25,27] (Table 13.2 and Figure 13.1). Preoperative cognitive testing is important to establish a baseline with which postoperative status can be compared. Additionally, patients with impairment can be identified and potentially further evaluated or referred for specialist workup. Finally, evidence of cognitive impairment is important in determining the patient's functional capacity and ability to follow medication regimen and maintain quality of life.

The assessment of a patient's competence, or their decision-making capacity, is recommended by the guidelines and is important in determining a patient's ability to provide informed consent for surgery and anesthesia [23]. Legal criteria for capacity are defined as the ability to demonstrate understanding, appreciation, reasoning, and choice as they pertain to medical decisions. That is, a patient must be able to understand the information communicated to them, appreciate their clinical situation and consequences, reason through various options, and choose from among the options. A discussion of approaches to capacity assessment is beyond the scope of this chapter but is covered in an excellent review [28].

Screening for depression and alcohol or substance dependence or abuse is recommended by the guidelines and can be accomplished via the use of validated questionnaires [23]. The Patient Health Questionnaire-2 (PHQ-2) is a simple, rapid, and recommended tool to screen for depression [23] (Table 13.3); patients screening positive can be referred for further evaluation or workup. Screening for alcohol or substance dependence or abuse can be accomplished through the CAGE (Cut down, Annoyed, Guilty, Eye-opener) questionnaire, with any "yes" answer considered a positive result [23,25]. Patients screening positive for substance dependence or abuse should be considered for perioperative withdrawal

Table 13.1 Risk Factors for Postoperative Delirium

Cognitive and behavioral disorders

- Dementia and cognitive impairment[a]
- Depression
- Alcohol use[b]
- Sleep deprivation or disturbance
- Coma[b]

Disease or illness related

- Aortic procedures
- Current hip fracture
- Severe illness or comorbidity burden[b]
- Presence of infection
- Renal insufficiency
- Inadequately controlled pain
- Anemia
- Hypoxia or hypercarbia
- History of hypertension[b]

Metabolic

- Poor nutrition
- Dehydration
- Electrolyte abnormalities (hypernatremia or hyponatremia)

Functional impairments

- Hearing or vision impairment
- Poor functional status
- Immobilization or limited mobility

Other

- Age greater than 65 years
- Polypharmacy and use of psychotropic medications (benzodiazepines, anticholinergics, antihistamines, antipsychotics)[b]
- Risk of urinary retention or constipation
- Presence of urinary catheter

[a] Strongest predisposing factor according to ACS NSQIP/AGS and SCCM guidelines.
[b] Significant risk factor according to SCCM guidelines.
(*Sources:* Refs. [1–4].)

prophylaxis, perioperative vitamin supplementation (e.g., thiamine and folic acid), and – time permitting – referral for abstinence or detoxification programs [23].

The preoperative cardiac assessment of the geriatric ICU patient should follow American College of Cardiology (ACC) and American Heart Association (AHA) guidelines. These guidelines were updated in 2014 and now include a Web-based perioperative risk calculator that replaces the Revised Cardiac Risk Index [29,30]. This new cardiac risk calculator estimates probability for perioperative myocardial infarction or cardiac arrest based on five criteria: age, ASA class, creatinine level, functional status with respect to ADLs,

Table 13.2 Cognitive Assessment with the Mini-Cog: Three-Item Recall and Clock Draw

1. Get the patient's attention, then say:
   - "I am going to say three words that I want you to remember now and later. The words are banana, sunrise, and chair. Please say them for me now."
   - Give the patient three tries to repeat the words. If unable after three tries, go to the next item.

2. Say all the following phrases in the order indicated:
   - "Please draw a clock in the space below. Start by drawing a large circle. Put all the numbers in the circle and set the hands to show 11:10 (10 past 11)."
   - If the patient has not finished the clock drawing in 3 minutes, discontinue and ask for recall items.

3. Say: "What were the three words I asked you to remember?"

(*Sources:* Refs. [1,2].)

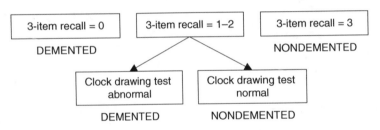

Figure 13.1 Mini-Cog scoring algorithm (www.ncbi.nlm.nih.gov/pubmed/11113982).

and type of surgery [29, 30]. This estimate may be helpful in guiding informed consent, prognosis, and risk/benefit discussions.

In assessing the pulmonary status of geriatric ICU patients, the guidelines recommend identifying a patient's risk factors for postoperative pulmonary complications and implementing strategies for risk mitigation where possible [23]. These strategies may not be possible for the trauma patients admitted to the ICU emergently, but for elective ICU patients, they include smoking cessation, optimization of asthma and chronic obstructive pulmonary disease (COPD) control, intensive inspiratory muscle training, and selective pulmonary function testing and chest radiography [23]. Similar to the Web-based cardiac risk calculator adopted by 2014 ACC/AHA guidelines, there exists a Web-based risk calculator for postoperative respiratory failure (PRF), defined as failure to wean from mechanical ventilation within 48 hours of surgery or unplanned intubation or reintubation within 30 days of surgery [31]. Risk of PRF is estimated based on five criteria: ASA class, presence or absence of sepsis, emergency (versus nonemergent) case, functional status with respect to ADLs, and type of surgery [31]. Other risk factors for postoperative pulmonary complications (including pneumonia) as identified by the guidelines are outlined in Table 13.4.

Table 13.3 The Patient Health Questionnaire-2

1. In the past 12 months, have you ever had a time when you felt sad, blue, depressed, or down for most of the time for at least 2 weeks?
2. In the past 12 months, have you ever had a time, lasting at least 2 weeks, when you did not care about the things that you usually cared about or when you did not enjoy the things that you usually enjoyed?

Note: If the patient answers "yes" to either question, then further evaluation by a primary care physician or specialist is recommended.
(*Sources:* Refs. [1,2].)

Table 13.4 Risk Factors for Postoperative Pulmonary Complications

Patient-related factors

- Age > 60 years
- Chronic obstructive pulmonary disease
- ASA class ≥ II[a]
- Functional dependence[a]
- Congestive heart failure
- Obstructive sleep apnea
- Pulmonary hypertension
- Current cigarette use
- Impaired sensorium
- Preoperative sepsis[a]
- Weight loss > 10 percent in 6 months
- Serum albumin level < 3.5 mg/dl
- Blood urea nitrogen level ≥ 7.5 mmol/liter (21 mg/dl)
- Serum creatinine level > 133 mol/liter (1.5 mg/dl)

Surgery-related factors

- Prolonged operation (>3 hours)
- Surgical site[a]
- Emergency operation[a]
- General anesthesia
- Perioperative transfusion
- Residual neuromuscular blockade after an operation

[a] Criteria for estimating postoperative pulmonary failure risk according to the Gupta risk calculator.
(*Sources:* Refs. [1,2,5].)

Functional status and performance status are now recognized as important predictors of postoperative outcomes, including delirium, surgical-site infections, discharge institutionalization, and 30-day and 6-month mortality [23]. Functional status can be easily assessed with a short series of screening questions assessing a patient's ability to independently get out of bed or a chair, dress, bathe, prepare meals, and shop (e.g., for groceries) [23]. Any "no" answer should prompt a more in-depth evaluation and consideration of physical and/

Table 13.5 Frailty Score

Criteria	Definition
Weight loss	Unintentional weight loss > 10 pounds in the last year
Exhaustion	Self-reported poor energy and endurance
Low physical activity	Low weekly energy expenditure
Slowness	Slow walking
Weakness	Decreased grip strength

Interpretation: The patient receives 1 point for each criterion met. 0–1 = not frail;
2–3 = intermediate or pre-frail; 4–5 = frail.
(*Sources:* Refs. [2,6].)

or occupational therapy referral as well as highlight a potential need for proactive discharge planning. Deficits in hearing, vision, swallowing, gait, or mobility also should be documented, as well as screening for falls or risk of falling [23,32]. The Timed Up and Go Test (TUGT) is another suggested screening tool for elderly surgical patients [23,32]. It is a timed test in which a seated patient rises from a standard armchair, walks forward in a straight line for 10 feet, turns around, and returns to a seated position in the chair [23]. Any patient who experiences difficulty completing the test or needs more than 15 seconds to complete the test is at high risk for falls and should be considered for physical therapy referral [23].

Frailty is a syndrome independent of disability and comorbidity that is highly prevalent in the geriatric population; some estimate that up to 50 percent of those over 85 years of age may be frail [23,25]. Multiple measures of frailty exist, but one widely recognized definition was put forth by Fried et al. [23,33].This definition evaluates patients on five criteria: weight loss, exhaustion, low physical activity, slowness, and weakness (Table 13.5); patients meeting two to three of the criteria are considered to be intermediate or prefrail, and those meeting four to five of the criteria are considered to be frail [23,33]. Frailty has important negative implications for postoperative outcomes [34]. Because frailty and decreased functional status are associated with worse outcomes, the notion of "prehabilitation" as a way to optimize patients in preparation for surgery has been proposed. Currently, there are studies that suggest that an exercise program aimed to improve the functional status of patients before surgery might improve recovery and overall outcomes, including in the geriatric population [35,36]. Such studies also suggest benefits in the cognitive domain as well [37].

Nutritional evaluation of geriatric ICU patients should include documenting baseline height, weight, body mass index (BMI), and serum albumin and prealbumin and inquiring about unintentional weight loss in the last year [23]. Risk factors for severe nutritional risk include a BMI of less than 18.5 kg/m², a serum albumin of less than 3.0 g/dl (with no evidence of renal or hepatic dysfunction), and unintentional weight loss of greater than 10 to 15 percent within 6 months [23]. It is recommended that patients who meet any of these criteria should undergo a full nutritional assessment by a dietitian and be considered for preoperative nutritional support [23]. Malnutrition is a surprisingly common entity among elderly patients, with rates ranging from 5.8 percent in the community to 38.7 percent in hospitals and 50.5 percent in rehabilitation [23]. Since poor nutritional status is a known risk factor for infectious and wound complications, assessing and addressing this issue is important to improve outcomes[23,25].

Medication management in the elderly can be challenging due to polypharmacy, increased patient sensitivity to medications and their side effects, as well as difficulty in determining existing medication regimen due to cognitive impairment or dementia [23,25]. Perioperative medication management in this population merits a careful and tailored approach. In addition to a careful review and documentation of all prescription and nonprescription medications, guidelines recommend the preoperative discontinuation of medications including: nonessential medications, medications on the Beers Criteria list, that are potentially inappropriate for older adults (last updated in 2015 [38]) and herbal medications [23,25]. Medications that should be reduced or avoided include benzodiazepines, meperidine, H_1 antagonists (in particular diphenhydramine) and other anticholinergic medications [23]. ACC/AHA guidelines should be followed for the initiation and dosing of perioperative beta blockers and statins [23,25]. Medications cleared by the kidneys, should be dosed based on glomerular filtration rate, since creatinine alone can be an inadequate estimate of renal function in older adults [23].

Finally, where possible, attempts at counseling the geriatric ICU patient should be made. Counseling efforts include ensuring that the patient has designated a health care proxy, has advanced directives, has adequate social support and understands treatment goals, plans and complications including possible functional decline and/or need for institutionalization if relevant [23]. Patients without adequate social support systems should be considered for referral to a social worker [23].

Intraoperative Management

Intraoperative management of older adults should take into account the preoperative concerns highlighted earlier and the generally decreased physiologic reserve of elderly patients. Lower doses of hypnotic, sedative, and analgesic agents can be used for geriatric patients due to the increased sensitivity of the elderly brain to any given drug level, decreased rate of redistribution leading to higher comparative blood levels of drug, and decreased metabolism of drug by the liver or kidney, leading to a longer drug half-life [39]. Ongoing controversy exists as to the superiority of regional over general anesthesia techniques (when a choice between the two is possible). Theoretically, when compared with general anesthesia, regional techniques should result in at least a decreased incidence of postoperative cognitive complications. However, studies comparing regional versus general anesthesia techniques have shown conflicting results on outcomes such as cognition, pulmonary complications, and mortality, and further research is required before a firm recommendation can be made [34].

From a cardiovascular standpoint, as patients age, stiffening of blood vessels and myocardium leads to systolic hypertension, venous stiffening, myocardial hypertrophy, and increased diastolic dysfunction compared with the younger population [40]. Furthermore, increased sympathetic tone leads to higher circulating levels of catecholamines and decreased myocardial sensitivity to catecholamines, hypotension, and exercise [40]. As a result of these cardiovascular changes, elderly patients are more dependent on atrial function for cardiac output, experience greater hypotension and blood pressure lability intraoperatively, and are less able to respond with intrinsic changes in venous capacitance, vascular tone, and heart rate or contractility changes [40].

With aging comes changes in pulmonary physiology that result in impaired respiratory mechanics and gas exchange. Elderly patients experience an age-dependent decrease in elastic recoil, respiratory muscle strength, functional residual capacity, residual volume, vital capacity, diffusion capacity, and forced expiratory volume in 1 second (FEV_1) [40]. As a result, compared with younger patients, geriatric patients are more prone to upper airway obstruction, aspiration, atelectasis, and postoperative pulmonary complications [40]. As such, additional care should be taken to minimize the risk of pulmonary complications postoperatively, including minimizing use of orogastric or nasogastric tubes, mechanical ventilation with positive end-expiratory pressure (PEEP), and consideration of recruitment maneuvers, minimizing sedatives or using short-acting agents, and vigilant monitoring for residual postoperative neuromuscular blockade.

Other organ systems also show an age-related decline in function, including the gastrointestinal, renal, and endocrine systems. Prolonged gastric emptying and impaired esophageal function are found in older adults [40]. Hepatic drug metabolism may decline, although this is a variable finding [40]. Renal function declines, with decreases in both creatinine clearance and glomerular filtration rate, resulting in a decrease in the clearance of renally metabolized or excreted drugs as well as impaired electrolyte homeostasis [40]. There is a decrease in production and responsiveness to hormones, including insulin and thyroid hormone [40]. As a result, geriatric patients will generally require increased attention in terms of physiologic monitoring and careful titration of medication dosing to effect.

Postoperative Considerations in the ICU

Postoperative critical care issues in older adults are adult are not dissimilar from those who are admitted for nonsurgical reasons. Issues in the neurologic, respiratory, cardiac, and renal systems, as well as end-of-life issues, are described elsewhere in this text. However, it is pertinent to discuss frailty as a predictor of outcomes in critically ill older adults.

The use of frailty as a predictor of outcomes in older critical care patients has been reported recently. A multicenter, prospective observational study conducted in France analyzed the impact of frailty on mortality rates [41]. The authors used two different frailty scoring systems – the frailty phenotype (FP) and the clinical frailty score (CFS). They reported that risk of mortality in the ICU was associated with a frailty phenotype of 3 or greater (hazard ratio [HR] 3.3, 95% CI 1.6–6.6, $p < 0.001$) and that 6-month mortality was associated with a CFS of 5 or greater (HR 2.4, 95% CI 1.49–3.87, $p < 0.001$). Zeng et al. found a correlation between a frailty index (derived from a proportion of health deficit accumulation) and mortality [42]. In this study, patients who died within 30 days had higher mean frailty index scores (0.41 ± 0.11) than those who survived to 300 days (0.22 ± 0.11, $F = 38.91$, $p < 0.001$). Additionally, each 1 percent increase in the index from the previous level was associated with an 11 percent increase in the 30-day mortality risk (95% CI 7–15 percent). No one with a frailty index score greater than 0.46 survived past 90 days.

More recently another group published their findings on a cohort of 122 patients. In a prospective study, the authors used a frailty index derived from a comprehensive geriatric assessment [43]. They characterized patients as robust if their frailty index score was 0.25 or less, prefrail if the score was 0.25 to 0.40, and as frail if the score was greater than 0.40. Their findings suggest a lower median overall survival in the frail group compared with prefrail and robust subjects (23, 31, and 140 days, $p = 0.013$, respectively). In the long term, frail patients also had a significantly higher mortality rate than others at 3 months

(80.8 percent) and 6 months (84.6 percent). Despite the fact that these studies used different frailty scoring systems, it seems clear that frailty can be used as a predictor of outcome in critically ill older adults. As such, it may provide guidance to the ICU team to make end-of-life decisions regarding withholding or withdrawing life support [44]. Finally, because preoperative frailty has been strongly correlated with postoperative outcomes in this population [45,46], a strong argument can be made for obtaining frailty scores preoperatively to predict perioperative outcomes and guide care in the ICU in elderly patients.

Conclusion

Management of the geriatric patient in the perioperative period should be aimed at the prevention of problems that might lead to complications and death. The concept of the PSH applies well to this population because better coordination and standardization of care will likely lead to achievement of the triple aim: improved patient experience, improved outcomes, and reduced cost of care. In terms of preoperative evaluation, novel concepts such as frailty are an excellent outcome predictor, and "prehabilitation" to optimize patients presenting for surgery and anesthesia is emerging in the literature. Tailoring the anesthetic care intraoperatively to physiologic changes that occur in the elderly and to specific patient needs is important as well. If the patient needs ICU care, this text provides chapters referring to those issues. Similar to the preoperative period, frailty seems to correlate well in predicting postoperative outcomes in geriatric patients who continue to require more and more critical care services.

References

1. Blot S, et al. Epidemiology and outcome of nosocomial bloodstream infection in elderly critically ill patients: a comparison between middle-aged, old, and very old patients. *Crit Care Med* 2009; **37**:1634–41.

2. Bagshaw SM, et al. Very old patients admitted to intensive care in Australia and New Zealand: a multi-centre cohort analysis. *Crit Care* 2009; **13**:R45.

3. Marik PE. Management of the critically ill geriatric patient. *Crit Care Med* 2006; **34**: S176–82.

4. Lewis MC. In *Manual of Geriatric Anesthesia*. New York, NY: Springer, 2013: 3–13.

5. Teno JM, et al. Change in end-of-life care for Medicare beneficiaries: site of death, place of care, and health care transitions in 2000, 2005, and 2009. *JAMA* 2013; **309**:470–77.

6. Barrett ML, Smith MW, Elixhauser A., Honigman LS. Utilization of intensive care services, 2011. *HCUP Statistical Brief* (Dec. 2011).

7. Wallace DJ, Angus DC, Seymour CW, Barnato AE, Kahn JM. Critical care bed growth in the United States: a comparison of regional and national trends. *Am J Respir Crit Care Med* 2015; **191**:410–16.

8. De Rooij SE. et al. Cognitive, functional, and quality-of-life outcomes of patients aged 80 and older who survived at least 1 year after planned or unplanned surgery or medical intensive care treatment. *J Am Geriatr Soc* 2008; **56**:816–22.

9. Tabah A, et al. Quality of life in patients aged 80 or over after ICU discharge. *Crit Care* 2010; **14**:R2.

10. Monk TG, Saini V, Weldon BC, Sigl JC. Anesthetic management and one-year mortality after noncardiac surgery. *Anesth Analg* 2005; **100**:4–10.

11. Li G, Warner M, Lang BH, Huang L, Sun LS. Epidemiology of anesthesia-related mortality in the United States, 1999–2005. *Anesthesiology* 2009; **110**:759–65.

12. Turrentine FE, Wang H, Simpson VB, Jones RS. Surgical risk factors, morbidity, and mortality in elderly patients. *J Am Coll Surg* 2006; **203**:865–77.

13. Manku K, Bacchetti P, Leung JM. Prognostic significance of postoperative in-hospital complications in elderly

patients: I. Long-term survival. *Anesth Analg* 2003; **96**:583–89.

14. Manku K, Leung JM. Prognostic significance of postoperative in-hospital complications in elderly patients: II. Long-term quality of life. *Anesth Analg* 2003; **96**:590–94.

15. Hamel MB, Henderson WG, Khuri SF, Daley J. Surgical outcomes for patients aged 80 and older: morbidity and mortality from major noncardiac surgery. *J Am Geriatr Soc* 2005; **53**:424–29.

16. Wunsch H, et al. Three-year outcomes for Medicare beneficiaries who survive intensive care. *JAMA* 2010; **303**:849–56.

17. Berwick DM, Nolan TW, Whittington J. The triple aim: care, health, and cost. *Health Aff* 2008; **27**:759–69.

18. Institute for Healthcare Improvement (IHI). *The IHI Triple Aim*, 2008, available at www.ihi.org/engage/initiatives/tripleaim/pages/default.aspx (accessed April 19, 2016).

19. Vetter TR, et al. The Perioperative Surgical Home: how can it make the case so everyone wins? *BMC Anesthesiol* 2013; **13**:1–11.

20. Vetter TR, Jones KA. Perioperative Surgical Home: perspective II. *Anesthesiol Clin* 2015; **33**:771–84.

21. Kain ZN, et al. The Perioperative Surgical Home as a future perioperative practice model. *Anesth Analg* 2014; **118**:1126–30.

22. Mello MT, Azocar RJ, Lewis MC. Geriatrics and the Perioperative Surgical Home. *Anesthesiol Clin* 2015; **33**:439–45.

23. Chow WB, et al. Optimal preoperative assessment of the geriatric surgical patient: a best practices guideline from the American College of Surgeons National Surgical Quality Improvement Program and the American Geriatrics Society. *J Am Coll Surg* 2012; **215**:453–66.

24. American Geriatrics Society Expert Panel on Postoperative Delirium in Older Adults. American Geriatrics Society abstracted clinical practice guideline for postoperative delirium in older adults. *J Am Geriatr Soc* 2015; **63**:142–50.

25. Nakhaie M, Tsai A. Preoperative assessment of geriatric patients. *Anesthesiol Clin* 2015; **33**:471–80.

26. Barr J, et al. Clinical practice guidelines for the management of pain, agitation, and delirium in adult patients in the intensive care unit. *Crit Care Med* 2013; **41**:263–306.

27. Borson S, Scanlan J, Brush M, Vitaliano P, Dokmak A. The Mini-Cog: a cognitive "vital signs" measure for dementia screening in multi-lingual elderly. *Int J Geriatr Psychiatry* 2000; **15**:1021–27.

28. Appelbaum PS. Assessment of patients' competence to consent to treatment. *N Engl J Med* 2007; **357**:1834–40.

29. Fleisher LA, et al. 2014 ACC/AHA guideline on perioperative cardiovascular evaluation and management of patients undergoing noncardiac surgery: executive summary. A report of the American College of Cardiology/American Heart Association Task Force on Practice Guidelines. *Circulation* 2014; **130**:2215–45.

30. Gupta PK, et al. Development and validation of a risk calculator for prediction of cardiac risk after surgery. *Circulation* 2011; **124**:381–87.

31. Gupta H, et al. Development and validation of a risk calculator predicting postoperative respiratory failure. *Chest* 2011; **140**:1207–15.

32. Panel on Prevention of Falls in Older Persons, American Geriatrics Society and British Geriatrics Society. Summary of the updated American Geriatrics Society/British Geriatrics Society clinical practice guideline for prevention of falls in older persons. *J Am Geriatr Soc* 2011; **59**:148–57.

33. Fried LP, et al. Frailty in older adults: evidence for a phenotype. *J Gerontol A Biol Sci Med Sci* 2001; **56**:M146–56.

34. Murthy S, Hepner DL, Cooper Z, Bader AM, Neuman MD. Controversies in anaesthesia for noncardiac surgery in older adults. *Br J Anaesth* 2015; **115**(Suppl 2):ii, 15–25.

35. Oosting E, et al. Preoperative home-based physical therapy versus usual care to improve functional health of frail older adults scheduled for elective total hip arthroplasty: a pilot randomized controlled

trial. *Arch Phys Med Rehabil* 2012; **93**: 610–16.

36. Dronkers JJ, et al. Preoperative therapeutic programme for elderly patients scheduled for elective abdominal oncological surgery: a randomized controlled pilot study. *Clin. Rehabil* 2010; **24**:614–22.

37. Saleh AJ, et al. Preoperative cognitive intervention reduces cognitive dysfunction in elderly patients after gastrointestinal surgery: a randomized controlled trial. *Med Sci Monit* 2015; **21**:798–805.

38. American Geriatrics Society 2015 Beers Criteria Update Expert Panel. American Geriatrics Society 2015 updated Beers Criteria for potentially inappropriate medication use in older adults. *J Am Geriatr Soc* 2015; **63**:2227–46.

39. Barash PG. *Clinical Anesthesia* Baltimore, MD: Wolters Kluwer/Lippincott Williams & Wilkins 2009.

40. Alvis BD Hughes C G. Physiology considerations in geriatric patients. *Anesthesiol Clin* 2015; **33**:447–56.

41. Le Maguet P, et al. Prevalence and impact of frailty on mortality in elderly ICU patients: a prospective, multicenter, observational study. *Intensive Care Med* 2014; **40**:674–82.

42. Zeng A, et al. Mortality in relation to frailty in patients admitted to a specialized geriatric intensive care unit. *J Gerontol A Biol Sci Med Sci* 2015; **70**: 1586–94.

43. Kizilarslanoglu MC, et al. Is frailty a prognostic factor for critically ill elderly patients? *Aging Clin Exp Res* 2016; **70**: 1586–94.

44. McDermid RC, Stelfox HT, Bagshaw SM. Frailty in the critically ill: a novel concept. *Crit Care* 2011; **15**:301.

45. Makary MA, et al. Frailty as a predictor of surgical outcomes in older patients. *J Am Coll Surg* **210**, 901–908 (2010).

46. Robinson TN, et al. Simple frailty score predicts postoperative complications across surgical specialties. *Am J Surg* 2013; **206**:544–50.

Ethical Issues: Withdrawing, Withholding, and Futility

Gail A. Van Norman

Key Points

- In most Western jurisdictions, withdrawing or withholding life-sustaining treatment (LST) at a competent patient's request is considered morally equivalent and is supported ethically and legally.
- Decisions to withdraw or withhold therapies in opposition to patient/surrogate wishes may be supportable on futility arguments but is more complex and subject to legal challenge.
- The concept of futility may have limited usefulness at the bedside but is a critical concept in understanding the perspectives of multiples parties in withdraw or withhold decisions.
- Open communication and respectful discourse between the physician and patient or their surrogates are prerequisites for resolving differences in values and finding an appropriate therapeutic pathway.

Introduction

The intensive care unit (ICU) presents daily opportunities for ethical discussions, dilemmas, and resolutions. Issues run the gamut from competency and informed consent to surrogate decision making, futility, withdrawing and withholding of life sustaining treatments (LSTs), and vital organ donation. This chapter focuses on several ethical concerns in end-of-life decision making: withdrawing or withholding LSTs and futility.

Withholding or Withdrawing Life-Sustaining Treatments

Withholding a treatment refers to a decision to not start or escalate an intervention, and *withdrawing* a treatment refers to discontinuing therapy that has already begun. In the ICU, *withdraw and withhold decisions* concern a wide spectrum of interventions, e.g., artificial hydration and nutrition, ventilator therapy, cardiopulmonary resuscitation, and pacemaker or implantable cardioverter-defibrillator therapies. Regardless of the therapy involved, ethical considerations underlying a withdraw or withhold decision stand on similar moral reasoning. And despite long-standing consensus, there is still considerable disquiet among clinicians about whether ethically relevant differences exist between withholding and withdrawing decisions.

In the late twentieth century, about half of ICU deaths occurred after withholding or withdrawing LSTs [1]. Such decisions have increased over time (Figure 14.1) and now

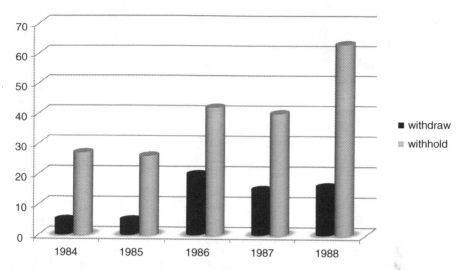

Figure 14.1 Change in pattern of decisions to withdraw/withhold life-sustaining therapies in an ICU over time. Withdraw decisions increased but remained significantly less common that withhold decisions. (*Source*: Koch et al. [1].)

precede death for 70 to 93 percent of patients dying in ICUs worldwide [2–8]. Studies indicate that a growing number of elderly patients across multiple cultures prefer to not have prolonged LSTs [3]. Older age is a significant factor for withdraw and withhold decisions by physicians and patients [10,11].

Moral Equivalency. Dominant Western ethical opinion concerning withdraw and withhold decisions is based in a *moral equivalence* thesis [12]; if there is no moral difference between withdrawing and withholding, then (all else being equal) there is no instance in which it would be allowable to withhold a treatment but not to discontinue the same treatment once it is started. Subjecting hopelessly ill patients to therapy that is unlikely to be beneficial potentially violates at least two basic principles of Western medical ethics: *beneficence* (doing good) and nonmaleficence (avoiding harm) [13,14]. Furthermore, if physicians cannot ethically withdraw LSTs once they are started, then they may be less willing to initiate treatments that have only a small potential for benefit out of concern that the patient may become trapped into therapy that cannot be discontinued if burdens turn out later to be too great [15]. Such *trial therapy* is an important strategy in treating and assessing prognosis in critically ill patients. Foregoing trial treatments because of misconceptions regarding the ethics of withdrawing them later could deny patients important potential benefits.

Many physicians believe that there is an important moral difference between withdrawing and withholding, although the more experienced the physician is with dying patients, the less likely they are to report either an ethical or a psychological difference between such decisions [16]. In a survey of 1,100 US physicians, over 90 percent agreed that requests from competent patients to withdraw treatments should be honored, but more than half the physicians also reported that withdrawing LSTs was significantly more difficult psychologically than withholding them [17]. The public appears much less willing than physicians to withhold therapy (40.2 versus 82.3 percent, respectively), although a strong majority (77.7 percent in one study) is willing to withdraw therapy [18]. Misgivings are not unique to US physicians. Studies have shown reluctance with regard to withdrawing compared with withholding of LSTs among German physicians [19] and that withdraw decisions are less common than withhold decisions among Indian [20], Lebanese [21], and Greek [22] intensivists.

Some argue that if a decision to start LSTS has been justly made, the patient has prima facie claim to have therapy continued on the basis of prior acquisition, unless they waive their claim [23]. This argument is based on the principle of physician fidelity to their patients – however, it does not command the conclusion that withdrawing LSTs is unethical—rather, to do so without the patient's consent would be unethical. The question remains as to what to do if therapy is determined to be "futile" and yet the patient refuses to have it withdrawn. Does a patient have a "right" to demand futile therapy indefinitely merely because it was begun under a later-disproven assumption that it would be beneficial? Concern over futility is at the heart of many withholding and withdrawing dilemmas, and yet it is a problematic concept, as will be discussed later.

Doing versus Allowing: Is There an Important Moral Difference? Another way of reasoning that there is an ethical difference between withholding and withdrawing LST is to draw a moral distinction between *acting* (or *doing*) and *allowing* [24]. Not initiating LST *allows* a patient to die of their disease, whereas withdrawing an established LST involves action by the physician, who has foresight that the action will likely lead to the patient's death. *Actions*, it is argued, place moral culpability on the actor, whereas inaction supposedly places responsibility for the outcomes on the patient or their health. This reasoning allows many physicians to be comfortable with withholding LSTs, but it does not support withdrawing treatment once it is begun. A problem with trying to distinguish *doing* from *allowing* is that *intention* is a powerful, if not determinative, moral aspect of human decisions, and if intentions and outcomes are the same, whether the physician decides to press a button (e.g., the "off" button of a ventilator in the case of withdrawing) or decides not to press a button (e.g., the "on" button of a ventilator in the case of withholding) seems morally irrelevant.

In discrediting arguments that the morality of a decision lies in a distinction between doing or merely allowing, ethicists have posed scenarios in which doing and allowing are equally morally wrong or, alternatively, in which identical actions and outcomes are in fact morally distinct. Rachels proposes that we consider Smith, who deliberately drowns his nephew in a bathtub by holding him underwater, versus Jones, who observes that his nephew is drowning in the bathtub and, though capable of rescuing him, deliberately stands by and lets him drown [25]. Both men are culpable. Brock asks us to consider a different scenario [26]. A disabled man who is ventilator dependent wishes to have the ventilator stopped; his physician turns off the ventilator, and the man dies. In another scenario, the man's greedy nephew, anticipating a large inheritance, sneaks into the room at night and turns off the ventilator, and the man dies. If the nephew's act is a killing, then the doctor's act is also – both involve identical actions and outcomes. Yet most ethicists agree that these scenarios are morally distinct. This is so is because not all features of an event are *morally relevant*. The morally relevant features of Brock's cases are not the actions that occur but the motives and intentions driving each actor

In most Western countries, ethicists favor the view that doing and allowing are not sufficient, and may even be immaterial, in identifying morally relevant differences of

Table 14.1 Some Medical Societies Confirming Ethical Equivalency of Withdraw/Withhold Treatment Decisions

American Medical Association
American College of Physicians
American College of Chest Physicians
American College of Critical Care Medicine
American Thoracic Society
The Australian and New Zealand Intensive Care Society
College of Intensive Care Medicine of Australia and New Zealand
Austrian Association of Intensive Care Medicine
Belgian Society of Intensive Care Medicine
Canadian Critical Care Society
The Dutch Intensive Care Society
French Society of Intensive Care
The UK General Medical Council

withholding and withdrawing treatments. The morally relevant features of withdrawing or withholding are the motives and intentions of reducing patient suffering and/or other burdens at end of life and of respect for patient autonomy. Since these motives are the same with both decisions, there is widespread agreement that, in most cases, withdrawing and withholding are morally equivalent [27–30]. This position has been supported by numerous professional and international organizations [2,27–30] (see Table 14.1).

Legal Considerations. Legal support for withdrawing or withholding LSTs is based in the United States on the ethical principle of respect for patient autonomy and in Constitutional provisions that limit government interference and protect the right of individuals to privacy. Between 1976 and 1990, the cases of Karen Ann Quinlan [31] and Nancy Cruzan [32] culminated in the codification of a patient's right to limit or refuse LST in the Federal Patient Self-Determination Act of 1990 [33]. This law states that competent patients have the right to refuse any medical therapy, including LST, and that hospitals must apprise patients of these rights and act accordingly and without discrimination toward them. US hospitals have been sanctioned for violations of this Act [34]. In 2005, the durability of this legal decision was repeatedly tested as the case of Terry Schiavo wound its way through state and federal courts [35]. *Every single court* determined that withdrawal of a feeding tube was legally permissible even though it would result in Terry's death. This principle survived attempts to legislate mandatory continuance of Terry's tube feedings by the Florida state legislature and the US Congress; the US Supreme Court refused requests to reconsider.

Cases have sometimes arisen in which physicians want to withdraw or withhold a patient's LSTs over objections by the patient or surrogates, as in the case of Helga Wanglie [36,37]. In that case, the court ordered family wishes to be followed. It is important to note that such cases do not question the legality of withdrawing or withholding LST but whether it can or should be done against the patient's or their surrogates' will.

Sometimes physicians argue that they can unilaterally withdraw therapy if it has become futile because it no longer constitutes legitimate medical therapy. Legal decisions in the United States are not always in favor of the physician and depend on issues such as patient perceptions of futility, confusion over definitions of brain death, and other complex considerations. Western countries other than the United States tend to favor withdraw/withhold practices, but legal decisions vary elsewhere; in Japan, for example, some withdraw decisions have led to investigations of homicide [38].

Futility

Futility is often raised as a justification for withdrawing and withholding decisions. Treatment that is perceived to be futile is common in the ICU setting; in one study, approximately 20 percent of patients in the ICU were adjudged to have received futile (11 percent) or probably futile (8.6 percent) care [39].

There is little, if any, disagreement among ethicists or clinicians that truly futile therapy need not be offered, should not be knowingly undertaken, and is probably actually unethical. Care that fails to meet a patient's goals or that maintains them in a suspended state of intensive therapy but minimal function is not only costly but also runs counter to professional values in medicine and creates serious moral conflicts for all concerned. Finding consensus regarding exactly what *futility* is, however, has proven problematic.

When a therapy presents a patient with more burdens than benefits, it should trigger a discussion about the goals of therapy. Defining a treatment as futile implies that there are few or no benefits to consider (or that at least the primary goal of the therapy will not be met) and therefore the treatment will result primarily in harms. Offering such treatment would be unethical because it would violate principles of beneficence and nonmaleficence, both of which are pillar concepts in Western medical ethics. Intentionally providing futile therapy furthermore threatens the value of veracity in medical practice; offering or pursuing futile treatment encourages false hopes – which is akin to lying.

Limits of Physician Authority. Physician refusal to comply with patient and family requests regarding treatments was not a prominent issue in medical ethics until the 1980s. The mid- to late twentieth century saw an evolution of medical decision making in the United States from being physician-centric (paternalistic) to being patient-centric. This change was driven by multiple factors: seemingly limitless advances in medical technology that raised complex moral questions about the nature of medical care, a political climate in the shadow of the Vietnam War in which antiauthoritarian philosophy flourished, and the increasing prominence of personal autonomy as a cultural value [40,41].

At first, the primary limitation of physician authority arose over patients' rights to refuse medical therapies, as in the Quinlan [31] and Cruzan [32] cases, rather than on rights of patients to demand specific treatments. Before long, however, such *positive rights* cases did arise, as in the case of Helga Wanglie [36,37]. Although physicians were compelled to continue to treat Mrs. Wanglie, the case raised questions about the limits of patient autonomy in demanding LST.

Medical professionalism demands that therapy be based on sound medical theory and supported by medical evidence of efficacy or at least a rational belief that the therapy has potential to work. Physicians have ethical obligations recognized as far back as Plato to refuse requested treatment that cannot restore health or meet realistic patient goals "even if they were richer than Midas" [42]. Such obligations differentiate the physician's role from that of a mere technician who is compensated for delivering a service on demand. The principle of respect for patient autonomy must be balanced against core principles and values that define what medical practice is – and what it isn't. Futility discussions have been important in elucidating physician concerns over "inappropriate" patient demands and in reclaiming authority regarding the value of professional education and judgment in the decision to treat.

The Cost of Patient Autonomy. Autonomy arguments are most convincing when the harms from treatment are limited to the individual patient. However, for many medical therapies, benefits and burdens are not limited to individuals but shared among communities. Financial costs are often spread out over some *risk pool*, such as an insurance cohort or government payers, and thus become borne by society as a whole. Huynh et al. estimated that the cost of care that was deemed futile in a study of five ICUs was in excess of $2.6 million over one 90-day period. More concerning was the additional finding that because of futile care being provided for a single patient in the study, treatment was delayed significantly for 33 other patients who needed critical care, and *at least two patients died* while waiting for transfer to other ICUs [39].

Defining Futility. Labeling a treatment as *futile* is powerful; many physicians assume that it ostensibly allows them to unilaterally withhold or withdraw LSTs, since it is tantamount to saying that to provide it is not compatible with the ethical practice of medicine [43]. The reality, however, is not so simple. One problem (if not *the* problem) in preventing or discontinuing futile treatments lies in defining exactly what *futile* therapy is. As Tonelli states, "despite the apparent acceptance of the existence of medically futile interventions, physicians simply cannot agree on when they have a futile case in front of them" [44].

Clinical outcomes of therapy can only be tallied retrospectively. Defining futility prospectively (e.g., should we withhold this treatment because it *will* be futile) rests in predicting that treatment is *unlikely* to deliver desired results. But how improbable must a positive outcome be to be considered futile? A commonly employed definition of futility is that a physician must conclude that it will succeed in fewer than 1 of 100 cases [45]. This number appears to have been extrapolated from assertions that a 1 percent difference in outcomes in clinical research ($p < 0.01$) is usually considered insignificant [46]. However, in one study, when physicians were asked to propose a probability of success below which a treatment should be considered futile, the answers ranged from 0 to 60 percent. One of five physicians chose a cutoff of 20 percent or higher [46]. Even after they were educated that *futility* is a probability of success of less than 0.01, one-third of medical residents defined futility as a probability of success of 5 percent [47].

What outcome should be determinative in defining futility? Even using a "straightforward" outcome such as mortality presents problems because mortality is notoriously difficult for physicians to predict accurately in hospitalized patients. Several scoring systems (APACHE IV, SAPS 3, MPM III) have been shown to discriminate groups of patients with elevated *risks* of mortality, but all of them overestimate final mortality rates [48]. Physicians also overpredict mortality when using clinical judgment. In one study, the positive predictive value of physicians' 2-year mortality estimates was only 57.4 percent – although, interestingly, this was comparable to the APACHE II and PREDICT risk-scoring systems [49]. Predicting future outcomes is furthermore operator dependent; the less experienced the physician, the less accurate is the prediction [50]. Neville et al. found that ICU fellows determined LST was futile on average 2 days earlier than attendings, weren't able to cite as many reasons for their determination and were less accurate than attendings in identifying patients who would die in hospital. Of note, overall accuracy of all physicians in the study was poor, irrespective of experience; a surprisingly high number of patients adjudged to be receiving futile treatment (38 and 15 percent for fellows and attendings, respectively) ended up surviving for more than 6 months [50]. Imbus and Zawaki reported their experience in the Burn Center at UCLA, underscoring this point: "No burn is certainly fatal until the patient dies … unable to prophesy and unwilling to strip the patient of any hope he may cherish, we prefer to diagnose burns as 'fatal' or 'hopeless' only in retrospect" [51]. This is not to say that they shrank from telling severely burned patients the truth. They told their most severely injured patients that while they could not predict the future, to their knowledge, "no one in the past of your age and with your size of burn has ever survived this injury, either with or without maximal treatment."

Is a therapy automatically futile if it fails to deliver the desired medical result? Or is it only futile if it fails to meet the social and health goals of the patient and their family? Patients and physicians often disagree about what makes a treatment futile and what benefits are worth pursuing, even if survival is unlikely. A treatment that is unlikely to extend life by more than a couple of days may be futile in the physician's eyes, whereas the patient may believe that even a few hours of extended time with family is a valuable goal [52]. In such cases, the physician and patient are defining benefits and futility with different measuring sticks – the physician is defining futility quantitatively, while the patient's surrogates are using qualitative definitions. Jecker describes the differences between quantitative and qualitative futility as follows: *quantitative* futility is the overwhelming probability that a treatment will fail to produce a desired physiologic effect, whereas *qualitative* futility describes a situation in which, whether or not the physiologic effect can be achieved, it does not offer a significant *benefit* to the patient [37]. In the former formulation of futility, evidence and physician experience predominate. In the latter formulation of futility, patient perception and values prevail.

Disagreements between physicians and patients regarding futility are based on differences in *values* between the patient and physician [53]. Disentangling values disagreements requires discussion, mutual respect, and negotiation [54], and persistent disagreements sometimes reach the courts. Some legislative efforts, such as the Texas Advance Directive Act (TADA), try to strike a balance between patient and physician interests by codifying a physician's authority to withhold or withdraw treatments they deem futile, despite disagreement with the patient or their surrogates [55,56].

Should the Concept of Futility Be Retired? Futility is a critical notion when exploring the philosophical nature of healthcare decision making. However, without consensus on a definition of futility that is useful at the bedside for directing medical care and resolving values disputes, many ethicists now believe that the term should be set aside, at least in clinical care situations [41,52]. Gallagher et al. suggest that futility is not an appropriate concept on which to base treatment discussions [57]. They and others propose that the issue of whether a medical treatment should be initiated or continued, regardless of whether requested or desired by the patient, the family, or the physician, should rest in understanding where that treatment lies "on the continuum of medical appropriateness" [57,58]. A determination of what treatments are appropriate will vary depending on the disease, the treatment, the anticipated outcomes, and the values of the patient, family, and physicians involved. Thus the "appropriateness" of initiating or continuing a medical treatment is unique to each patient.

Recommendations for Practice: Approaching the Patient about Futility

Susan Rubin suggests that when faced with a conflict between physician and patient about the futility of a treatment, it can be helpful to stop and ask the following two-part question: "Treatment is futile with respect to what goal? And whose goal is that?" [43]. This may invite conversations about the goals and values of both the patient and physician that are more meaningful in moving toward resolution.

Imbus and Zawacki based their approach to severely burned patients in their conviction that "the decision to begin or withhold maximal therapeutic effort is more of an ethical than a medical judgment" [51]. They employed a nonjudgmental system of shared decision making with critically burned patients that recognized and honored the fact that different people value and respond to medical data differently. Most of their patients, when faced with a decision regarding treatment for burns from which there had been no reported survivors, declined aggressive therapy and opted for palliative care. But an occasional patient chose the "minority" option to pursue maximal intervention, and as Rubin points out, this should serve to remind us that we err if we believe that a "singular vision of a good death" applies to everyone regardless of his or her values [43]. In the words of Weisman, "[t]he pervasive dread in dying seems not only to be the extinction of consciousness, but the fear that the death we die may not be our own. This is the singular distinction between death as a property of life and being put to death" [59].

References

1. Prendergast TJ, Claessens MT, Luce JM. A national survey of end-of-life care for critically ill patients. *Am J Respir Crit Care Med* 1998; **158**(4):1163–67.

2. Sprung C, Paruk F, Kissoon N, et al. The Durban World Congress ethics round table conference report: I. Differences between withholding and withdrawing life-sustaining treatments. *J Crit Care* 2014; **29**:890–95.

3. Azoulay E, Metnitz B, Sprung CL. End-of-life practices in 282 intensive care units: data from the SAPS 3 database. *Intensive Care Med* 2009; **35**:623–30.

4. Vincent JL, Parquier JN, Preiser JC, Brimioulle S, Kahn RJ. Terminal events in the intensive care unit: review of 258 fatal cases in one year. *Crit Care Med* 1989; **17**:530–33.

5. Koch K, Rodeffer HD, Wears RL. Changing patterns of terminal care management in an intensive care unit. *Crit Care Med* 1994; **22**: 233–43.

6. Keenan SP, Busche KD, Chen LM, et al. A retrospective review of a large cohort of patients undergoing the process of withholding or withdrawal of life support. *Crit Care Med* 1997; **25**:1324–31.

7. Hall RI, Rocker GM. End-of-life care in the ICU: treatments provided when life support was or was not withdrawn. *Chest* 2000; **118**:1424–30.

8. Sise MJ, Sise CB, Thorndike JF, et al. Withdrawal of care: a 10-year perspective at a Level I trauma center. *J Trauma Acute Care Surg* 2012; **72**:1186–89.

9. Aita K, Miyata H, Takahashi M, Kai I. Japanese physicians' practice of withholding and withdrawing mechanical ventilation and artificial nutrition and hydration from older adults with very severe stroke. *Arch Gerontol Geriatr* 2008; **3**:263–72.

10. Hoel H, Skjaker SA, Haagensen R, Stavem K. Decisions to withhold or withdraw life-sustaining treatment in a Norwegian intensive care unit. *Acta Anaesthesiol Scand* 2014; **58**:329–36.

11. Guidet B, Hodgson E, Feldman C, et al. The Durban World Congress ethics roundtable conference report: II.

Withholding or withdrawing of treatment in elderly patients admitted to the intensive care unit. *J Crit Care* 2014; **29**:896–901.

12. Wilkinson D, Savulescu J. A costly separation between withdrawing and withholding treatment in intensive care. *Bioethics* 2014; **28**:127–37.

13. President' Commission for the Study of Ethical Problems in Medicine and Biomedical and Behavioral Research. *Deciding to Forego Life-Sustaining Treatment: A Report on the Technical Medical and Legal Issues in Treatment Decisions.* Washington, DC, US Government Printing Office, 1983: 73–77.

14. Vincent JL. Withdrawing may be preferable to withholding. *Crit Care* 2005; **9**:226–29.

15. Truog RD, Cambell M, Curtis JR, et al. Recommendations for end-of-life care in the intensive care unit: a consensus statement by the American College of Critical Care Medicine. *Crit Care Med* 2008; **36**:953–63.

16. Chung GS, Yoon JD, Rsinski KA, Curlin FA. US Physicians' opinions about distinctions between withdrawing and withholding life-sustaining treatment. *J Relig Health* 2016; **55**:1596–606.

17. Melthorp G, Nistun T. The difference between withholding and withdrawing life-sustaining treatment. *Intens Care Med* 1997; **23**:1264–87.

18. Rydvall A, Lynoe N. Withholding and withdrawing life-sustaining treatment: a comparative study of the ethical reasoning of physicians and the general public. *Crit Care* 2008; **12**:R13.

19. Beck S, van de Loo A, Reiter-Theil S. A "little bit illegal"? Withholding and withdrawing of mechanical ventilation in the eyes of German intensive care physicians. *Med Health Care Philos* 2008; **11**:7–16.

20. Mani RK, Mandal AK, Bal S, et al. End-of]-life decisions in an Indian intensive care unit. *Intensive Care Med* 2009; **35**:1713–19.

21. Yazigi A, Riachi M, Dabbar G. Withholding and withdrawal of life-sustaining treatment in a Lebanese intensive care unit: a prospective observational study. *Intensive Care Med* 2005; **31**:562–67.

22. Krandidiotis G, Gerovasili V, Tasoulis A, et al. End-of-life decisions in Greek intensive care units: a multicenter cohort study. *Crit Care* 2010; **14**:R228.

23. Sulmassy DP, Sugarman J. Are withholding and withdrawing therapy always morally equivalent? *J Med Ethics* 1994; **20**:218–22.

24. Huddle TS. Moral fiction or moral fact? the distinction between doing and allowing in medical ethics. *Bioethics* 2013; **27**:257–62.

25. Rachels J. Active and passive euthanasia. *N Engl J Med* 1975; **292**:78–80.

26. Brock D. Taking human life. *Ethics.* 1985; **95**:851–65.

27. Sprung CL, Paruk F, Kissoon N, et al. The Durban World Congress ethics round table conference report: I. Differences between withholding and withdrawing life-sustaining treatments. *J Crit Care* 2014; **29**:890–95.

28. AMA Council on Ethical and Judicial Affairs. *Code of Medical Ethics of the American Medical Association.* Chicago, IL: AMA, 2014–15.

29. Snyder L. American College of Physicians Ethics Manual, 6th Edition. *Ann Intern Med* 2012; **156**:73–104.

30. General Medical Council. *Withholding and Withdrawing: Guidance for Doctors.* London: GMC, July 2010.

31. *In Re* Quinlan, 355 A.2d 647 (NJ 1976).

32. *Cruzan v. Director, Missouri Department of Health,* 497 U.S. 261 (1990).

33. H.R. 4449. Patient Self-Determination Act of 1990, 101st Congress (1989–90).

34. Sawicki N. A new life for wrongful living. In *LAW eCommons: Faculty Publications and Other Works.* Chicago, IL: Loyola University of Chicago School of Law, 2014, available at http://lawecommons.luc.edu/cgi/viewcontent.cgi?article=1472&context=facpubs (accessed April 27, 2016).

35. *Jeb BUSH, Governor of Florida, et al., Appellants* v. *Michael SCHIAVO, Guardian*

of Theresa Schiavo, Appellee. No. SC04–925 (Supreme Court of Florida, 2004).

36. Cranford RE. Helga Wanglie's ventilator. *Hastings Ctr Rep* 1991; **21**:23–24.

37. Jecker NS. Medical futility: a paradigm analysis. *HEC Forum* 2007; **19**:13–32.

38. Aita K, Kai L. Withdrawal of care in Japan. *Lancet* 2006; **368**:12–14.

39. Huynh TN, Kleerup EC, Wiley JF, et al. The frequency and cost of treatment perceived to be futile in critical care. *JAMA Intern Med* 2013; **173**:1887–94.

40. Pelligrino ED. The metamorphosis of medical ethics: a 30-year retrospective. *JAMA* 1993; **269**:1158–62.

41. Paris JJ, Hawkins A. "Futility" is a failed concept in medical decision making: its use should be abandoned. *Am J Bioethics* 2015; **15**:50–52.

42. Plato. *The Republic*, trans. G. M. A. Grube. Indianapolis, IN, Hacket, 1974.

43. Rubin SB. If we think it's futile, can't we just say no? *HEC Forum* 2007; **19**:45–65.

44. Toneill MR. What medical futility means to clinicians. *HEC Forum* 2007; **19**:83–93.

45. Schneiderman LJ, Jecker NS, Jonsen AR. Medical futility: its meaning and ethical implications. *Ann Intern Med* 1990; **112**:949–54.

46. McCrary S, Swanson J, Young S, et al. Physicians' quantitative assessments of medical futility. *J Clin Ethics* 1994; **5**:100–5.

47. Curtis JR Park DR, Krone MR, et al. Use of the medical futility rationale in do-not-attempt resuscitation orders. *JAMA* 1995; **273**:124–28.

48. Nassar AP, Mocelin AO Nunes ALB, et al. Caution when using prognostic models: a prospective comparison of 3 recent prognostic models. *J Crit Care* 2012; **4**:423, e1–7.

49. Litton E, Kwok M, Webb SA. Comparison of physician prediction with 2 prognostic scoring systems in predicting 2-year mortality after intensive care admission: a linked-data cohort study. *J Crit Care* 2012; **27**:423, e9–15.

50. Neville TH, Wiley JF, Holm ES, et al. Differences between attendings' and fellows' perceptions of futile treatment in the intensive care unit at one academic health center: implications for training. *Acad Med* 2015; **90**:324–30.

51. Imbus SH, Zawacki BE. Autonomy for burned patients when survival is unprecedented. *N Engl J Med* 1977; **297**: 308–11.

52. Lantos JD, Singer PA, Walker RM, et al. The illusion of futility in clinical practice. *Am J Med* 1989; **87**:81–84.

53. Weijer C, Singer PA, Dickens BM, Workman S. Dealing with demands for inappropriate treatment. *CMAJ* 1998; **159**: 817–21.

54. Bruni T, Weijer C. A misunderstanding concerning futilily. *Am J Bioeth* 2015; **15**:59–60.

55. Gallagher CM, Farroni JS, Moore JA, Nates JL, Rodriguez MA. The misleading vividness of a physician requesting futile treatment. *Am J Bioeth* 2015; **8**:54–56.

56. Texas Legislature. 2015. Senate Bill 1163: An act relating to advance directives and health care and treatment decisions. Available at www.legis.state.tx.us/tlodocs/ 84 R/billtext/pdf/SB01163I.pdf#nav panes=0 (accessed April 27, 2016).

57. Jecker NS. Futility and fairness: a defense of the Texas advance directive law. *Am J Bioeth*. 2015; **15**:43–64.

58. Ewer MS. The definition of medical futility: are we trying to define the wrong term? *Heart Lung* 2001; **30**:3–4.

59. Weiman AD. *On Dying and Denying: A Psychiatric Study of Terminality*. New York, NY: Behavioral Publications, 1972.

Chapter 15

Geriatric Critical Care Units: Model for Interdisciplinary Approach

Steven R. Allen and Lewis J. Kaplan

Key Points

- The interdisciplinary team members of a geriatric critical care unit (GCCU) should include physician, nurses, registered dietitian, physical and occupational therapy, respiratory therapy, pharmacist, and family members.
- Structural elements of a geriatric-focused intensive care unit (ICU) are meticulously designed to ensure optimal and efficient use of the space that also targets the specific needs of the elderly patients.
- A quiet environment at all times of the day is essential to the adequate rest and recovery of elderly patients.
- Monitor alarms should be adjusted to patient's baseline status, and frequency of alarms must be minimized to avoid unwarranted "noise," which can exacerbate sleep disturbances and potentially increase the frequency of delirium.
- Palliative care medicine (PCM) may be ideal to help manage a variety of nonmedical issues experienced by the family, such as guilt, anger, fear, sparse information, unrealistic expectations, misperceptions, life circumstance adjustment, and conflict resolution. Indeed, having a PCM team member regularly round with the ICU team in a geriatric-focused ICU helps enable appropriate medical care.
- Postdischarge medication should be resumed as soon as possible because failure to resume preadmission medications leads to untoward events, ranging from withdrawal syndromes, to hyper- or hypoglycemia, to heart failure.

Introduction

The geriatric population, defined as patients 65 years of age and older, is growing at an unprecedented rate within the United States and other Western nations. This population has experienced a nearly 25 percent increase from 2003 to 2013 (35.9 million in 2003 to 44.7 million in 2013). This population is expected to double to nearly 98 million by 2060. The geriatric population will make up 21.4 percent of the US population by 2040. The "older" geriatric population (85 years of age and older) is expected to triple from 6.1 million in 2013 to 14.6 million in 2040 [1]. As this "Silver Tsunami" approaches, it is critical to thoroughly understand this population and the medical complexities inherent to it in order to optimize care of critically ill elderly patients.

The correlation between chronologic and physiologic age is not necessarily linear. By way of example, Ma et al. investigated the correlation between aging and insulin secretion and demonstrated a decline from maturation to approximately 45 years of age, with stabilization in decline until after 55 years of age, followed by a further decline [2]. The accumulation of various physiologic conditions and medical diseases that may be either spontaneous (genetic mutations) or acquired (external exposures) may accelerate one's physiologic age in relation to chronologic age. The interactions and processes that influence how an individual is affected by the accumulation of physiologic insults is complex and poorly understood. Accelerated physiologic age is likely to diminish the reserve with which one may address further challenges such as septic shock, injury, or stroke; of course, the inverse is also true and may augment recovery at an unexpectedly rapid pace. This discrepancy in both chronologic and physiologic ages results in differences in morbidity and mortality among cohorts and appears to be more pronounced among the elderly.

Elderly patients with a more advanced physiologic age may be described as being more frail than those with a "younger" physiologic age. Frailty has a variety of dimensions and definitions, but common features of frailty include weight loss, decreased strength, exhaustion, slowness, and reduced activity level [3]. Other dimensions associated with frailty include cognitive impairment, falls, anemia, and increased numbers of identified comorbidities [4]. This state of weakness leads one to be vulnerable to various stressors and may be manifested as healthcare-related morbidity and mortality, including worse perioperative outcomes [5–8]. Multiple instruments that assess frailty have been developed to objectively assess for frailty. The Comprehensive Geriatric Assessment (CGA) encompasses all areas of geriatric frailty, including cognitive function, mobility, activities of daily living (ADLs) functioning, mood, and nutrition. Because the CGA is labor intensive, other shorter questionnaires have been developed to assess frailty in elderly individuals and include the Hopkins Frailty Score, the Edmonton Frail Scale, and the Groningen Frailty Indicator (GFI). One study demonstrated that a score of greater than 3 on the GFI is associated with increased in-hospital mortality, increased serious complications, and increased hospital length of stay [9]. These instruments to assess frailty are invaluable in assessing operative risk so as to appropriately inform patients and families of associated risks with operative intervention.

Due to the unique aspects of the elderly population, including significant differences in physiologic age that may not correspond to chronologic age and the associated frailty, the elderly population requires special consideration to optimize outcomes after illness or surgical interventions and avoid nonbeneficial outcomes such as organ failure, nursing home residence, cognitive failure, chronic pain, failed obligations, long length of stay, and death in a chronic care facility [10]. Much as in other domains where targeted teams with focused areas of excellence have improved outcomes, geriatric critical care follows suit.

Components of a Successful Interdisciplinary Geriatric Critical Care Unit (GCCU)

Team Members. The interdisciplinary team members of a GCCU are nearly indistinguishable from those that comprise any other high-functioning critical care unit with an important exception. A GCCU also specifically incorporates additional key team members possessing specific expertise in geriatric medical and surgical care. These unique team members are the key in addressing the spectrum of care needs seen in critically ill geriatric

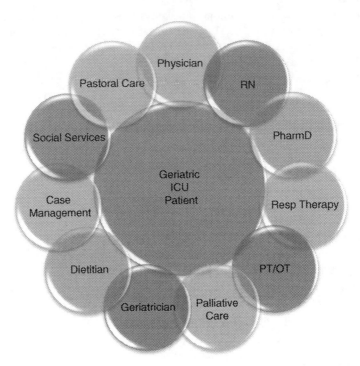

Figure 15.1 Geriatric ICU multiprofessional team. This diagram demonstrates the multiplicity of team members who interact with geriatric ICU patients for optimal outcomes.

patients in contrast to their more youthful counterparts. We will discuss the team members and their specific roles, as well as the structural components on the ICU in which they practice, in further detail below. It is important to recognize that most facilities will *not* have a separate and specifically designated GCCU but will instead have a functional one, as defined by the presence of the GCCU team in a more general ICU setting (Figure 15.1).

Structural Elements of a Geriatric-Focused ICU. The physical organization that makes up the geriatric-focused ICU is just as critical as the team that surrounds and cares for the patient. This unit must be meticulously designed to ensure optimal and efficient use of the space that also targets the specific needs of the elderly patients. As with all ICUs, the rooms should be arranged so that patients are easily visible from multiple vantage points within the unit. This ensures that all patients are adequately observed, given the high potential for delirium in the elderly. All rooms should have direct access to large windows with outside views and access to bright natural light. This will optimize attempts to normalize the sleep-wake cycle for these patients, in whom sleep hygiene is critical. Additionally, each room should have large sliding-glass doors that allow adequate noise control while closed and allow adequate visualization of the patient while drawn. A quiet environment at all times of the day is essential to the adequate rest and recovery of elderly patients. Additionally, monitor alarms should be adjusted to patient's baseline status and frequency of alarms must be minimized. This unwarranted "noise" can exacerbate sleep disturbances, in a population that is critically dependent on restful sleep to minimize frequency of delirium.

Hygiene is also an essential element of patients within a geriatric specific ICU. Patients and care providers must have ready access to sinks, soap and hand sanitizer upon entry and exit from each of the patient's room. Each patient room must be equipped with a shower and toilet, that are accessible and safety hand-rails, non-slip flooring, and sturdy seating for safety. Showers should be ideally large enough to accommodate the patient and a care provider for hygiene assistance, as well as physical or occupational therapy, for training in the use of assistive devices for hygiene. Toilets should be raised to ensure the patient's ability to sit comfortably and stand up, without leading to imbalance and inadvertent fall. The room should also be large enough to accommodate family members. Of necessity, a respite area for the family is also ideal, especially during prolonged periods of critical illness. A variety of ICU designs that specifically address these elements are available from different critical care organizations.

Other elements to optimize the effectiveness of a geriatric specific intensive care unit include large font, high contrast signage, within the rooms that facilitate frequent re-orientation. A mechanism to update the day, date and time as well as the shift based care provider are essential to enhance orientation; attention should be paid to ensuring accuracy and frequent updating as necessary, especially with provider changes. A mechanism to communicate daily goals and the changing treatment plan to both the patient and the patient's family members helps shape expectations and provides opportunities for family input and education. Specific attention is required to ensure that information is visible and large enough to be readable by the potentially visually impaired patient.

Functional Elements of a Geriatric-Focused ICU. There are multiple functional elements within a geriatric-specific ICU that must come together to ensure effective and efficient care and to optimize outcomes. These elements include physical therapy on site, as well as various elements that facilitate adequate communication between care providers, patients, and their families. Assistive devices such as prescription glasses, electronic devices that speak for the patient or translate between languages, hearing aids that enable effective communication with those who may have impaired auditory or vocal capabilities should not be ignored. A large number of apps and other programs are available for laptops, tablets, and handheld devices. Larger television monitors and controls that accommodate decreased grip strength, as well as reduced digital dexterity from arthritis and related conditions, further enable comfort and communication and reduce frustration for patients with impairments. They further provide geriatric patients with some control over their environment at a time when they have become dependent in an unfamiliar hospital/critical care environment.

The physical plant of the ICU designed for geriatric patients should have adequate conference room space that is accessible to all team members. This space should be linked to the electronic health record (including imaging), be suitable for educational conference presentations, and be able to display Web-based educational presentations as well. The space is ideally tasked as a confidential space for care transition handoffs and inter-disciplinary care planning. A separate space that is more comfortable and less formal may be ideal for family meetings, but the conference space may be used in this way for larger meetings as well. Of course, daily plans and goals of care also may be part of the rounding process to continue to engage the patient in those plans when appropriate.

Daily Operations

Due to the complexities of the elderly surgical patient who requires intensive care in the perioperative period, multiple teams and care providers are crucial to the comprehensive care of these patients. This team approach ensures that every aspect of the patient's care is optimized. Ideally, a representative from each discipline having an impact on care would be present on rounds to ensure that their domain issues are addressed and incorporated seamlessly into the daily overall care plan. Recognizing that some members may be incorporated into teams in more than one ICU, a mechanism to communicate plans and queries to team members who cannot attend rounds is essential. White boards, glass door panels, and goals sheets (electronic and paper) have all been used successfully.

Interprofessional rounds should include, but are not limited to, physician, nurses, registered dietitian, physical and occupational therapy, respiratory therapy, pharmacist, and family members who are integral to the care of each elderly patient. Input from each team member is necessary to ensure that a single, congruent plan is developed. This prevents potential breakdowns in communication between different team members, allows each team member to voice their specific plans for the day, and addresses any questions/concerns associated with each patient's care plan.

Family involvement in daily rounds as members of the care team is also beneficial. Incorporation of the family not only ensures that the daily care plan is clearly communicated but also allows real-time discussion and problem solving among other members of the team and the family. The elaboration of goals of care is facilitated by having an engaged and informed family. In fact, such discussions may be incorporated into rounds and eliminate the potential stigma associated with the "afternoon family meeting." Moreover, having direct family communication on rounds appears to reduce the number of nurse phone calls during the day for information gathering, thus allowing more time for the bedside care. Designating a spokesperson helps facilitate intrafamily communication as well. Since the geriatric-focused ICU will likely use several consultants on a regular basis, having the abundance of information funneled to the family at a regular time is not only efficient but also sets reasonable expectations for the patient (when they can participate), the family, and team members. Teams expand when there are concomitant medical conditions requiring specialist evaluation that are not the primary reason for admission.

Elderly patients who require intensive care for various surgical issues often have a long list of preexisting medical conditions that complicate the care of the presenting problem. Additionally, patients with serious surgical disease processes may do so with little to no previous medical attention, leading to new diagnoses of a variety of preexisting but undiagnosed conditions. Therefore, the newly diagnosed medical comorbidities are often poorly controlled and make management of the presenting surgical disease process much more difficult. That the elderly, even at an advanced age, substantially engage with surgical services is illustrated by an exploration of Medicare decedents who in 2008 ($n = 1,802,029$ patients) were parsed by those who had surgery within 1 year (31.9 percent), 1 month (18.8 percent), and 1 week (8 percent) of their death [11]. Decedents spanned 65 to 98 years of age. Not surprisingly, those who were operated on had a longer ICU stay and hospital length of stay, were more frequently readmitted, and did so at a higher total cost. The ability to tolerate and recover from surgical management is influenced by comorbidities and their impact on the elderly patient – an analysis that can potentially be assessed using a frailty metric.

Assessment of Frailty. *Frailty*, defined as physiologic decline across multiple organ systems, making the patient vulnerable to even minor external stressors [12], has a prevalence of nearly 15 percent in those 65 years of age and older and up to 30 percent in patient older than 85 years. Chronic illnesses have been found to worsen frailty significantly, as demonstrated in a study by Bandeen-Roche et al [13]. Within this study, for each chronic condition there was a steep prevalence gradient from robust (or nonfrail) to frail. This increase was most striking for diabetes, heart disease, pulmonary disease, osteoporosis, and stroke. Additionally, those who require assistance in ADLs were significantly more likely to be considered frail than those who lived independently. Non-nursing-home patients who live in residential care settings are twice as likely to be frail than their independent counterparts [13].

Frail older adults are at major risk for postoperative complications. Hence the geriatric population should be assessed, if possible, in the preoperative setting for frailty. There are several instruments to measure frailty. Examples include the timed Up and Go (TUG) test, the Groningen Frailty Index (Table 15.1), and the Edmonton Frailty Scale (EFS), which has been validated in the preoperative setting for elective surgery. An exhaustive review by de Vries et al. identified the Frailty Index as the most suitable instrument as an evaluative outcome measure although there are a large number of other instruments that may be useful [14]. Based on the sound evidence that frail surgical patients do worse than more robust patients, preoperative evaluation should include assessment of frailty for both prognostic and therapeutic considerations. With this evaluation of frailty, patients and families can be appropriately counseled as to realistic outcomes and potential complications. Additionally, from a functional stand-point, those deemed frail may be referred for early and intensive physical therapy evaluation and treatment (i.e., optimization) to improve acute postsurgical outcomes and improve long-term quality of life. Therefore, frailty assessment in geriatric-specific ICUs should be performed on every patient when appropriate to determine a baseline and a care plan consistent with those findings to improve outcomes.

Treatment of Preexisting Conditions. Many elderly patients present with chronic .preexisting conditions, and many more are found to have previously unrecognized medical conditions such as poorly controlled diabetes, chronic obstructive pulmonary disease (COPD), and coronary artery disease on admission to the ICU. For those with known disease, the intensivist must decide on the advisability of continuing or revising the preexisting regimen. One must weigh the risks and benefits for each medication as well as assess the potential interactions of home medications with the therapeutic agents being used to treat the acute processes that led to the admission. Prime examples include vitamin K antagonists or antiplatelet agents being used for atrial fibrillation or other thromboembolism prevention. Often the decision has already been made prior to elective admission, and the intensivist must instead decide on the timing of resumption of those

Table 15.1 Domains Assessed by the Groningen Frailty Index

Mobility	Can the person perform the following tasks without assistance: 1. Grocery shopping 2. Walking outside the house 3. Getting (un)dressed 4. Visiting restroom
Vision	Does the patient encounter problems due to impaired vision?
Hearing	Does the patient encounter problems due to impaired hearing?
Nutrition	Has the patient undergone unintentional weight loss over the past 6 months (6 kg/6 months or 3 kg/3 months)?
Comorbidity	Does the patient use four or more types of medications?
Cognition	Does the patient have problems or complaints about memory?
Psychosocial	1. Does the patient feel emptiness? 2. Does the patient ever miss the presence of people? 3. Does the patient feel left alone? 4. Has the patient felt down or depressed lately? 5. Has the patient felt nervous or anxious?
Physical fitness	How would the patient rate their own physical fitness (0–10; 0=very bad, 10=very good)?

(*Source:* Adapted from Bielderman et al. [43].)

agents. Having an integrated team structure in the geriatric-focused ICU that includes the surgical team helps facilitate discussions such as those in the table.

Due to the complexities of medication management among the elderly population, a geriatric-focused pharmacist is an ideal ICU team member. The specialized pharmacist may assist in medication reconciliation and appropriate dosing. Pharmacists who specialize in the care of critically ill elderly patients understand the physiologic and pharmacologic changes that accompany aging. Understanding the changes in renal and hepatic function and the effect of these changes on medication clearance assist in the appropriate dosing of such medications. These pharmacists may assist with negative medication interactions and counsel physicians and the care team about adverse reactions that may occur with certain medications among older patients (i.e., benzodiazepines and any number of medications contained on the Beers list). In a study of 90 patients taking five or more medications (excluding those with heart failure), the home medication list was compared with the list proposed by the acute care facility. A total of 1,045 home medications were reviewed, of which 290 discrepancies were noted between what the patients were prescribed preadmission and what the providers believed the patients were prescribed, with the most common discrepancy being dose optimization (45.5 percent). The remainder of the discrepancies included adding therapy (27.6 percent), other (15.2 percent), and discontinuing therapy (11.7 percent). Pharmacists intervened in nearly 50 percent of the cohort with a projected cost saving of more than $2 million in a single facility, assuming an average of 1.6 interventions per patient and an average cost of $8,750 per preventable adverse drug event [15].

Postdischarge medication resumption is a key event that benefits from a systems-based approach. Failure to resume preadmission medications leads to untoward events ranging from withdrawal syndromes, to hyper- or hypoglycemia, to heart failure [16]. Factors associated with this unique failure include rushed discharges, sparse discharge orders, compromised patient or caregiver cognition, and lack of discharge medication counseling and medication reconciliation. A dedicated pharmacist or advanced practice providers can be anticipated to play a key role in the successful transition from inpatient to outpatient for those receiving care in a geriatric-focused ICU [17].

Assessment of Pain and Delirium

Delirium. *Delirium* is defined as an acute change in mental status that waxes and wanes and is due to a generalized medical condition. The incidence of delirium ranges from 14 to 56 percent of all hospitalized patients, and it affects up to 80 percent of patients in ICUs, with a higher incidence among the elderly population. Additionally, delirium is associated with a nearly 33 percent mortality [18].

There are multiple classifications of delirium that include hyperactive, hypoactive, and mixed forms. While hyperactive delirium is easy to identify based on the patient's frequently agitated state, hypoactive may be more difficult to identify and diagnose. In hypoactive delirium, patients often appear to be sleeping or have a depressed mental status. Thus this form of delirium goes unrecognized and untreated. For these reasons and because delirium is so prevalent among the geriatric population, patients should be assessed for delirium every shift by the nursing staff. Objective measures of delirium should be used to make a formal diagnosis. To diagnose delirium of all types, the patients must maintain a reasonable level of consciousness, as assessed by the Richmond Agitation and Sedation Scale (RASS). Once this has been established, objective methods to evaluate for delirium include the Delirium Rating Scale–Revised (DRS-R), the Intensive Care Delirium Symptoms Checklist (ICDSC), and the Memorial Delirium Assessment Scale (MDAS). However, the Confusion Assessment Method–ICU (CAM-ICU) has become the assessment method of choice in many ICUs due to its ease of administration. These instruments were discussed in greater detail in Chapter 5.

Logically, the best treatment for delirium is the prevention of delirium. There are multiple measures that can be implemented in the geriatric-specific ICU to prevent delirium. Patients with hearing or visual deficits should have access to their hearing aids and eyeglasses. This allows an easier time with patient communication and reorientation as needed. Patients should be routinely reoriented to person, place, date, and time instead of when they are recognized to be disoriented; reclaiming orientation is more difficult than maintaining it in the first place.

Another nonpharmacologic means of delirium prevention is the maintenance of a normal sleep-wake cycle. This can be accomplished with environmental interventions such as shades that can block out ambient light during the evening hours. Televisions should be turned off at night, and when appropriate, doors should be closed to reduce noise from within the nursing station of the ICU. Staff should make a conscious effort to minimize the noise level in the unit to allow for better sleep hygiene. Additionally, adjusting nursing workflow to avoid a scheduled hourly interaction with the patient allows for sleep instead of establishing a night of broken sleep as part of the workflow plan. For example, avoid changing intravenous (IV) tubing at 11 P.M., IV site evaluation and relabeling at 2 A.M., bed bath at 4 A.M., and others and instead move tasks that can be scheduled to occur during waking hours instead of at night. Similarly, morning chest x-rays can be obtained at 6 A.M. instead of 5 A.M., and laboratory draws can occur after the chest x-ray. This may require altering shifts for allied health personnel or adopting some of the work by the unit staff, but it should be an essential part of an overall plan for the geriatric-focused ICU.

Should delirium develop within a geriatric patient, life-threatening yet reversible medical conditions such as hypoxia, sepsis, myocardial infarction, and so on should be quickly identified. Pharmacologic treatment ideally should be a last resort to minimize further consequences of delirium. Staff should differentiate between pain, anxiety, and agitation. Pain should be treated with an appropriate analgesic regimen that may include acetaminophen, opiates, or nonsteroidal agents. Anxiety should be treated with anxiolytics when necessary. Of note, some elderly patients may demonstrate paradoxical agitation instead of sedation when treated with benzodiazepine agents; the at-risk population cannot be more precisely defined at present. Therefore, many recommend using typical or atypical antipsychotic agents as the preferred alternative to benzodiazepines in the elderly. One notable exception is the elderly patient who is already on a regular dose of benzodiazepine, for whom cessation may precipitate withdrawal symptoms; it is unlikely that this patient population will demonstrate paradoxical agitation to continuation therapy [19]. Finally, agitation should be addressed with reassurance and reorientation, with sedatives administered for failure of nonpharmacologic therapy, or to preserve patient or staff safety.

Pain Management. Pain is a common accompaniment to surgical and nonsurgical therapy. Edema is an often-overlooked source of constant discomfort from cutaneous nerve stretch and activation of nociceptors. Nonetheless, older patients may not report nor perceive pain in the same way as younger patients. Elderly patients may have a difficult time in describing or acknowledging pain. Patients may manifest signs of pain with increased heart rate or other arrhythmias or hypertension. Patients with chronic cognitive impairment such as Alzheimer's dementia may be nonverbal and difficult to assess. Subtle signs such as those described in addition to facial signs (grimacing or wincing on abdominal examination) or voluntary or even involuntary guarding may be the only indication that the patient is in pain.

Best practices for pain control in elderly patients are to ensure adequate pain control from the onset. One must attempt to minimize opioid usage. This may be accomplished by adding standing acetaminophen to the pain regimen if there are no contraindications. Furthermore, if the patient has normal renal function, one may consider a short course of nonsteroidal anti-inflammatory drugs (NSAIDs) such as ibuprofen or ketorolac to further minimize opioid usage. Among elderly patients with injuries such as rib fractures, the aggressive use of paravertebral blocks or thoracic epidurals is invaluable to optimize pain control without inadvertent sedation. Adequate pain control is crucial to ensure good pulmonary toilet to minimize the risk of pneumonia and atelectasis [20,21], as well as support early mobilization and ambulation to prevent venous thromboembolic events. Opioids and bed rest can exacerbate constipation, which can cause pain and significant discomfort. Constipation should be prevented with a regular bowel regimen. Stool hydrants are essential due to the decreased thirst sensing that accompanies aging and should be paired with an agent to enhance stool flow; recall that the colon excels at salt and water absorption to aid in the repair of plasma hyperosmolar states such as dehydration. Lavage solutions help to avoid the sequelae of laxative abuse and do provide some water for stool rehydration.

Effects of Delirium and Pain on Underlying Cognitive Deficits and Dementia. Medications often administered to surgical and critically ill patients include sedatives, opioids, and neuromuscular blocking (NMB) agents, all of which have profound effects on long-term neuropsychological function and have been shown to lead to *long-term cognitive impairment after a critical illness* (LTCI-CI). Each of these medications has been shown to be associated with worsened delirium in these populations, especially the elderly. While NMB agents are less frequently used in the ICU than in previous decades, they may be used in the management of acute respiratory distress syndrome (ARDS). NMB agents are associated with persistent weakness that may be difficult to distinguish from the polyneuropathy of critical illness or the weakness that accompanies the post–intensive care syndrome. Daily sedation interruption to assess the integrity of the neuroaxis has been demonstrated to be beneficial in all populations and should be incorporated into geriatric-focused ICU care [22].

Preexisting cognitive impairment and dementia have been shown to worsen in the face of even a single episode of delirium. These effects seem to have long-term consequences that span up to 6 years after the index hospitalization [23–25]. It is unclear whether daily or every-shift sedation holidays will have a salutary impact on the occurrence of delirium, but they have been noted to reduce the number of days on the ventilator. Relatedly, delirium has been recently demonstrated to be increased in patients who are cared for in a remote ICU compared with the parent ICU of the managing team [26]; multiple factors likely influence this observation, including remote care by telephone, sequenced care that is at the end of rounds, and others that have yet to be established that directly relate to causality. However, these observations argue quite strongly for cohorting geriatric patients in an ICU focused on their care and the systematic abrogation of confounders to their care.

Pulmonary Support in the Elderly

Pulmonary support in the elderly is essentially the same as that for their younger counterparts with a few notable exceptions. The exceptions may be conveniently grouped into the following categories:

1. Due to decreased muscle mass that accompanies aging, for any given amount of lean body mass loss, there will be a disproportionate decrease in strength and endurance.
2. Loss of muscle mass as well as changes in dentition may hinder obtaining an adequate seal when using full-face-mask noninvasive ventilation.

3. Increases is oral biofilm due to prostheses, dehydration, and diabetes may change the flora associated with aspiration-related pneumonia and should be considered when selecting empirical antibiotics for new pulmonary infections.

Because of these three elements, a concentrated effort at liberation from mechanical ventilation as rapidly as possible makes intuitive sense, as do efforts at maintenance of lean body mass. Accordingly, intensive physical therapy, including, but not limited to, early ambulation, ambulation and exercise while mechanically ventilated, early nutritional support, and oral hygiene are interventions that are internally consistent and improve outcomes [27]. Recent efforts have dispelled many of the myths that pervaded the previous practice of immobilization of ICU patients, demonstrating that it is indeed feasible to ambulate and exercise patients while mechanically ventilated or on ventricular assist devices [28]. A recent review of biofilm is available for the interested reader that outlines essential features of biofilms and current approaches to management [29].

Nutritional Support for the Elderly

Nutritional support is critical to maintain lean body mass as well as enable host defenses. It is important to note that most trials will specifically exclude very elderly patients from inclusion. Therefore, little data exist to guide decision making in an evidence-based medicine fashion. However, there are certain elements from trial-derived data that may be translated to the geriatric population. According to the Choosing Wisely Campaign recommendations for critical care practitioners, nutritional support need not be provided prior to day 7 in the nutritionally replete – this recommendation, albeit in a backwards fashion, supports early nutritional support of the elderly because they are infrequently nutritionally replete [30]. Given the inherent decreases in host defense competency that accompany aging – comorbidities, malnutrition, and, of course, critical illness – use of the gastrointestinal tract for nutritional support reduces infections in the elderly in the ICU. Moreover, luminal nutritional support also serves to nourish the gut mucosa and preserves the mucosal barrier function that is important in limiting translocation [31]. Preservation of the glycocalyx also enables the use of nonelemental luminal feeds as opposed to elemental formulations that provide substances that are directly absorbed across the lumen without needing further processing. Of course, using nonelemental feeds in a patient whose glycocalyx is not intact (i.e., NPO > 3 days) may lead to diarrhea, and luminal support should be decreased or stopped while the increased stool flow is evaluated [32,33].

Recognizing that low albumin may be a reflection of dilution, consumption, or a response to increases in plasma negative charge, other measures of nutritional health are appropriate [34]. Prealbumin is a better indicator but needs to be measured in conjunction with C-reactive protein (CRP) because these two measures covary inversely; indeed, the fidelity of prealbumin as a measure of nutritional health requires a normal CRP level for accurate interpretation [35]. For patients with long ICU stays, it is also appropriate to assess whether the targeted nutritional prescription is meeting the patient's protein needs by using assays such as the urinary urea nitrogen assay, with the goal of positive nitrogen balance [36]. It is important to recall that critical illness should not be accompanied by dietary restriction of protein, even while non-protein-caloric intake may be reduced (i.e., 22 cal/kg per day) to avoid hepatic steatosis [37]. Commonly, increased protein targets such as 1.5 to 2.0 g protein/kg per day are appropriate for those with critical illness, especially those with septic shock or multitrauma. Consultation with a registered dietitian is key to establishing a program that incorporates assessment, prescription, and monitoring in a consistent framework [38]. Furthermore, often overlooked are vitamin and micronutrient deficiencies such as those of iron, vitamin D, vitamin B_{12}, zinc, selenium, and other micronutrients. Empirical therapy approaches as well as those that engage in specific level monitoring have been successfully deployed to enhance outcomes in the elderly [39,40].

Palliative Care Program

While it would be ideal to have the goals of care established for every patient on ICU admission, this is not realistic. For many, the ICU admission is unexpected and is coupled with serious illness, whose outcome is unable to be reliably anticipated. Furthermore, even if the condition is treatable, the interventions required to do so may not be acceptable to the patient, if their thoughts regarding those interventions were able to be known. Critical illness is often accompanied by the need for endotracheal intubation, analgesics, and sedatives and is frequently the result of infection and other conditions that affect neurologic status. Therefore, the patient is often unable to articulate their desires about their situation and their goals of care. Consequently, the clinician is driven to accept surrogate judgment from family members or others (ideally the individual with the healthcare power of attorney) regarding goals of care. Since discussions regarding a critically ill individual are often complex and, in the case of an elder, may be complicated by a variety of nonmedical issues, including but not limited to guilt, anger, fear, sparse information, unrealistic expectations, and misperceptions, aid in navigating many of these issues is optimal. Palliative care medicine (PCM) may be ideal to help sort out these issues and serve as a liaison for the family. Indeed, having a PCM team member regularly round with the ICU team in a geriatric-focused ICU makes not only intuitive sense but also helps enable appropriate medical care.

While palliative care is most often asked to address end-of-life issues, such teams also engage in multiple other functions, including life circumstance adjustment and conflict resolution. New diagnoses of cancer, progression to dialysis requiring renal failure, limb loss, transition to supervised living, and nursing home entry are but a few of the life circumstance adjustments with which palliative care medicine may be of service. Pain, anxiety, and depression commonly accompany such life changes, and the expertise of the PCM team is invaluable in navigating not only the inpatient care, but care coordination in the outpatient arena as well. Indeed, PCM engagement in the ICU is linked with improved resource utilization, increased life span, and enhanced patient satisfaction [41]. Despite many intensivists possessing expertise at managing acute pain, their involvement with the patient often ends with transfer out of the ICU. PCM continues to engage with the patient and family, as appropriate, beyond the confines of the ICU, providing a necessary link between all the care providers and the patient-family unit, an important element because palliative care extends beyond the hospital inpatient care domain.

All too often end-of-life discussions are fraught with differences of opinion, misaligned expectations, and seemingly irreconcilable differences in perspective between patients and families, among family members, and between clinicians and different clinical teams. PCM team members often serve as intermediaries between the teams or individuals in conflict. By having spent considerable time with each of the individuals involved, PCM team members are often able to understand each of the perspectives that color the varying positions and help those in conflict to reach a resolution. However, such a role places the

PCM team member in a potentially awkward position because they are involved in direct care as well. Instead, a conflict-management team may be helpful as an alternative approach to conflict resolution because such an approach allows PCM team members to retain their role as part of the treatment instead of becoming a mediator.

Conflict-Management Teams in the ICU

As an alternative to using PCM team members to pursue apparently intractable conflict resolution in the ICU, conflict mediation and conflict mediators provide an underutilized alternative. Conflict mediation is not a new concept, and many teams exist outside of medicine, especially in law enforcement and the legal system. These teams are ideal when parties in conflict cannot resolve their conflicts on their own.

Mediators may be physicians or may come from other medical or nonmedical fields, as noted earlier. While adhering to ethical principles, mediators are not engaged in answering ethical questions – that is the purview of a clinical ethics consultation team. Note is made that there are relatively few true ethical questions to be answered in the context of a conflict and that clinical ethics consultants are not ideally suited for typical conflict resolution as a result.

A key aspect of the conflict mediator is that the mediator has no stake in either side of a conflict but is instead invested in helping the parties come to a mutually acceptable resolution – regardless of what that resolution may be. Therefore, the mediator should not be a member of a care team or directly involved with the patient or family and remains a neutral intermediary, unaligned with either side. By the nature of finding a position to which both parties may agree, mediators engage in what may be characterized as an *integrative form of bargaining* because, in general, both sides engage in compromise to reach resolution. Because communication failure often underpins conflict in the ICU, active listening as well as rephrasing skills are essential elements to be brought to the table by the mediator. These skills may be learned and are not generally intuitive. A recent review of conflict-management teams in the ICU provides additional in-depth reading and direction in crafting and deploying a conflict-management team in the ICU [42].

Conclusion

The population is aging at an unprecedented rate. As the population ages, physicians and other healthcare professionals will see an increasing number of elderly patients who are injured or become critically ill from various disease processes. Additionally, the care of older patients may be made more difficult by any number of preexisting medical conditions that not only complicate their care but contribute to their frailty. These chronic medical conditions and significant frailty adversely affect both short- and long-term outcomes in this population of patients. Older patients require specialized care to optimize their outcomes. Specialized GCCUs, or units that have on-demand geriatric expertise, may allow patient-centered optimization of care for this special population.

References

1. *A Profile of Older Americans: 2014*. Available at www.acl.gov/sites/default/files/Aging%20 and%20Disability%20in%20America/2014 (accessed November 18, 2015).

2. Ma XH, Muzumdar R, Yang XM, et al. Aging is associated with resistance to effects of leptin on fat distribution and insulin action. *J Gerontol A Biol Sci Med Sci* 2002; 57:B225–31.

3. Scandrett KG, Zuckerbraun BS, Peitzman AB. Operative risk stratification in the older adult. *Surg Clin North Am* 2015; **95**:149–72.

4. Robinson TN, Wu DS, Pointer L, et al. Simple frailty score predicts postoperative complications across surgical specialties. *Am J Surg* 2013; **206**:544–50.

5. Dasgupta M, Rolfson DB, Stolee P, Borrie MJ, Speechley M. Frailty is associated with postoperative complications in older adults with medical problems. *Arch Gerontol Geriatr* 2009; **48**:78–83.

6. Makary MA, Segev DL, Pronovost PJ, et al. Frailty as a predictor of surgical outcomes in older patients. *J Am Coll Surg* 2010; **210**: 901–8.

7. Robinson TN, Eiseman B, Wallace JI, et al. Redefining geriatric preoperative assessment using frailty, disability and co-morbidity. *Ann Surg* 2009; **250**: 449–55.

8. Oresanya LB, Lyons WL, Finlayson E. Preoperative assessment of the older patient: a narrative review. *JAMA* 2014; **311**:2110–20.

9. Theou O, Brothers TD, Pena FG, Mitnitski A, Rockwood K. Identifying common characteristics of frailty across seven scales. *J Am Geriatr Soc* 2014; **62**:901–6.

10. Cooper Z, Courtwright A, Karlage A, Gawande A, Block S. Pitfalls in communication that lead to nonbeneficial emergency surgery in elderly patients with serious illness: description of the problem and elements of a solution. *Ann Surg* 2014; **260**:949–57.

11. Kwok AC, Semel ME, Lipsitz SR, et al. The intensity and variation of surgical care at the end of life: a retrospective cohort study. *Lancet* 2011; **378**:1408–13.

12. Partridge JS, Fuller M, Harari D, et al. Frailty and poor functional status are common in arterial vascular surgical patients and affect postoperative outcomes. *Int J Surg* 2015; **18**:57–63.

13. Bandeen-Roche K, Seplaki CL, Huang J, et al. Frailty in older adults: a nationally representative profile in the United States. *J Gerontol A Biol Sci Med Sci* 2015; **70**: 1427–34.

14. de Vries NM, Staal JB, van Ravensberg CD, et al. Outcome instruments to measure frailty: a systematic review. *Ageing Res Rev* 2011; **10**:104–14.

15. Smith L, Mosley J, Lott S, et al. Impact of pharmacy-led medication reconciliation on medication errors during transition in the hospital setting. *Pharm Pract (Granada)* 2015; **13**:634.

16. Lovig KO, Horwitz L, Lipska K, et al. Discontinuation of antihyperglycemic therapy after acute myocardial infarction: medical necessity or medical error? *Jt Comm J Qual Patient Saf* 2012; **38**:403–7.

17. Tan WA. *The Role of a Pharmacist in a Transdisciplinary Geriatric Surgery Team*. New York, NY: Springer, 2015.

18. Collinsworth AW, Priest EL, Campbell CR, Vasilevskis EE, Masica AL. A review of multifaceted care approaches for the prevention and mitigation of delirium in intensive care units. *J Intensive Care Med* 2016; **31**:127–41.

19. Luijendijk HJ, Tiemeier H, Hofman A, Heeringa J, Stricker BH. Determinants of chronic benzodiazepine use in the elderly: a longitudinal study. *Br J Clin Pharmacol* 2008; **65**:593–99.

20. Gage A, Rivara F, Wang J, Jurkovich GJ, Arbabi S. The effect of epidural placement in patients after blunt thoracic trauma. *J Trauma Acute Care Surg* 2014; **76**:39–45; discussion 46.

21. Yeh DD, Kutcher ME, Knudson MM, Tang JF. Epidural analgesia for blunt thoracic injury–which patients benefit most? *Injury* 2012; **43**:1667–71.

22. Brummel NE, Balas MC, Morandi A, et al. Understanding and reducing disability in older adults following critical illness. *Crit Care Med* 2015; **43**:1265–75.

23. Rothenhausler HB, Ehrentraut S, Stoll C, Schelling G, Kapfhammer HP. The relationship between cognitive performance and employment and health status in long-term survivors of the acute respiratory distress syndrome: results of an exploratory study. *Gen Hosp Psychiatry* 2001; **23**:90–96.

24. Morandi A, Pandharipande PP, Jackson JC, et al. Understanding terminology of delirium and long-term cognitive impairment in critically ill patients. *Best Pract Res Clin Anaesthesiol* 2012; **26**:267–76.

25. Hopkins RO, Suchyta MR, Farrer TJ, Needham D. Improving post–intensive care unit neuropsychiatric outcomes: understanding cognitive effects of physical activity. *Am J Respir Crit Care Med* 2012; **186**:1220–28.

26. Pascual JL, Blank NW, Holena DN, et al. There's no place like home: boarding surgical ICU patients in other ICUs and the effect of distances from the home unit. *J Trauma Acute Care Surg* 2014; **76**:1096–102.

27. Girard TD, Kress JP, Fuchs BD, et al. Efficacy and safety of a paired sedation and ventilator weaning protocol for mechanically ventilated patients in intensive care (Awakening and Breathing Controlled trial): a randomised controlled trial. *Lancet* 2008; **371**:126–34.

28. King MS, Render ML, Ely EW, Watson PL. Liberation and animation: strategies to minimize brain dysfunction in critically ill patients. *Semin Respir Crit Care Med* 2010; **31**:87–96.

29. Hall MR, McGillicuddy E, Kaplan LJ. Biofilm: basic principles, pathophysiology, and implications for clinicians. *Surg Infect (Larchmt)* 2014; **15**:1–7.

30. Halpern SD, Becker D, Curtis JR, et al. An official American Thoracic Society/ American Association of Critical-Care Nurses/American College of Chest Physicians/Society of Critical Care Medicine policy statement: the Choosing Wisely Top 5 list in critical care medicine. *Am J Respir Crit Care Med* 2014; **190**:818–26.

31. Wade CE, Kozar RA, Dyer CB, et al. Evaluation of nutrition deficits in adult and elderly trauma patients. *JPEN J Parenter Enteral Nutr* 2015; **39**:449–55.

32. Poley JR. The scanning electron microscope: how valuable in the evaluation of small bowel mucosal pathology in chronic childhood diarrhea? *Scanning Microsc* 1991; **5**:1037–62; discussion 62–63.

33. Zonta S, Doni M, Alessiani M, et al. Elemental enteral nutrition preserves the mucosal barrier and improves the trophism of the villi after small bowel transplantation in piglets. *Transplant Proc* 2007; **39**:2024–27.

34. Piper GL, Kaplan LJ. Fluid and electrolyte management for the surgical patient. *Surg Clin North Am* 2012; **92**:189–205, vii.

35. Chiari MM, Bagnoli R, De Luca PD, Monti M, Rampoldi E, Cunietti E. Influence of acute inflammation on iron and nutritional status indexes in older inpatients. *J Am Geriatr Soc* 1995; **43**:767–71.

36. Gaillard C, Alix E, Boirie Y, Berrut G, Ritz P. Are elderly hospitalized patients getting enough protein? *J Am Geriatr Soc* 2008; **56**:1045–49.

37. Hennebelle M, Roy M, St-Pierre V, et al. Energy restriction does not prevent insulin resistance but does prevent liver steatosis in aging rats on a Western-style diet. *Nutrition* 2015; **31**:523–30.

38. Directors, Clinical Guidelines Task Force. Guidelines for the use of parenteral and enteral nutrition in adult and pediatric patients. *JPEN J Parenter Enteral Nutr* 2002; **26**:1SA–138SA.

39. Bunker VW, Clayton BE. Research review: studies in the nutrition of elderly people with particular reference to essential trace elements. *Age Ageing* 1989; **18**:422–29.

40. Manal B, Suzana S, Singh DK. Nutrition and frailty: a review of clinical intervention studies. *J Frailty Aging* 2015; **4**:100–6.

41. Barnett MD, Williams BR, Tucker RO. Sudden advanced illness: an emerging concept among palliative care and surgical critical care physicians. *Am J Hosp Palliat Care* 2016; **33**:321–26.

42. Maung AA, Toevs CC, Kayser JB, Kaplan LJ. Conflict management teams in the intensive care unit: a concise definitive review. *J Trauma Acute Care Surg* 2015; **79**:314–20.

43. Bielderman A, van der Schans CP, van Lieshout MR, et al. Multidimensional structure of the Groningen Frailty Indicator in community-dwelling older people. *BMC Geriatr* 2013; **13**:86.

Index

Printed in the United States
By Bookmasters